29.95

NEWMARKET PUBLIC LIBRARY

AIDS in the Twenty-First Century

D0110643

AIDS in the Twenty-First Century

Century

Disease and Globalization

Tony Barnett

and

Alan Whiteside

NEWMARKET PUBLIC LIBRARY

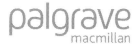

© Tony Barnett and Alan Whiteside 2002

All rights reserved. No reproduction, copy or transmission of this publication may be made without permission.

No paragraph of this publication may be reproduced, copied or transmitted save with written permission or in accordance with the provisions of the Copyright, Designs and Patents Act 1988, or under the terms of any licence permitting limited copying issued by the Copyright Licensing Agency, 90 Tottenham Court Road, London W1T 4LP.

Any person who does any unauthorised act in relation to this publication may be liable to criminal prosecution and civil claims for damages.

The authors have asserted their rights to be identified as the authors of this work in accordance with the Copyright, Designs and Patents Act 1988.

First published 2002 by
PALGRAVE MACMILLAN
Houndmills, Basingstoke, Hampshire RG21 6XS and
175 Fifth Avenue, New York, N.Y. 10010
Companies and representatives throughout the world

Reprinted 2003

PALGRAVE MACMILLAN is the new global academic imprint of St. Martin's Press LLC Scholarly and Reference Division and Palgrave Macmillan Ltd (formerly Macmillan Press Ltd).

ISBN 1–4039–0005–1 hardback
ISBN 1–4039–0006–X paperback

This book is printed on paper suitable for recycling and made from fully managed and sustained forest sources.

A catalogue record for this book is available from the British Library.

Library of Congress Cataloging-in-Publication Data
Barnett Tony.
    AIDS in the twenty–first century / Tony Barnett and Alan Whiteside.
        p. cm.
    Includes bibliographical references and index.
    ISBN 1–4039–0005–1 (hbk.) — ISBN 1–4039–0006–X (pbk.)
        1. AIDS (Disease)—Social aspects. 2. AIDS (Disease)—Economic aspects. I. Whiteside, Alan. II. Title.
    RA643.8 .B37 2002
    362.1'969792—dc21   DEC 2 3 2003

                                                      2002072399

Printed and bound in Great Britain by
Antony Rowe Ltd, Chippenham and Eastbourne

Contents

List of Tables and Figures

Tables

Figures

Acknowledgements

Together and separately we have researched the social and economic impact of the HIV/AIDS epidemic since 1986. Although there is still much to learn about the processes of disease impact, now is the time to bring together in one place some of what we have learned so far.

Each of us has argued in many fora that HIV/AIDS has for too long received insufficient attention because its implications are difficult to comprehend and more difficult to confront. We hope that this book will spur others to take the issue seriously and work towards better understanding and effective action. We believe that the world community has a limited comprehension of what the HIV/AIDS epidemic means for us all. We fear that many people in positions of power may not really care. We suspect that social and economic theorists do not find the problem of sufficient intellectual interest to think the novel thoughts that are required if we are properly to respond to this event.

In writing this book we have incurred many debts. Most immediately, we are grateful to the Association François-Xavier Bagnoud for enabling us to pursue this and providing generous funding that allowed us to take time out from our universities to read, think and finally to write. Its President, Albina du Boisrouvray, who has done so much to draw the world's attention to the implications of the HIV/AIDS epidemic, was supportive throughout the process of writing. She gave us encouragement from the time we first met to the point of publication and took the time to read and comment on various drafts.

Over the last 12 years, we have jointly facilitated a large number of policy research workshops for senior policy makers and activists. At these we tried to develop a common understanding of the social and economic impact of the epidemic. The global nature of the problem will be clear from the location of these workshops: in Norwich, UK; Durban, South Africa; Jaipur, Raichak and Delhi, India; Pokhara, Nepal; Penang, Malaysia; Manila in the Philippines; and in Kyiv, Ukraine. We have learned much from these meetings and thank each of the thousand or so participants who have worked with us. The workshops required considerable funding and in particular we must thank the European Union, the Swedish International Development Agency, the British Council and the United Kingdom Department for International Development for their support. We owe particular debts to Lieve

Fransen of the European Union whose commitment meant that the policy research workshop programme was able to grow with the assurance of core funding over a number of years, and to Veena Lakhumalani of the British Council in Calcutta who, after participating in our Norwich workshop, devoted her considerable energies to arranging a four-year series of workshops in India.

At various stages and in many different ways, others have been important in facilitating and encouraging our work. They include: Martha Ainsworth, Anita Alban, Peter Badcock-Walters, Olga Balakeriva, Joe Collins, K.K. Choo, Josef Decosas, Paul Delay, Chris Desmond, Charlie Gilks, Tsetsele Fantan, Paul Farmer, Liz Floyd, Susan Foster, Stephen Forsythe, Yulia Fustian, George Gardner, Robert Greener, Merle Holden, Ishrat Husain, Lev Khodakevich, John King, Yuri Kruglov, Daniel Low-Beer, Anthony Lumby , Mattias Lundberg, the late Jonathan Mann, the late Dan Mudoola, Mead Over, Suzi Peel, Wendy Roseberry, Gabriel Rugalema, Rose Smart, David Sokal, Karen Stanecki, Valentina Steshenko, Rand Stoneburner, Bradford Strickland, Daniel Tarantola, Sandy Thurman, Jane Tomlinson, Peter Way and Samantha Willan.

A number of colleagues were kind enough to read drafts of the whole book or of individual chapters. Their comments were often critical but always helpful and kind. Among those who deserve special thanks are: John Stover, Shula Marks, William Rau, Catherine Dolan, Mildred Blaxter and Jane Wirgman. Of course we have not been able to make all the changes that they suggested, but we have endeavoured to take account of their comments.

The book benefited from the work of a number of research assistants. At the University of Natal, we would like to thank Su Erskine and Nicole Pahl of HEARD, for their meticulous work. In addition Jaine Roberts and Gavin George provided valuable inputs. At the School of Development Studies, University of East Anglia, Helen O'Driscoll and Richard Dean of University College, Cork, Ireland, worked as research assistants in the summer of 2000. Also in Durban thanks are due to Samantha Willan and Madeline Freeman.

Tony Barnett would in particular like to thank Martin Wallis whose life, ideas and ideals have been such an inspiration to a long-term project that had its origins in a conversation with Martin in Norwich in 1986.

Where we have used material published elsewhere the source has been acknowledged within the caption and permission to reprint was sought. If we have inadvertently infringed copyright we will be happy to make amends in future printings of the book.

The staff of KLM and of the KLM Royal Wing Lounge at Schiphol Airport in Amsterdam deserve a special mention. Parts of the book were written and discussed there and on various KLM flights around the world.

Last but not least our families deserve special thanks for their support: Tony Barnett is grateful to his wife, Sarah Knights, who read most of the chapters more than once in early draft and made very useful critical comments, and to his son Rafael Barnett-Knights. Alan Whiteside is grateful to Ailsa Marcham and to their children, Rowan and Douglas Whiteside, for their constant support.

It is conventional in a book dealing with a subject like this to thank all those who struggle individually with the personal impact of a horrendous illness. While we hesitate to extend such broad thanks to millions of people because it may appear an empty gesture, we are both deeply aware of and moved by what we have seen and learned from many people in Uganda, Tanzania, Zambia, South Africa, Ukraine, India, the Philippines, Nepal, Malaysia and elsewhere.

That is why we have written what follows.

Tony Barnett
University of East Anglia
Norwich, UK

Alan Whiteside
University of Natal
Durban, South Africa

Part I
Introduction

1
Disease, Change, Consciousness and Denial

People are dying

Abantu Abaafa! – People are dying![1] An elderly woman calls to us from a village in Uganda. She says what everybody knows. People *are* dying from AIDS. Her thin arms are held out imploringly. She is distraught. The skin hangs in folds where once there was flesh. She is in her eighties and cares for her many orphaned grandchildren. People are dying – they are and were and will be her children and grandchildren. She cares for them, but when she dies they are orphaned once again. They grow up. They too may become infected and die of AIDS. No one listens.

HIV/AIDS is predominantly a sexually transmitted disease. It causes illness and death among mature adults. The groups at greatest risk are those between 15 and 50 years of age, often described as the 'sexually active'. These are the most productive people in any society.

This book is about the social and economic impact of HIV and AIDS, the failure to respond, what we must learn from this global epidemic, and what we must do. It is about the need to look beyond the individual to social and economic conditions, to see health as more than medicine, to understand concepts of 'well-being'. It is about the long-term effects of large-scale death and illness as they will echo through our common history. 'Despite millennia of epidemics, war and famine, never before in history have death rates of this magnitude been seen among young adults of both sexes and from all walks of life.'[2]

AIDS teaches us lessons

Even if we do listen, what can or should we do? There are lessons we can learn from this epidemic that has – for the moment – hit Africa

3

more dramatically than any other part of the world. There are lessons that go beyond the bare facts that this is a disease which has affected every continent and every country. There are lessons we can take forward to the next stage, the evolving Asian epidemic. There are lessons for our understanding of the social and economic significance of infectious diseases and the importance of public health. There are lessons about the implications of the new globalisation and international relations.

This is not the first epidemic disease to have spread around the world over long distances and between diverse societies. After 600 years, plague occupies a special and horrific place in the European imagination. Plague is long gone from Europe and North America but remains endemic in some poorer countries. By and large it is ignored, except by those whom it affects directly and those whom it threatens when it escapes from India, Madagascar or its other refuges. HIV/AIDS shows us – albeit dimly – that as a species we have to take urgent account of the needs of our common welfare. Infectious disease epidemics are deeply rooted in the global social and economic life that we share.

We can no longer push the afflicted into plague hospitals and retreat like medieval burghers behind the high walls of our city's defences. We must begin by recognising that welfare is a global common good. AIDS is the first epidemic of globalisation. It has spread rapidly because of the massive acceleration of communication, the rapidity with which desire is reconstructed and marketed globally, and the flagrant inequality that exists within and between societies.

Common consciousness

HIV/AIDS has succeeded in joining people around the world in a common consciousness about its threats and implications. It is the only disease to have a dedicated United Nations organisation – UNAIDS – charged with the single aim of confronting it. It is the first epidemic where the long-term implications could be recognised as they happen. Global climate change has taught that human action has long-term consequences. This provides a better appreciation of the nature of risk and its social, spatial and temporal distribution. We recognise that risk is distributed unequally between poor and rich, between one place and another, and that actions by a few may create risks and hazards for the many. HIV/AIDS has struck at a time when we are able to perceive such events within very long-term scientific perspectives without taking refuge in millennial or apocalyptic responses.

In place of irrational responses, we ask:

- What will this epidemic do to people's lives over many years and decades?
- What does it mean for our collective future as it throws into sharp relief world inequities in welfare and well-being?

This epidemic pointedly questions how 'we' value other human beings. It asks whether such humanistic valuing is a thing of the past, replaced by 'the market' (Frank, 2001); a market that omits the valuing of social goods, reflects only competing preferences for goods and services, and threatens to become the sole determinant of values as well as of value.

The glacial response to impact

For the last 20 years a few academics and policy makers have debated whether or not HIV/AIDS has social and economic impacts and what they might be. Most have preferred to ignore and deny the problem. The authors have spent much of this period researching these issues. We have looked at what HIV/AIDS does to the lives of individuals, communities, companies and societies. It is surprising how few senior policy makers and even fewer politicians have been prepared to consider the potential consequences of the epidemic and what should be done about them. In part this has been the result of the glacial pace at which governments and international organisations are able to move and change. But this is not the whole story. There has been a full measure of denial. Some, perhaps the majority, seeing no way in which to engage with what has appeared to be and has become an overwhelming problem, withdraw from any engagement with the long-term impact of the epidemic. Others fear the disease stigma may besmirch their professional lives.

Politicians, policy makers, community leaders and academics have all denied what was patently obvious – that the epidemic of HIV/AIDS would affect not only the health of individuals but also the welfare and well-being of households, communities and, in the end, entire societies. The effects of disease are rarely considered beyond the clinical impact on individuals.

It is difficult to see what is happening, harder to measure, easiest to deny

There is a problem of course. Politicians, policy makers, opinion formers and the media inhabit the world of today. They find it

---

Box 1.1   Vignettes of denial

In 1987 the Deputy Director-General of United Nations' Food and Agriculture Organisation wrote explaining that the UN system could only concern itself with medical aspects of HIV/AIDS, and: 'Until there are credible medical data on the present and projected incidence of AIDS it is virtually impossible for an intergovernmental organisation like FAO to make a serious assessment of the implications for development' (Walton, 1987). This at a time when the evidence of the extent of the epidemic from parts of central Africa was already overwhelming and the Fortieth World Health Assembly had declared that it was 'Deeply concerned that this disease ... has assumed pandemic proportions affecting all regions of the world and ... represents a threat to the attainment of health for all' (World Health Assembly, 1987, p. 1).

The conversations with officials from the WHO in 1988 in which the idea that social and economic impact was an important issue was dismissed in the face of the urgent need for prevention.

The Barbican Hall, London, 1988: the First (and to date also the last!) International Conference on the Global Impact of HIV/AIDS. Medical participants almost to a man opening their newspapers – or leaving the conference hall – at the start of the session on social and economic impact.

The Tanzanian civil servants and ministers who, confronted with the implications of the epidemic for agriculture, retreated rapidly into the reassuring belief that 'the village' and 'the extended family' would soak up the problem. This in 1993 when seroprevalence levels in Tanzania were rising dramatically and impact was already evident in Kagera.

Delhi in 1998: the Indian academics and civil servants who could not envisage that HIV/AIDS would ever have an effect on a country with a population of 1 billion, and for whom the issues were insufficiently 'interesting' to merit attention.

---

difficult to look beyond the immediacy of the present. There are undoubted technical problems of how to measure social and economic impact of excess death and illness. Gradual processes of attrition – and in most cases that is the nature of impact – elicit responses, but these responses are often hidden in the lives of ordinary people. People cope; they cope until a step change occurs in their circumstances and their lives and their societies take a dramatic new turn. A poor household sells its animals, its implements and then the thatch from its roof in the hopeless quest for treatment. Then they cease to farm or to herd and go to the city. When those individual changes become communal and then social, history's trajectory has been irreversibly altered. The individual lives that go to make up that history have disappeared, been impoverished or, in a few cases, enriched.[3] It is hard to perceive or to measure very slow events. Other than in historical retrospect they are difficult to see. It is hard to measure things – quality of life, quality of relationships, pain of loss – for which measures are partial or non-existent. If it is hard to see these things, it is all the easier to deny them.

Part of the cost of losing a community's teacher or nurse can be estimated in money terms, but not all losses and costs can be afforded a money value. How do we value parenting? What is the cost of a cuddle forgone? What is the cost to an organisation of the loss of institutional memory? How do we estimate the value of lost community morale? The impacts of HIV and AIDS are felt by those who experience them. Those who try to measure and research the impacts find them difficult to pin down.

In the end, when the epidemic has gone on long enough and things have changed, people forget how they once were.

The wretched of the earth

Abantu Abaafa! – People are dying! People are dying. Children are being orphaned. The elderly are left uncared for. Already disgraceful poverty is made worse. HIV/AIDS marks exclusions that can be found not only across the gross geography of continents, but also in the more subtle geography of social networks and city blocks. It is marked in the ebb and flow of global and local labour markets, where the quest for work and livelihoods may take on a sexual complexion.

With the development of anti-retroviral therapies (ARTs), the epidemic defines who is saved ... and who is left to die from the disease and its impacts. In its distribution across the continents and in relation to access to drugs that can save lives, it is a global epidemic that defines the excluded of the world – the wretched of the earth. Above all, HIV/AIDS defines those who can purchase well-being and those who cannot.

In the world a core of people hold the power to count those who do not count. Kenichi Ohmae (1985, p. xvi–xvii) uses the term 'triad' countries to refer to the core of the global economy and society, those areas of the Europe, North America and the Pacific Asia region where many people can and do live well. He argues that 600 million middle-class consumers make up the global market: they are the people who count. Unfortunately for the rest of the world's 5.5 billion people, it is the people who count who do the counting for the others. They count the money and the medicines. They release the rights to these only in return for the work and the resources of those who do not count and who only have value as 'labour' on the globalised market. Distribution of wealth, income and assets is not simply a matter of 'north' or 'south', of 'developed' or 'underdeveloped', 'undeveloped' or 'develop-ing' or any of the other pairs which describe the nature of poverty in the world. The 'excluded', the 'third world' can be on the doorstep of the 'first world'. In New York, the Bronx is close to Manhattan; in London, St John's Wood is not far from Whitechapel; in Paris, the 16th arrondissement – the richest in Paris – is next door to Seine Saint Denis, areas where life is acutely constrained by poverty, migrant status and social exclusion.

This epidemic kills people in the prime of their lives. But why should we be concerned? There are, after all, in the view of some, too many people in the world. Apart from the purely humanitarian aspects – that we do not want to see others suffer and our heartstrings are torn by the sight of the deprivations among swathes of the world's population – on cool reflection, labour is not required in the quantities that once it was. This is the age of the information economy, of just-in-time production, of delayering, of contracting out and subcontracting. All of these terms are indicative of a drive to economise on the use of labour. Once it was necessary for employers to offer training, pensions, jobs for life, to build up a workforce with skills at many levels and retain it within the company. In the second half of the twentieth century this changed dramatically.

Where low-level labour became all that was required this could be obtained wherever it was cheapest, most docile and easily available. In contrast stood the highly skilled labour of the information and managerial workers (often one and the same) who organised the unskilled, low-quality labour. In the closing decades of the twentieth century it was the former who were members of the 600 million. The latter were among the excluded. They had little to offer the 600 million beyond their occasional labour. And it is among these excluded that most of the world's HIV infections and AIDS cases are to be found (World Bank, 1997b, pp. 27–8; Cohen, 1999).

HIV/AIDS – the current situation

HIV/AIDS has been reported from every inhabited continent and from every country. Box 1.2 provides an overview of the situation at the end of the year 2001.[4]

Box 1.2   HIV/AIDS: The Global Situation

In 2001, approximately 36 million individuals were living with HIV/AIDS. Assuming that each HIV/AIDS case directly influences the lives of four other individuals, a total of more than 150 million people are being affected by the disease. Sub-Saharan Africa is the region most affected by HIV/AIDS – now that area's leading cause of adult morbidity and mortality. Most, if not all, of the 25 million people in sub-Saharan Africa who are living with HIV/AIDS will have died by the year 2020, in addition to the 13.7 million Africans already claimed by the epidemic.

HIV/AIDS is also spreading dramatically in Asia. India leads the region in absolute numbers of HIV infections, estimated at 3–5 million. China, too, has a growing HIV/AIDS problem, with approximately 0.5 million AIDS cases and, according to private estimates by Chinese specialists, up to 10 million HIV infections. Asia will overtake sub-Saharan Africa in absolute numbers before 2010; by 2020 Asia will be the HIV/AIDS epicentre.[5]

The epidemic has hit hardest in Africa south of the Sahara and it is still gaining speed there (Box 1.3). Parts of Latin America are severely affected (Box 1.4). In the rich countries about 1.5 million people are estimated to be HIV positive (Box 1.5). Eastern Europe and the former Soviet Union confront a diverse but potentially major epidemic rooted in drug use and the break-down of public health and social security (Box 1.6). In Asia, Thailand has been dealing with an epidemic of around 1 million infected in a population of about 61 million. The

Table 1.1   Global summary of the HIV/AIDS epidemic, end 2000

People newly infected with HIV in 1999	Total	**5.4 million**
	Adults	4.7 million
	Women	*2.3 million*
	Children < 15 years	620,000
Number of people living with HIV/AIDS	Total	**34.3 million**
	Adults	33.0 million
	Women	*15.7 million*
	Children < 15 years	1.3 million
AIDS deaths in 1999	Total	**2.8 million**
	Adults	2.3 million
	Women	*1.2 million*
	Children < 15 years	500,000
Total number of AIDS deaths since the beginning of the epidemic	Total	**18.8 million**
	Adults	15.0 million
	Women	*7.7 million*
	Children < 15 years	3.8 million
Total number of AIDS orphans* since the beginning of the epidemic		**13.2 million**

* Defined as children who lost their mother or both parents to AIDS when they were under the age of 15 but see Chapter 8.

Box 1.3   HIV/AIDS in Africa

In Africa, AIDS now kills ten times more people a year than does war.

- In 16 African countries more than one-tenth of the adult population (aged 15–49) is infected with HIV.
- In the six countries of southern Africa, AIDS is expected to claim the lives of between 8% and 25% of today's practising doctors by the year 2005.
- In seven countries, all in the southern cone of the continent, at least one adult in five is living with HIV. In countries where 10% of the adult population has HIV infection, almost 80% of all deaths in young adults aged 25–45 will be associated with HIV.
- Infection rates in young African women are far higher than young men. The average rates of infection in teenage girls were over five times higher than in teenage boys. Among young people in their early twenties, the rates were three times higher in women.

- In 1997, public health spending for AIDS alone already exceeded 2% of gross domestic product (GDP) in 7 African countries – and total health spending accounts for 3–5% of GDP.
- In Zimbabwe, by 1997 the likelihood of a 15-year-old woman dying before the end of her reproductive years quadrupled from around 11% in the early 1980s to over 40%. More than 2000 Zimbabweans die of AIDS each week.
- In Botswana, 35.8% of adults are now infected with HIV, while in South Africa, 19.9% are infected, up from 12.9% just two years ago. The adult HIV prevalence rate in Botswana has more than tripled since 1992.

Box 1.4   HIV/AIDS in Latin America

- The HIV epidemic in Latin America is highly diverse. Several Caribbean island states have worse epidemics than any country outside of sub-Saharan Africa.
- In Central American countries and Latin American countries on the Caribbean coast, HIV is spreading mainly through sex between men and women.
- Brazil is experiencing a major heterosexual epidemic, but there are very high rates of infection among injecting drug users and men who have sex with men. In Mexico, Argentina and Colombia, HIV infection is confined largely to these groups. The Andean countries are currently among those least affected by HIV infection.
- The countries with the highest HIV rates in the region are found on the Caribbean side of the continent. According to the most recent figures, over 7% of pregnant women in urban Guyana tested positive for HIV.
- In Honduras, Guatemala and Belize there is also a fast-growing heterosexual epidemic, with HIV prevalence rates of between 1% and 2% among adults in the general population. In 1994, less than 1% of pregnant women using antenatal services in Belize District tested positive for HIV, while one year later the prevalence had risen to 2.5%.
- In the Honduras city of San Pedro Sula, the rate of HIV infection among pregnant women has fluctuated between 2% and 5% for several years. This is mainly teenagers, suggesting that the worst is still to come.

- Heterosexual transmission of HIV is rarer in other countries of Central America. In Costa Rica, for example, HIV is transmitted mainly during unprotected sex between men. In Mexico, too, HIV has affected mainly men who have sex with men, more than 14% of whom are currently infected. According to one study, fewer than 1 in every 1,000 women of childbearing age is infected.

Box 1.5   HIV/AIDS in the rich world

The industrial countries of North America, Europe, Australia and New Zealand have only about 1.5 million adults and children living with HIV/AIDS, less than 5% of the global burden of infection. (UNAIDS, 2000g). By far the largest number are in the US where about 850,000 people live with HIV/AIDS. In Western Europe the largest number of infections are in France (130,000), followed by Spain (120,000) and Italy (95,000). The UK has 31,000 infections (UNAIDS, June 2000f). The epidemics in these countries are concentrated in specific populations, primarily men who have sex with men, and injecting drug users. Recent data from the UK indicate that rates of heterosexual infection may be increasing and some of these infections are resistant to ARTs.

Numbers of infected persons in these parts of the world have increased for two main reasons: first, the introduction of new treatments (see Chapter 13 for a fuller discussion) has improved survival and reduced mortality; second, there is increasing evidence that in some populations reductions in risk behaviours are being reversed. 'These developments may be the result of a false sense of security following a perception that HIV is now a "normal" treatable disease. It might also be the result of a general fatigue in continuing with safe behaviours. Whatever the reasons, such trends are alarming and show the risks of complacency' (Monitoring the AIDS Pandemic, 2000, p. 20).

The challenge for the rich world is to reverse the trend of slow and steady increases in new infections, especially among the most susceptible groups. The future of anti-retroviral treatments must also be called into question with the growth in drug resistance and this needs to be carefully monitored.

Box 1.6   Eastern Europe and the former Soviet Union

In the states of Eastern Europe and the former Soviet Union the epidemic is characterised by rapid spread among intravenous drug users (IVDUs). Up to the early 1990s, despite massive surveillance, very few cases of HIV infection were recorded in these countries. Ukraine found only 24 HIV positive results from the 25 million tests it carried out between 1987 and 1994. Most infected people were foreigners.

The HIV epidemic took off among IVDUs in the mid-1990s.

At present it is known that high levels of infection exist among drug users and that the epidemic continues to spread in this group. A major problem is the lack of surveillance data from other groups. It is known that other sexually transmitted infections (STIs) are spreading. Between 200,000 and 400,000 new cases of syphilis are reported annually from Russia alone. When this is linked with the collapse of the public health service it is evident that the potential for the spread of the epidemic into the general community is marked. These countries are at the 'concentrated' stage; there is no guarantee that this will remain the case and there is need for urgent and targeted action.

Estimates indicate the largest number of infections are in the Ukraine with 240,000 infections followed by the Russian Federation with 130,000 and Belarus with 14,000. All other countries have fewer than 10,000 while in some cases – the central Asian countries – there are reported to be less than 100.

---

coming decade promises two potential hot-spots: the world's most populous countries, India and China (Box 1.7).

HIV/AIDS has changed the lives of individuals, ruined their health, caused their deaths, left survivors to mourn. HIV/AIDS is the first epidemic of which we have been globally conscious because we can and do know about the disease's origins and structure. It is changing not only individual lives but also the trajectories of whole societies. Yet

Box 1.7   The Asian epidemics

The Asian epidemics vary greatly. In some countries, such as the Philippines and Taiwan, HIV is under control and the number of cases is small. In others there has been a significant epidemic, but prevalence appears to have peaked and actually be declining. Best-known is Thailand, which currently has an estimated adult prevalence of 2.15% and 755,000 people living with HIV/AIDS. However over the past year there are the first signs that Cambodia is getting its epidemic under control; here prevalence peaked at 4.04% of adults and 220,000 infections in 2000.

There are small but growing epidemics in other countries – mainly in marginalised groups. Examples here include Pakistan, Bangladesh, Malaysia, Indonesia and Sri Lanka.

Another group of countries include those where there is little data but there seems to be potential for an epidemic. These include Nepal, Burma, Vietnam and Laos.

The rich countries of the region have the same scale of epidemics as do Europe and the US – small and under control. These include Japan, Brunei Darussalam, Singapore and South Korea.

The greatest concern is with regard to the epidemic in India and China. Together these two countries account for nearly half the world's population. It is estimated that there are about 4 million infections in India and half a million in China, but there are few data on either country. It is certain that both countries have the potential for explosive epidemics with highly mobile populations, untreated STIs and gender inequality. Certainly the pattern is for epidemics to spread across national borders. If the south of China, east India and northern Burma and Thailand constituted a single country then it would have one of the highest HIV prevalence rates in Asia, certainly much higher than in each of the constituent countries.

Speaking in Melbourne, Australia, in October 2001, the Executive Director of UNAIDS, Dr Peter Piot, said: 'We are kidding ourselves if we think Asia is not at risk from a major AIDS epidemic, it is already here ... Today I think that about a third or 40% of the world's people with HIV are living in Asia' (*Guardian*, 2001, p. 18).

**Adults and children estimated to be living
with HIV/AIDS as of end 1999**

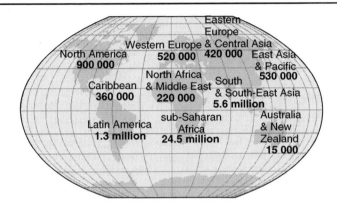

Total: 34.3 million

Figure 1.1   Global summary of the HIV/AIDS epidemic, end 1999
Source: UNAIDS (2000f), p. 6.

we choose, globally, in a world more closely shared than ever before, to deny what is happening. We choose to deny what is happening and not to recognise the global implications of this epidemic for the welfare and well-being of others.

The origins and the impact of a disease epidemic such as HIV/AIDS are linked at the root – they only appear to be different plants. The conditions that facilitate rapid spread of an infectious disease are also, by and large, those that make it hard for societies to respond and ensure that impact will be severe. Rapid spread and harsh impact are only apparently distinct symptoms of the same conditions, inequality and poverty. The relationship between inequality, poverty and infectious disease is observable. It is not straightforward and there will be many confounding variables in any particular situation. However, the link between poverty, inequality and HIV infection has recently been made clearer by Eileen Stillwaggon's work (Stillwaggon, 2000). Her comparative study of HIV epidemics in Africa and Latin America shows the link between malnutrition, parasitosis and susceptibility to infection in general and to HIV in particular. This analysis provides solid evidence that there is a strong relationship between poverty and epidemic spread and that the chain of causation between poverty and epidemic infection passes through a link of poor nutrition and related subsequent immunosuppression – this even before a person is infected by HIV (Stillwaggon, 2000, p. 1,006). The relationship between poverty, inequality and infection is discussed at greater length in Chapters 3–5 and elsewhere in this book.

A long-wave event – HIV/AIDS and time

People's existential perspectives relate to their own lifetimes and those of people around them. Some specialists, for example, historians, geologists and climatologists, consider long time periods: centuries or millennia; much longer than a human lifetime. Other human beings may be so tested to survive that their perspective is survival from week to week or month to month. Different actors, people but also organisations and institutions, have differing perspectives on time and the epidemic. We are aware of and inhabit differing timescapes (Adams, 1998).

The individual who is sick seeks a cure or relief of symptoms now; an epidemiologist sees the epidemic as it develops over many months or years; while a historian may consider it in the context of centuries. To understand the impact of this epidemic, we must adopt a perspective that spans several decades. And here is a paradox: the longer the required perspective, the easier it is to deny and not take responsibility. While we may all feel urgency and compassion in the face of immediately apparent need – the begging child, the dying victim of famine, the refugee fleeing from certain death – few of us have the time to respond to the long-term roots of a situation and its long-term implications.

The socio-economic impact of the epidemic operates at different ends of the range of time perspectives – the very short and the very long. Illness strikes. It weakens an individual; it weakens the household and the community. This is a timescape of maybe five years. At the other end of the continuum, there is the very long timescape of 'history'. In this book we are concerned with both ends of the spectrum.

It can take years of infection before debilitating symptoms become apparent in the individual. The HIV/AIDS epidemic spans many years. By the time the wave of HIV infection makes itself felt in the form of AIDS illnesses in individuals, the torrent of the epidemic is about to overwhelm medical services, households, communities. This can be illustrated with two examples.

Figure 1.2 shows the long-term nature of the epidemic in relation to South Africa in terms of normal death, actual and projected AIDS deaths and existing and projected HIV infections. By the time AIDS cases were seen in clinics in the late 1980s, the people already infected but not yet sick were forming a wave of future suffering, cost and death. This is now being seen across South African society with its estimated 4.7 million people HIV positive.

Figure 1.3 is an example of an impact that was already apparent in the early 1990s; the impact of AIDS-related death on the population structure of Uganda as it actually happened. This is history now but it is also a vision of the future. The three age–gender pyramids are derived from the Ugandan census of 1991. The first pyramid (a) shows the national situation. It is broad at the base and narrow at the top, reflecting the high birth rate and low life expectancy characteristic of many African and other poor countries. Pyramid (b) shows the demographic impact of HIV/AIDS at the District level (an administrative unit with a population of hundreds of thousands). This gives a slight hint of the excess deaths that had occurred in the most susceptible age groups. Pyramid (d) shows the marked impact of the epidemic on the population at the Parish level (an administrative unit with a population of between 2,500 and 6,500) where unusual numbers of deaths in the 15–30-year age cohorts and in the under-fives are all too apparent, as are the results of this on birth rates.

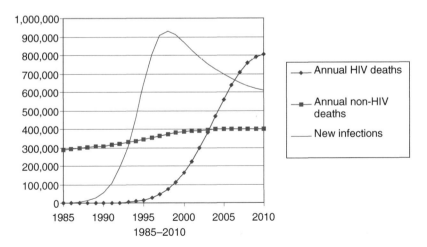

Figure 1.2   HIV infections, AIDS deaths and 'normal' deaths, South Africa
Source: Dorrington and Johnson (2001).

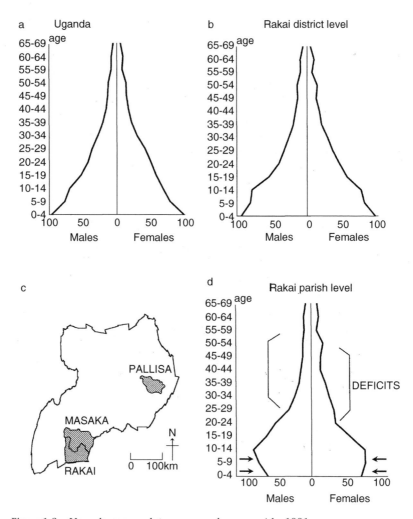

Figure 1.3   Uganda census data: age–gender pyramids, 1991
Source: Low-Beer et al. (1997).

These demographic data from Uganda show how this epidemic will reverberate through the history of Africa for many generations to come. While it shows us a picture of the recent past and the present, it also presents a longer vision, a perspective on the changed future of a society.

Time, gender and the individual

For the individual, the time perspective is naturally shorter but no less pressing. A young woman from a small village in Uganda speaking shortly before her death in 1989 said: 'I do not mind dying, but to die without having a child is most painful because I shall go to my grave knowing that nobody will remember my name.'[6] She faced death with courage. She was ill and desperately uncomfortable. But her mind was clear and she saw her death in the context of lives beyond her own which was soon to end. She feared her name would disappear. She saw her death as a withering of the branch of her lineage, and the end of her unique identity.

'Live for the present' is the motto of some young men. Also in 1989, a young fisherman/smuggler in Kasensero, a fishing village on Lake Victoria in Rakai District, Uganda, said: 'I cannot think about this AIDS business. I could drown tomorrow. There are too many girls here.'[7]

There are numerous records of women in particular who say that they cannot think of the long-term risks of illness and death when they have to undertake commercial sex work without a condom so as to feed themselves and their children over the next few days. A 16-year-old Ghanaian sex worker said: 'All die be die' – a statement that translates as 'every death is death', implying that each person is going to die and the cause of death does not much matter. She needed to survive and she could die from anything, including AIDS. 'In her view dying from AIDS through commercial sex was no different from dying from any other disease, including hunger' (Awusabo-Asare et al., 1999, p. 134).

Time is not neutral, ticking away in the background, measuring out each life in equal amounts. Time is relative. Consider the real implications of differing life expectancies. A young adult aged 20 in a country where life expectancy is only 40 has only 20 more years to look forward to, 20 years in which to fulfil herself. Contrast this with 20-year-olds in a society where life expectancy is 75 years. They have time to play, to learn, to experiment, to grow old. This is a real contrast which should make us look anew at the two words *life* and *expectancy* when we come upon them again in Chapter 6, and reflect on what they mean for real people with real expectations – or not.

Such different expectations affect orientations and decisions made in the present. There are also differences between the expectations of men and women. Time, indeed, is gendered and so is the risk of infection – see Table 1.2.

In relation to this, Preston-Whyte (1999) explores some of the cultural barriers to condom use and draws attention to the connection

Table 1.2 Time is gendered – women's lives, women's risks

HIV positive child of HIV positive mother	Life and death	TIME	HIV negative child of an HIV positive mother	Life and death
Age 0	Birth – found HIV positive	2000	Age 0	Birth, HIV negative
0–10	Dies	2000–10	0–10	Grows, helps at home, cares for infected mother and father
		2007–10	7–10	Parents die: placed as orphan with grandparent
		2010–12	10–12	Grandparent dies; goes to uncle's household
		2012–50	12–50	Enters adolescence and adulthood – must avoid infection
		2017–50	17–50	Sexual relationship(s) – may become infected.
				Has children
		2020–50	20–50	Helps children avoid infection nurses those who are HIV positive
		2036–70	36–70	Becomes a grandmother, cares for grandchildren when her own children die

Source: Hunter (2000)

between social position and time perception in relation to what she calls 'the fertility conundrum'. She describes how women are socially positioned and culturally defined to expect to be fertile and, in many societies, to achieve this speedily. Fertility confirms social identity as a woman and also ensures care in old age. Condom use thus confronts women with a problem in the present and in relation to the future. Men and women both expect women to have children. Marriage in the present is seen as an investment in the future. In parts of South Africa, they say: 'Children are what we give iLobolo (bridewealth) for' (Preston-Whyte, 1999, p. 143). This perspective on fertility in Africa has been extensively explored by the Caldwells and their colleague (Caldwell et al., 1989), who argue that: 'The core of African society is its emphasis on ancestry and descent' (Caldwell and Caldwell, 1990, p. 83). Thus lineage time and safe sex do not hold the same power, they cannot be equated – the former must win. People may want to avoid HIV infection; they may want to defer marriage or childbearing; but the pressures of lineage, family, gender roles and short life expectancy may often be for sex now (preferably reproductive, fertile sex) rather than for deferred sex and the use of a condom.

While the sick Ugandan woman was worried about her individuality, that may be less important than her lineage which provided a vital aspect of her identity. People's *lifetime* homes may be their lineages but their lifetimes are much shorter than that of the lineages which are in principle infinitely existing entities and perceived as such by those who are part of them. Looked at in this way, decisions about individual infection and risk take on a different complexion. This is particularly so when the timeline is bisected by the gender line and each partner in the decision as to condom use has a different perspective on which points in time and personhood are most important to protect: the present or the future, the individual or the group.

AIDS and development

Development is about hope for the future and changing social and economic trajectories for the better. AIDS will alter the history of many of the world's poorest societies. In the absence of effective and available vaccines or economically feasible and effective treatments, AIDS may be expected to wipe out half a century of development gains as measured by life expectancy at birth. In least developed countries, such as sub-Saharan Africa, global life expectancy of 36 years in the early 1950s rose to 52 in the early 1990s (United Nations, 1996). Yet this progress should not mask the fact that health conditions remain grim in these parts of the world. A child born in the worst affected countries between 2005 and 2010 can expect to die before his or her 40th birthday.

Figure 1.4 looks at life expectancy through the lens of some of today's 15-year-olds. These projections assume that AIDS prevention programmes will be successful enough to halve the risk of becoming HIV infected over the next 15 years. They do not take into account possible improvements in treatment or the availability of an HIV vaccine.

According to these conservative analyses, in countries where 15% of adults are currently infected, around one-third of today's 15-year-olds will die of AIDS. Where adult prevalence rates exceed 15%, the lifetime risk of dying of AIDS is much greater. In countries such as South Africa and Zimbabwe, where one-fifth or one-quarter of the adult population is infected, AIDS is set to claim the lives of around half of all 15-year-olds. And, in Botswana, where about one in three adults is already HIV infected – the highest prevalence rate in the world – it is estimated that two-thirds of today's 15-year-old boys will die prematurely of AIDS.

Life expectancy and child mortality rates have been widely used as markers for improvements in the welfare of populations. In Botswana, life expectancy at birth is now estimated to be 39 years, instead of 71 without AIDS. In Zimbabwe, life expectancy is 38 instead of 70. In fact, children born today in several southern and east African countries have life expectancies below 40.

In Latin America and the Caribbean, the impact on life expectancy is not as great as in sub-Saharan Africa because of lower HIV prevalence

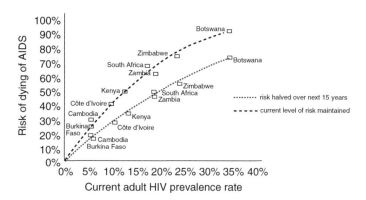

Figure 1.4   Lifetime risk of AIDS death for 15-year-old boys, assuming unchanged or halved risk of becoming infected with HIV, selected countries
Source: Data from B. Zaba published in UNAIDS (2000f) p. 26

levels. Even here impacts can be seen. In the Bahamas, life expectancy at birth is 71 years instead of 80, and in Haiti, life expectancy is 49 instead of 57. In Asia, people living in countries such as Thailand, Cambodia and Burma have lost three years of life expectancy.

The impact of HIV/AIDS on child mortality is highest in those countries that had significantly reduced child mortality due to other causes. Many HIV infected children survive beyond their first birthdays only to die before the age of five. In Zimbabwe, 70% of all deaths among children younger than five are due to AIDS. In the Bahamas, 60% of deaths among children younger than five are due to AIDS. As a result of AIDS, only 5 out of 51 countries in sub-Saharan Africa will reach the International Conference on Population and Development goals for decreased child mortality. This means that for many countries, particularly in Africa, 'development' becomes virtually impossible in the era of AIDS.

For all of the above reasons, development must now be seen against the background of four long-wave events associated with the HIV/AIDS epidemic:

1. the wave of HIV infection
2. the wave of tuberculosis (some of it multi-drug resistant) which, because it is the most common opportunistic infection, is usually the first visible wave of the epidemic
3. the wave of AIDS illness and death
4. the wave of impact – which includes household poverty, orphaning and many other effects which will be discussed in this book.

Taken together, this long-wave event extends over many decades and probably as long as a century. The global HIV/AIDS epidemic has deep roots in social and economic inequalities. It is a long-wave event, the effects of unusual levels of illness and death will profoundly affect the lives of many individuals and many societies for decades to come.

2
The Disease and its Epidemiology

HIV/AIDS is not the first global epidemic, and it certainly won't be the last: it is a disease that is changing human history. HIV/AIDS shows up global inequalities. Its presence and impacts are felt most profoundly in poor countries and communities. Here we look at its origins, how it is transmitted and the particular characteristics which make consideration of its social and economic roots and impacts necessary. Because of its scale and the international and local concern it evokes, we are confronted by quantities of information that may threaten to overwhelm us. Thus, in the last part of the chapter we look at data: what we know about AIDS and HIV, and how we know it, and how those data are used to construct particular accounts of the epidemic process.

Communicable diseases have been responsible for past epidemics and pandemics. They played an important role in human history and we had few defences against them. Bubonic plague, which spread from the Mediterranean ports of southern Europe in 1347, changed the course of European, and thus of world, history.

> Most historians now accept the plague's role in destroying feudal barriers to economic growth, and creating an instant demand for labour which had to be satisfied from a drastically reduced work force. In effect, the fourteenth century bubonic plague intensified the action of powerful structural forces which were turning Europe toward modernity. (McGrew, 1985, p. 40)

During the first outbreak of plague in Europe from 1347 to 1351, mortality varied at between one-eighth and two-thirds of the population. Overall, three out of ten Europeans may have died, some 24 million

24

people (Watts, 1999 in Cook, 1999). Some historians have argued that consequent labour scarcity led to technical, social and religious innovation, and ultimately to capitalism.

Box 2.1   Definitions

An **epidemic** is a rate of disease that reaches unexpectedly high levels, affecting a large number of people in a relatively short time. Epidemic is a relative concept: a small absolute number of cases of a disease is considered an epidemic if the disease incidence is usually very low. In contrast, a disease (such as malaria) is considered **endemic** if it is continuously present in a population but at low or moderate levels, while a **pandemic** describes epidemics of worldwide proportions, such as influenza in 1918 or HIV/AIDS today (Barfield, 1997, p. 150).

While Europe was affected by epidemics, they devastated other regions of the world. From the middle of the last millennium contact between Europe, the Americas, Australasia and parts of Africa proved disastrous for immunologically naive indigenous populations. Lacking defences against common European diseases such as smallpox, typhus, measles and influenza, these populations fell ill faster and diseases were more virulent. Diseases spread easily and mortality rates were very high. The result was massive depopulation: whole peoples disappeared; others were so seriously depleted as to have been written out of history.

Documentation of this process begins with Columbus's landfall on the Caribbean island of Hispaniola. In 1492 at the time of his arrival, there were at least a million Taino people. A disease akin to smallpox appeared in 1519 and by 1550 the Taino were extinct (Watts 1997, p. 88). This pattern of devastation was repeated throughout the Caribbean islands. The Aztec and Inca kingdoms of mainland South and Central America were next. The troops of the Spanish conquistador Hernán Cortès brought smallpox. It is estimated that the population of Mexico fell from 25.2 million in 1518 to 1.1 million in 1605. Similarly affected were the Inca to the south and Native American populations to the north. There, Spanish explorers had encountered a vibrant culture with towns and temples in the Mississippi valley. By the early 1700s this had vanished along with most of the people.

The role of disease in human history has been charted by a number of authors: initially by McNeil (1976) and most recently by Diamond (1999). McNeil began by posing the question, 'How did Cortès and his tiny band of less than 600 Spaniards conquer the mighty Aztec empire, whose subjects numbered many millions?' (McNeil, 1976, p. 1). Diamond's perspective is informed by a question posed by a Papua New Guinean: 'Why is it that you white people developed so much cargo and brought it to New Guinea, but we black people had little cargo of our own?' (Diamond, 1999, p. 14). For McNeil the disease was the key. Diamond, however, saw disease as part of a broader geographical determinism.

By the end of the nineteenth century the principles of disease transmission were generally known in Europe. The first well-known public health intervention was in 1854 when Dr John Snow tracked the source of an outbreak of cholera in London to a water pump in Broad Street. Closing the public pump brought the outbreak under control. However it was not until 1883 that Robert Koch identified the cholera bacillus. The first identified 'germs' or disease-causing organisms were the bacilli of anthrax and tuberculosis discovered by Louis Pasteur in the 1870s. In the latter part of the nineteenth century a flurry of activity (often associated with expansion of European empires) led to the identification of more 'germs' and linked them with specific diseases. Thus began scientifically based public health interventions.

Among these was the US-funded Yellow Fever Commission, which in 1900 identified the mosquito as the vector for disease transmission. In Havana anti-mosquito measures reduced the number of cases from 1,400 in 1900 to none in 1902. Public health interventions were being developed and seen to work.

Medical advances lead to the development of vaccines initially for polio, and by the 1960s for most other major childhood illnesses. Global smallpox vaccination resulted in eradication of the virus; the last case was reported in Somalia in 1977. By the mid-twentieth century, drug and vaccine development suggested to many that the world might be entering a period when the battle against infectious disease could be won. The next challenge was viral disease.

Prior to the emergence of HIV/AIDS, the last global epidemic had been influenza in 1918–19, so long ago that there was little 'institutional memory' of global epidemics. In the wealthy world there was also little memory of any killer epidemics. Poliomyelitis ceased to be a major concern with the introduction of a vaccine in 1955. Between 1946 and 1955 in the US there were on average 32,890 cases per year and 1,742 deaths. After the introduction of vaccination the number of cases fell to 5,749 and deaths to 268 (Oldstone, 1998, p. 109). In the rich world preventable diseases are generally prevented. Most people have clean water, heat, decent housing, nutritious diets and access to health care. The diseases that kill the rich are diseases of affluence such as heart disease. Outside of the rich world there have been major successes in immunisation against childhood diseases, although large numbers of children are still not reached and they die.

Where epidemics do emerge, scientific and medical responses are mobilised and emergencies are contained. However all is not well. Public health systems are underfunded; politically they attract few votes, and in parts of the world they are close to collapse. For the moment, there is only a mere intimation of any system of *global* public health.

Neither public health nor clinical medicine pays sufficient attention to what does improve health – escaping from poverty, access to good food, clean water, sanitation, shelter, education and preventative care. Clinical medicine has only marginal effects on people's long-term health. In the US – which spends the largest proportion of GNP on medical care of any country – 'less than 4% of the total improvements in life expectancy can be credited to twentieth century advances in medical care' (Garrett, 2000, p. 10). Preventive medicine is often piece-meal. For example, measles immunisation may be undertaken in slums where diarrhoeal disease is rife. Social and economic conditions negate many gains made by any particular intervention. Health is not only about confronting individual diseases. Well-being, of which health is a part, is a reflection of general social and economic conditions.

The 1990s has seen the recognition of many 'emergent' diseases – Ebola, Lassa fever, Marburg fever are well-known and hit the headlines. More serious is multi-drug resistant TB. Also of concern are the rise of antibiotic resistant bacteria, new strains of salmonella and most recently bovine spongiform encephalopathy and the related human form, new variant Creuzfeld-Jakob Disease (nvCJD).

HIV/AIDS has emerged into this setting. It is the first global epidemic for 60 years. Working from past experience, many hoped that the solutions lay in a quick technical fix – drugs or a vaccine. But there has been no medical-scientific solution. With the exception of its first manifestations in the US, this disease is linked to poverty and inequality and the ways that globalisation exacerbates these. Its consequences will be felt for decades to come, and its origins lie far back in time and deep within the structures of social, economic and cultural life. The epidemic is not just about medicine or even public health.

The emergence of the new epidemic: the discovery of AIDS and HIV

The story of HIV/AIDS begins in 1979 and 1980 when doctors in the US observed clusters of previously extremely rare diseases. These included a type of pneumonia carried by birds (*pneumocystis carinii*) and a cancer called Kaposi's sarcoma. The phenomenon was first reported in the *Morbidity and Mortality Weekly Report* (*MMWR*) of 5 June 1981, published by the US Center for Disease Control in Atlanta. The *MMWR* recorded five cases of *pneumocystis carinii*. A month later it reported a clustering of cases of Kaposi's sarcoma in New York. Subsequently, the number of cases of both diseases – which were mainly centred around New York and San Francisco – rose rapidly, and scientists realised that they were dealing with something new.

   The first cases were among homosexual men. As a result the disease was called Gay-Related Immune Deficiency Syndrome (GRID). American epidemiologists began to see cases among other groups, initially mainly haemophiliacs and recipients of blood transfusions. Subsequently the syndrome was identified among injecting drug users, and infants born to mothers who used drugs. It was apparent that this was not a 'gay' disease. It was renamed 'Acquired Immunodeficiency Syndrome', shortened to the acronym AIDS:

- The 'A' stands for Acquired. This means that the virus is not spread through casual or inadvertent contact like flu or chickenpox. In order to be infected, a person has do something (or have something done to him or her) which exposes him or her to the virus.
- 'I' and 'D' stand for Immunodeficiency. The virus attacks a person's immune system and makes it less capable of fighting infections. Thus, the immune system becomes deficient.
- 'S' is for Syndrome. AIDS is not one disease but rather presents itself as a number of diseases that come about as the immune system fails. Hence, it is regarded as a syndrome.

The illness was seen simultaneously in a number of locations outside the US. In Zambia, Dr Anne Bayley, Professor of Surgery at the University Teaching Hospital in Lusaka, reported a significant rise in the number of Kaposi's sarcoma cases (Bayley, 1984). In 1982, reports of a significant wave of deaths in the south of the country began to reach the Ugandan Ministry of Health. In 1983 the ministry sent a team to investigate this new disease in the Lake Victoria fishing village of Kasensero. They concluded that it was AIDS (Kaleeba et al., 2000; Hooper, 1990). Hooper (1999) documents similar recognition of the disease in Tanzania, Congo and Rwanda.

In October 1983 a team of American and European doctors travelled to Kigali and Zaire where they identified and described cases of AIDS. Of course many hundreds of African doctors were well aware that a new disease was killing their patients. However these frontline health care workers do not write for learned journals such as the *Lancet* or *Science and Nature*, so the cases and the disease remained unreported.

Outside Africa AIDS cases were identified in all Western countries and in Australia, New Zealand and some Latin American countries – most notably Brazil and Mexico. From 1981 there was global recognition of the syndrome; clinicians and others now knew what to look for and that it could be given a name. Immediately there was a question of where HIV/AIDS was seen, by whom and what it meant. What it meant and how it was represented in the press and the popular consciousness was of the greatest significance for people affected by a disease linking sex, sexuality, death, ethnicity and status. Inevitably it became a vehicle for stigma (Farmer, 1992).

Once the new syndrome had been identified, the pace of scientific and epidemiological activity to identify the cause of the disease increased. In 1983 a team lead by French scientist Luc Montagnier identified the virus we now know as HIV-1 (the Human Immunodeficiency Virus). In 1985, a second Human Immunodeficiency Virus, HIV-2, was identified. This is more difficult to transmit and is slower acting and less virulent than HIV-1. Initially HIV-2 was found in west Africa with the greatest number of infections outside this area in Angola, Mozambique, France and Portugal. 'Overall, the most striking feature about the global epidemiology of HIV-2 is its lack of epidemic spread internationally' (De Cock and Brun-Vézinet, 1996).

Viruses have been defined as 'a piece of nucleic acid surrounded by bad news' (Oldstone, 1998, p. 8). They are genetic material covered with a coat of protein molecules. They do not have cell walls, are parasitic, and can only replicate by entering host cells. The genetic material of viruses is commonly DNA, or less frequently RNA. Viruses have few genes compared with other organisms: HIV has fewer than 10 genes (as does Ebola and measles); smallpox has between 200 and 400 genes. The smallest bacteria has 5,000–10,000 genes (Oldstone, 1998, p. 9). Humans have between 30,000 and 80,000 (Ridley, 2000, p. 5).

HIV belongs in the family of viruses known as retroviruses, scientifically called *Retroviridae*. The first retroviruses were only identified in the 1970s. All members of this family have the ability to produce latent infections. HIV is in a virus group called the lentiviruses. These develop over a long period, producing diseases, many of which affect the immune system and brain (Schoub, 1999). The viruses have a unique enzyme, reverse transcriptase. Outside the cells they infect, they consist of two strands of RNA. Once they infect a cell they make DNA copies of their own RNA and are able to reproduce. It is this feature as well as the ability of the virus to mutate rapidly which makes it hard to develop pharmaceutical responses.

How HIV works

For infection to occur, the virus has to enter the body and attach itself to host cells (see Figure 2.1). HIV attacks a particular set of cells in the human immune system known as CD4 cells. There are two main types of CD4 cells. The first type are CD4 positive T cells which organise the body's overall immune response to foreign bodies and infections. These T helper cells are the prime target of HIV. For a person to become infected, virus particles must enter the body and attach themselves to the CD4 cells. HIV also attacks immune cells called macrophages. These cells engulf foreign invaders and ensure that the body's immune system will recognise them in the future.

Once the virus has penetrated the wall of the CD4 cell it is safe from the immune system because it copies the cell's DNA, and therefore cannot be identified and destroyed by the body's defence mechanisms. Virus particles lurk in the cells until their replication is triggered. Once this happens they make new virus particles that bud from the surface of the host cell in vast numbers, destroying that cell as they do so. These viruses then go on to infect more CD4 cells.

When a person is infected a battle commences between the virus and the immune system. There is an initial burst of activity during which many cells are infected, but the immune system fights back, manufacturing immense numbers of antibodies. This period is marked by an unseen and unfelt war in a person's body. The viral load is high, the immune system is taking a knock, and the person's HIV status cannot be detected using standard tests. This is commonly called 'the window period' and lasts from several weeks to several months. At this stage a person is highly infectious as his or her viral load (the number of viral particles they are carrying) is considerable. This fact is of epidemiological importance. The more people there are in the early stage of infection, the greater the chance of effective transmission between people.

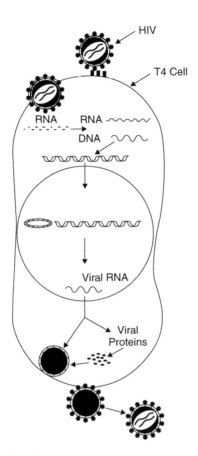

Figure 2.1   The virus in action
Source: Whiteside and Sunter (2000), p. 7.

An infected person will usually experience an episode of illness at the end of the window period – but this will often resemble flu and will not be seen as a marker for HIV.

The window period is followed by the long incubation stage. During this phase, the viruses and the cells they attack are reproducing rapidly and being destroyed as quickly by each other. Up to 5% of the body's CD4 cells (about 2,000 million cells) may be destroyed each day by the billions of virus particles (Schoub, 1999, p. 85). Eventually, the virus is able to destroy the immune cells more quickly than they can be replaced and slowly the number of CD4 cells falls. In a healthy person there are 1,200 CD4 cells per microlitre of blood. As infection progresses, the number will fall. When the CD4 cell count falls below 200, opportunistic infections begin to occur and a person is said to have AIDS. Infections will increase in frequency, severity and duration until the person dies. It is these opportunistic infections that cause the syndrome referred to as AIDS.

The period from HIV infection to illness and death is crucial. It was generally believed that, in the rich world, on average people lived for ten years before they began to fall ill. Without treatment, the normal period from the onset of AIDS to death was thought to be a further 12–24 months. With the development of effective anti-retroviral therapies, infected people can expect to live a reasonable life for a longer time. Indeed, it is hoped that AIDS can be turned into a manageable chronic disease like diabetes. In this event, people could expect to live longer though they would remain infected. However, recent evidence suggests that viral resistance to these drugs is growing, approximately 20% of new HIV diagnoses in the UK are of drug resistant mutations.[1] If, as is feared, this phenomenon is generalised, then the threat from the epidemic is as great in the future as it is in the present.

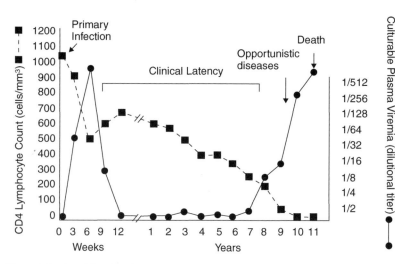

Figure 2.2   Viral load and CD4 cell counts over time
Source: Whiteside and Sunter (2000), p. 9.

Development and use of anti-retroviral therapies creates new problems:

- the virus mutates, there are over 120 sites in its structures which can mutate, and 'with hundreds of millions of virus particles being produced daily, it is not difficult to see how readily mutations occur which give rise to a wide range of biological variants even within the same individual' (Schoub, 1999, p. 87). This gives rise to drug resistance
- if people perceive AIDS as 'just' a chronic manageable condition they may be less inclined to take precautions against infection.

The incubation period in the developing world was thought to be shorter – between six and eight years. This was based on the assumption that people in the poor world had more challenges to their immune systems, poorer nutrition, and less access to health care. It seemed inevitable that they would progress to symptomatic AIDS faster. However of six African studies reported in 1996, four suggested progression rates similar to those in the industrial world, and two found shorter periods. Data then were 'scanty and are limited to sub-Saharan Africa' (Mulder, 1996, p. 15). Schoub (1999) notes, 'little is known as yet about the rate of progression in African patients where the prognosis appears to be considerably worse (than among homosexual men in Western countries)' (Schoub, 1999, p. 42; parentheses added).

One recent study found that the time from HIV illness to death is shorter for untreated patients in Uganda than in the rich world, and the spectrum of HIV/AIDS related disease is different. However the period from infection to illness did not seem to vary. This suggests that tropical diseases and infections such as TB or sexually transmitted infections do not hasten the progression of HIV to AIDS in Uganda (French et al., 1999, p. 509).

The issue of how long a period a person has between infection and illness is crucial for planning for the epidemic's economic and social impact. There is no one easy answer: time from infection to illness and from illness to death appears to be linked to disease environment, availability of health care and other factors. The period from onset of symptoms to death is shorter in poor countries. This has been borne out by a number of studies, most recently French et al. (1999) who speculate that it is because patients do not receive early and appropriate treatment – an obvious issue in resource-constrained environments.

The differences between the poor and rich worlds also apply to the rich and the poor worldwide, and come down to the following: people who are able to eat enough nutritious food, who lead stress-free lives and who are not exposed to multiple infections will stay healthy and live longer. This is true generally and does not apply just to those who are HIV infected. However HIV infection throws inequality into even starker relief. 'Extreme poverty deprives people of almost all means of managing risk themselves' (World Bank, *World Development Report*, 2000/01, p. 146). For the poor, HIV is more likely to be a death sentence than for those who can care for themselves and afford treatment.

Detecting HIV and describing AIDS

HIV was hard to locate because it is a retrovirus, hiding itself in the body's immune system. The first tests detected the *antibodies* to the virus rather than the virus itself. These might be compared to footprints on a sandy beach: they show a person has been there even though that person cannot be seen. Antibodies show that a person has been (and in the case of HIV, is) infected. Even today, most screening and diagnostic tests are based on discovery of antibodies rather than the virus. These tests have a high degree of sensitivity (which means that they do not miss positive results – if the person is infected then the tests will show this) and specificity (which means that they do not miss negative results – if the person is not infected the tests will not suggest that they are). The most advanced tests have reduced the window period to about three weeks. People are said to be HIV positive when the HIV antibodies are detected in their blood.

It is more difficult to define AIDS. In areas where CD4 counts and viral loads can be measured, people are regarded as having AIDS when their CD4 count falls below 200. In most settings, however, the capacity to carry out such sophisticated tests does not exist. In such places AIDS is defined clinically by examining the patient and making an assessment of his or her condition. A number of opportunistic infections, some of which are common in HIV infected people, take particular advantage of a depleted immune system. TB is one of these. Complicating matters further, new drug therapies make it possible for people to move from a state of AIDS, when they are very sick, to one of being HIV positive and leading a fairly normal life.

The origin of HIV

HIV derives from a virus that crossed the species barrier into humans. It is closely related to a number of Simian (monkey) Immunodeficiency

Viruses (SIVs) found in Africa. The evolution of the virus over time is traced through a 'family tree' as shown in Figure 2.3. This differs from the more familiar family tree because to read it you must start near the middle. In this case, the proximity of the different types of virus is an indication of how closely they are related. For example, HIV-1 is clearly related to chimpanzee SIV and HIV-2 to macaque SIV.

How did HIV enter the human population? Here we need to make a brief diversion to look at some other diseases. An important starting point is that the spread of diseases from animals to humans is not unique to HIV. Indeed we know that human diseases also spread to animals – but animals do not have access to science and the media, thus this goes unrealised and unremarked by most people. The influenza virus evolves in birds – waterfowl to be exact.[2] Virologists describe these birds as 'reservoirs' of infection. They carry nearly all known types of influenza, with no ill-effects, and spread them to the rest of the animal kingdom through their faeces. Hence, many kinds of animals can get flu – horses, ferrets, seals, pigs – as well as human beings.

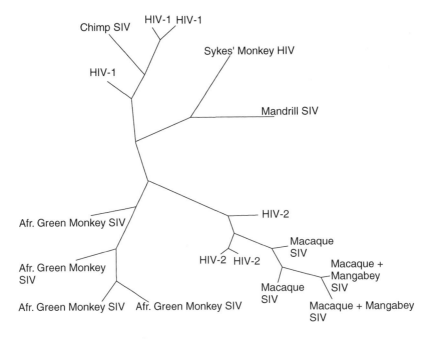

Figure 2.3   The HIV family tree
Source: Wills (1996)

However, viruses can only infect and take over a cell if it has a proper 'receptor'. Human cells do not have a receptor enabling them to contract avian flu directly. For human infection to occur another species must act as an intermediary; it can play this role by having a receptor for avian flu and humans in turn having a receptor for its flu. Pigs are one such species. The process can be as simple as a flu-contaminated duck dropping faeces into the dirt in which a pig then rolls. The pig is then infected and passes the virus on to a farmer. It can also be more complex. It is possible for a pig to be infected with one kind of flu, say human flu, only to contract another avian flu. The pig then has two types of flu simultaneously. When the pig re-infects the human, it passes on a pig-bird-human influenza. The Hong Kong flu, for example, held seven genes from a human virus and one gene from a duck virus: these met inside a pig, producing a new hybrid.

It is not just different viruses that can combine to create new and possibly more deadly diseases in the host. Viruses, and indeed all diseases, also replicate themselves within the host. This gives rise to variants of the virus within one person. These may in turn recombine to create new variants, some of which may be more virulent or drug resistant.

The speed with which HIV-1 replicates makes it a formidable enemy. There are two major strains of HIV-1. Group M causes over 99% of the world's HIV/AIDS infections. Groups O and the newly discovered N cause the remainder (Stine, 2001). Group M is divided into eleven subtypes or clades (A to K). The ability of the virus to mutate rapidly has significance in the quest for both a cure and a vaccine.

The question of when and how HIV entered human populations has been a source of great debate. We know that at some point the virus entered the blood of humans and then spread through sexual contact from person to person. In west Africa the less virulent HIV-2 spread from macaque monkeys. HIV-1 spread from chimpanzees into humans in central Africa. Four lines of evidence have been used to substantiate the zoonotic (transmission of a disease from one species to another) origin of AIDS:

1. similarities in organisation of the viral genome
2. phylogenic[3] relatedness of a particular HIV strain to that of SIV in the natural host
3. geographical coincidence between the SIV and particular HIV strains
4. plausible routes of transmission (Van Rensburg, 2000).

How did HIV cross the species barrier? We know that it is not an easily transmittable disease. It is carried in body fluids, with the highest concentration in blood, semen and vaginal secretions. For transmission to occur it had to enter the human body and reach the infectable cells. It thus had to breach the skin or mucosal barriers. There are a number of hypotheses as to how this might have happened:

- *Bush meat.* It is not hard to imagine a hunter killing, or someone butchering, an infected monkey and in the process contaminating a cut on his hand with the monkey's blood
- *Contaminated vaccine.* This is most elegantly (and lengthily) argued by Hooper (1999). He suggests that experimental polio vaccination campaigns in central Africa in the 1950s, using vaccine cultivated on chimpanzee kidneys, may have provided the opportunity for the virus to cross the species barrier
- *Contaminated needles.* The arguments above may explain how the virus crossed into humankind but they do not explain the rapid spread. It has been suggested that vaccine campaigns and poorly equipped clinics in rural Africa may have contributed to this through the use of unsterilised needles on one patient after another.
- *Ritual behaviour.* Finally, it has been suggested that use of monkey blood in certain rituals might have caused transmission. This hypothesis reflects a high degree of ethnographic ignorance and no little prejudice, as no one has described these rituals or given any examples as to where they take place.

The second and third hypotheses place the beginnings of the epidemic in the twentieth century. Hooper suggests that the polio campaigns of the late 1950s in Congo and Rwanda were the spark that ignited the fire. The cut hunter view has been used to suggest that the epidemic originated in infection across the species barrier in the 1930s.[4] Interestingly, in this case the transfer of the virus from an animal into a human may have happened on a number of previous occasions. However, because on those occasions each infected person did not in turn infect more than one other person, the potential epidemic petered out. There could have been a pool (or pools) of infection among isolated peoples in some parts of Africa for many years. What was different about the crossing of the species barriers in the 1930s (and the subsequent pattern of the epidemic) was the environment into which the virus was introduced. The upheavals of the colonial and post-colonial periods and development of modern transport infrastructure allowed HIV to spread quickly into the global community.

When all is said and done, the debate about the exact manner of zoonotic transmission is largely irrelevant. What matters today and in the future is that the virus has infected humans and is spreading fast.

Modes of infection

Fortunately for humankind, HIV is not a robust virus and it is hard to transmit. Unlike many diseases it can only be transmitted through contaminated body fluids. For a person to be infected, the virus has to enter the body in sufficient quantities. It must pass through an entry point in the skin and/or mucous membranes into the bloodstream. The main modes of transmission, in order of importance, are:

- unsafe sex
- transmission from infected mother to child
- use of infected blood or blood products
- intravenous drug use with contaminated needles
- other modes of transmission involving blood; for example, bleeding wounds.

Sexual transmission

The vast majority of HIV infections are the result of sexual transmission. Initially most cases were discovered among homosexual men. This was because HIV was first identified in this group in the West. Moreover, the chances of infection are higher during anal intercourse than vaginal sex. The relative probability of HIV infection per type of exposure is shown in Table 2.1. There is a small chance that HIV can be transmitted through oral sex, especially if a person has abrasions in the mouth or gum disease.

Table 2.1   Probability of HIV-1 infection per exposure

Mode of transmission	Infections per 1000 exposures
Female-to-male, unprotected vaginal sex	0.33–1
Male-to-female, unprotected vaginal sex	1–2
Male-to-male, unprotected anal sex	5–30
Needle stick	3
Mother-to-child transmission	130–480
Exposure to contaminated blood products	900–1000

Source: World Bank (1997a), p. 59.

The presence of sexually transmitted diseases (STDs), particularly those involving ulcers or discharges, will greatly increase the odds of HIV infection. An STD means that there is more chance of broken skin or membranes allowing the virus to enter the body. Furthermore, the very same cells that the virus is seeking to infect will be concentrated at the site of the STD because these cells are fighting the infection.

Mother-to-child transmission

After sexual transmission, the next most important cause of HIV infection is mother-to-child transmission (MTCT). It is known that the child can be infected with HIV prenatally, at the time of delivery, or postnatally through breastfeeding. Infection at delivery is the most common mode of transmission. A number of factors influence the risk of infection, particularly the viral load of the mother at birth – the higher the load, the higher the risk. A low CD4 count is also associated with increased risk. Anti-retroviral drugs may decrease the viral load and inhibit viral reproduction in the infant, thus decreasing the risk of MTCT. A number of studies of the use of anti-retroviral drugs to combat MTCT have shown that the chance of this transmission can be greatly reduced at a relatively low cost and using fairly simple treatment regimes.

An important issue requiring clarification is the role of breastfeeding. On the one hand, formula feeding reduces the risk of MTCT; on the other hand, it increases the risk of children dying of other causes, particularly when they live in poverty. Breastfeeding has been promoted in developing countries for many years as part of child health and survival strategies. There are many problems with formula feeding, including the cost and availability of the product in the short and long term, access to clean water, the means and fuel to boil the water and prepare the feed, and knowledge of how to mix the feed. The formula approach also means that women can be 'labelled' as being HIV positive, by virtue of their using replacement feed. Recent work suggests that the key to reducing risk is consistency in either breastfeeding or formula feeding an infant. Mixing the two is the most risky approach. 'A baby who is fed both the breast-milk of an HIV-positive mother and poorly made-up formula feeds is "getting the worst of both worlds"' (Chinnock, 1996, p. 15).

Infection through blood and blood products

Use of contaminated blood or blood products is the most effective way of transmitting the virus as it introduces the virus directly into the bloodstream. This is one of the reasons why so many haemophiliacs were infected during the early years of the epidemic: they received unscreened blood products. It also accounts for early infections among recipients of blood transfusions. Fortunately, in most countries, the risks of transmission through this route are now minimal. Blood banks seek to discourage those who might be infected from donating blood, and the technology is available to test all donations. However, because of the window period when people are infected but the antibodies are not detectable, the risk of infection cannot be entirely eliminated. The problem is greatest where blood is sold by donors and this gave the initial impetus to the epidemic in a number of Asian countries.

Intravenous drug use

Drug users who share needles are at risk of infection. If the equipment or drugs are contaminated, then the virus will be introduced directly into the body. This has driven the epidemic in Eastern Europe, the former Soviet Union and parts of Asia.

Other modes of transmission

There is a possibility that HIV may be transmitted in other ways. Medical or other instruments that are contaminated can transmit the virus. Examples include dental equipment, syringes and tattoo needles. Sterilisation procedures should ensure that this does not happen. Accidents through needlestick injury or during surgery are a concern for medical staff. Standard precautions, use of gloves and sterilising equipment, will protect doctors and nurses against HIV transmission from patients, and vice versa.

Responding to the disease

First prize with any disease is to prevent it. If prevention programmes had been successful, there would be no story to tell around HIV and AIDS. Unfortunately prevention programmes have not been successful in many parts of the world, and, where the epidemic has been controlled, no one is quite sure what actually worked (see Chapter 13).

Prevention

The principle of successful prevention is ensuring that people are not exposed to the disease or, if they are, that they are not susceptible to infection. Vaccines provide the latter form of protection but are not yet available for HIV. Preventing infections through blood transfusion depends on screening all donations and discouraging potentially infected donors from donating their blood. Occupational exposure can be reduced through adopting universally accepted precautions regarding safety and sterility. In the event that a health care worker is exposed, immediate treatment with anti-retroviral therapy can greatly reduce the risk of infection. In the case of injecting drug users, simple procedures such as the use of sterilised needles and needle exchange programmes have been very successful in some countries.

Preventing sexual transmission

As sex is the main mode of transmission, prevention strategies are most important here. One of the first responses to the epidemic was to call for the isolation of HIV infected people. This was seen by many as impracticable, oppressive and discriminatory. The one exception is Cuba. In the 1980s the authorities tested the entire population, isolating those found to be HIV positive in 'sanatoria'. This has contributed to the low level of HIV infection seen to date in that country. At the end of 1997, it was estimated that there were only 1,400 infected Cubans (UNAIDS/Pan American Health Organisation/WHO, 1998). However, for this approach to work, a high degree of governmental control is necessary, people entering the country who might be infected and/or spread the disease have to be tested, and there has to be good border control. In addition, there needs to be a programme of regular repeat testing. This was never an option for most countries and certainly not for poorer countries. Apart from the expense and difficulty of implementing such a programme, some argue that it is a violation of human rights.

To prevent sexual transmission there is a limited but potentially effective range of interventions. The first set of interventions is 'biomedical'; these aim to reduce sexual transmission. Good sexual health is paramount. This means that STDs should be treated immediately, and the availability of STD treatment in the rich world has probably played a major role in controlling HIV. Sexual practices that increase risk can be discouraged or made safer: a southern African example is 'dry sex' where a woman may use a drying agent in her vagina to increase friction during intercourse. This practice increases the risk of tears and abrasions, and can therefore facilitate the entry of the virus. The Filipino practice of inserting small metal balls into the penis, also in the belief that these *bolitas* increase pleasure, can create a portal for infection.

The most available biomedical intervention is the use of condoms. These provide a barrier to the virus and, if properly used, are effective. Both male and female condoms are available, but female condoms are more expensive and more difficult to use.

The second set of interventions seeks to prevent exposure to HIV by altering sexual behaviour; these are the Knowledge, Attitude and Practices and Behaviour (KAPB) interventions. First, people need to have *knowledge*, then they need to change their *attitudes* and finally alter their *practices* and *behaviour*. People are encouraged to stick to one partner, to delay first sexual intercourse, and to use condoms if they have more than one partner. This is the classic ABC message: A – abstain; B – be faithful; C – condom if necessary. The problem is that even if people have the knowledge, they may not have the incentive or the power to change their behaviour. If prevention is to move beyond knowledge to action, we must look at the socio-economic causes of the epidemic and intervene there too. (This is discussed in Chapters 3, 4 and 5.)

Treatment[5]

Enormous resources have gone into the search for a cure and a vaccine. Neither has yet been developed. However, there have been major advances in clinical treatment.

Developments in treatment have resulted in declining mortality rates from HIV among the rich. There are three stages in the treatment of HIV positive people. The first is when they are infected, but CD4 cell counts are high. At this point, the emphasis is on 'positive living' – staying healthy, eating the correct food, and so on. The second stage is when the CD4 cell count begins to drop. At this stage, prophylactic treatment to prevent TB and other common infections commences. The third stage is the use of anti-retroviral drugs to fight HIV directly.

Since the first anti-retroviral drugs were developed, many new generations of drugs have become available. At the moment anti-retroviral drugs may be used in single therapies (just one drug), double therapies (a combination of two drugs) or triple therapies (three drugs). The way the drugs act is shown in Figure 2.4. Single drug therapy is no longer used much because it causes fairly swift mutation of the virus into drug resistant strains. Dual therapy is cheaper than triple therapy, but the antiviral effect is less immediate as the viral load falls slowly and the viral control may be of a limited duration. Highly Active Anti-Retroviral Therapy (HAART) is any anti-retroviral regimen capable of suppressing HIV for many months and perhaps years in a significant number of individuals. Such is the case with triple therapy. It usually involves the

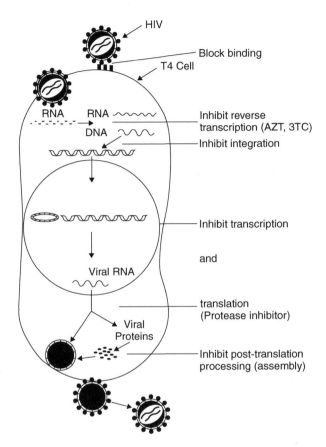

Figure 2.4   Where the drugs act
Source: Whiteside and Sunter (2000), p. 23.

use of two reverse transcriptase inhibitors and one protease inhibitor. Although not a cure, such treatments are effective in rapidly reducing the viral load to undetectable levels, thereby prolonging survival.

When to introduce a HAART regimen is of importance. Early treatment prevents damage to the body caused by high and prolonged viral loads – but it does use up the big guns sooner, which can decrease subsequent options if resistance builds up. That is why some clinicians prefer to step up the treatment gradually starting with single drug therapy. Cost is also a factor. The cost of anti-retroviral AIDS treatment in the rich world ranges between US$10,000 and US$20,000 per patient per year, although it can go much higher. Effective treatment of HIV/AIDS involves more than merely prescribing drugs: patients need regular consultations, testing for viral load and CD4 cell counts and, if treatment fails, testing for drug resistance. All this adds to costs.

Some Latin American countries (such as Brazil and Argentina) have been able to negotiate down the costs of the drugs. Argentina pays US$0.33 for AZT pills that previously cost US$2. Donations or subsidisation of drugs by the large pharmaceutical companies can reduce the costs of treatments. For example, in Senegal discounted drugs enable patients to have access to a range of therapeutic options costing between US$1,000 and US$1,800 per year (Gellman, 2000). It is not clear if the other costs are included.

The cheapest price on offer for the most advanced triple therapy at the beginning of 2001 was from drug company Cipla Ltd of Bombay who offered to sell drugs for US$600 per patient per year to the South African government and US$350 to non-governmental organisations (NGOs) (Swarms, 2001). The difference in cost may be based on whether the cost of observing patents is included or not. This is illustrated by comparing the costs of Flucanzole (used to treat AIDS-related meningitis) in Thailand (which does not observe patents), where the drug costs US$0.30 and Kenya (which does observe patents), where it costs US$18 (Kimani, 2000).

One study (Voelker, 2000) determined that for treatments to be affordable, HAART would need to be available at a monthly cost per person of US$10 for Zambia, US$20 for Botswana and US$45 for Mozambique. These figures assumed that it would be reasonable to spend 15% of the total health budget to treat 25% of the HIV positive population.

Anti-retroviral therapies are used when patient CD4 counts fall and their immune systems fail. Before this happens most HIV infected people will experience infection from other treatable diseases. These include candidiasis, meningitis and TB. In most of the poor world drugs to treat these infections are not available or are too expensive.

Of course, for the majority of AIDS sufferers all these treatments are out of reach because pharmaceutical companies are unprepared to make the drugs available at affordable prices. Furthermore most countries do not have the infrastructure to deliver the therapies.

Patient adherence is a real problem. Some triple drug therapies involve taking 18 pills a day in a particular sequence. Yet adherence to prescribed anti-HIV drug regimens is crucial for long-term success. Missing a single dose of medication may allow drug concentration in blood and tissues to drop below that needed for full HIV suppression. This decrease allows HIV replication to occur in the optimum environment for selection of drug resistant mutant strains. Combination pills are at present being developed to make adherence easier.

Vaccines

Intensive research is being carried out to develop a vaccine, so far with limited success. More than 15 years have passed since the first efforts, but as yet a vaccine remains elusive. Unfortunately the amount of money spent on researching AIDS vaccines is small (US$300–600 million a year) and is focused on strains found mainly in the US and Western Europe. The World Bank and the European Union, among others, have been involved in the search for new mechanisms and incentives to increase research and development of vaccines for developing countries. The International AIDS Vaccine Initiative (IAVI), based in New York, plays an increasingly important role in mustering resources and facilitating development.

HIV and other diseases

As their immune systems are progressively suppressed, other diseases will affect HIV positive people. Most of these are not a threat to uninfected people. But people with HIV are very much more likely to develop active TB.[6] In the absence of HIV, the chance of developing TB is low. In the event that a person is co-infected with HIV, the chance rises greatly. It is estimated that 40–50% of people with TB in South Africa are co-infected with HIV, and one-third of people with HIV are expected to contract TB. This has to be seen against a general background of high TB infection in South Africa. The annual incidence there in 1998 was 254 per 100,000 people – in Europe it is 19; in China, 113, and in India, 187.

TB can be treated. For instance, the DOTS regime (Directly Observed Treatment, short course) has dramatically raised cure rates. But this is for all patients. Prophylactic treatment for HIV positive people is far more costly and problematic. Not for nothing are HIV and TB variously referred to as 'the terrible twins' and 'Bonnie and Clyde'.

New evidence suggests that there are links between HIV and malaria. It is possible that people with HIV contract malaria more easily and certainly have a poorer prognosis.

So far we have described disease and processes in the individual body as a result of this particular virus. Disease is of social and economic significance. It causes groups of people to become infected, fall ill and die. HIV/AIDS is unique. The disease is sexually transmitted, therefore it affects prime-age adults; it is fatal and it is widespread. It is unusual for this group (prime-age adults) to be the target of any disease. This is why it has profound social and economic consequences. To understand the aggregate nature of disease, as a precursor to looking at these consequences, we need to understand something about HIV/AIDS epidemiology and epidemiology in general.

Epidemiology

Epidemiology has been defined as 'the study of the distribution and determinants of health-related conditions and events in populations, and the application of this study to the control of health problems' (Katzenellenbogen et al., 1997, p. 5).

Epidemiology examines patterns of disease in aggregate. It describes the social and geographical distribution and dynamics of disease. However, as we shall see, this is not at all straightforward, especially with regard to HIV/AIDS, because:

- data can be confusing, often people do not distinguish between HIV and AIDS
- data quality is variable
- data are *constructed* according to a variety of implicit or explicit assumptions
- data may be *interpreted* according to biases which people bring depending on their discipline, politics or paymaster.

Data are important. We need to know where the epidemic is located and where it might spread if we are to design effective prevention interventions. If we want to consider the potential social and economic impact of an HIV/AIDS epidemic, we need to have some idea of the numbers of people who are infected with the virus, and who and where they are. We need to be able to predict how many people will fall ill and die and when this will happen. For example, an education department needs to know how pupil numbers will change and what effects the epidemic will have on teacher availability and training needs. In this section we are concerned with how we know about the epidemic, how we obtain data on the disease, how we understand it and interpret it and the policy implications of this understanding.

Epidemiology provides only some of the required information. In later chapters we shall add to what epidemiology has to tell us by reviewing another set of questions about *why* epidemics take different forms in different societies. Our argument is that there are social and economic characteristics which make an epidemic grow more or less rapidly. They determine whether the epidemic is concentrated in a few 'high risk' or 'core' groups or whether it becomes generalised to the wider population. These determinants, which make a society more or less *susceptible* to epidemic spread, are closely tied to the characteristics which make that society more likely to suffer adverse consequences resulting from increased illness and death. We use the term *vulnerability* to talk about this greater or lesser likelihood of adverse impact. (Chapters 4 and 5 describe and discuss susceptibility, while Chapters 6–11 discuss vulnerability and impact.)

Epidemic curves

A key concept is the epidemic curve. HIV – indeed, any disease – will move through a susceptible population, infecting some and missing others. Epidemics follow an 'S' curve, as shown in Figure 2.5 They start slowly and gradually. At a certain stage, a critical mass of infected people is reached and the growth of new infections accelerates thereafter. The epidemic then spreads through the population until many of those who are susceptible to infection have been infected. Some are lucky because even though they are susceptible, they never come into contact with an infectious person. With modern transport networks there are few instances of isolated communities. Hence, epidemics can rapidly go global. The large and rising global population also means that many more people will be infected.

In the final phase of an epidemic – where the 'S' flattens off at the top and turns down – people are either getting better or deaths outnumber new cases so that the total number alive and infected passes its peak and begins to decline. With most diseases the curve will decline rapidly. HIV and AIDS are different.

What sets HIV and AIDS apart from other epidemics is that there are two curves, as shown in Figure 2.5. With most other diseases, infection is followed by illness within a few days or, at most, weeks. In the case of HIV the infection curve precedes the AIDS curve by between five and eight years. This reflects the long incubation period between infection and the onset of illness. This is why HIV/AIDS is in some ways such a lethal epidemic compared to, say, Ebola fever. In the latter case, victims of the disease quickly and visibly fall ill, putting the general population and public health professionals on their guard. The community takes precautions to halt spread and the infected person is rapidly immobilised, reducing his or her infective potential.

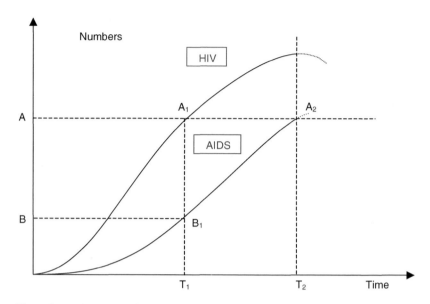

Figure 2.5   The two epidemic curves

HIV infection moves through a population giving little sign of its presence. It is only later, when substantial numbers are infected, that AIDS deaths begin to rise. People do not leave the infected pool by getting better because there is no cure. They leave by dying (of AIDS or other causes). The effect of life-prolonging ARTs is, ironically, to increase the pool of infected people.

Figure 2.5 illustrates this point clearly. The vertical axis represents numbers of infections or cases of illness and the horizontal represents axis time. At time T_1, when the level of HIV is at A_1, the number of AIDS cases will be very much lower, at B_1. AIDS cases will only reach A_2 (that is, the same level as A_1) at time T_2. By then years will have passed and the numbers of people who are infected with HIV will have risen even higher.

Figure 2.5 also shows that while prevention efforts may aim to lower the number of new infections, the reality is that without affordable and effective treatment, AIDS case numbers and deaths will continue to increase after the HIV tide has been turned.

Beyond the point T_2, the lines are dotted. This is because we do not know how either the HIV or the AIDS curves will proceed. In only two poorer countries, Uganda and Thailand, does national HIV prevalence (and incidence – see below) appear to have peaked and turned down.

Figure 2.5 shows an epidemic curve. But a national epidemic is made up of many sub-epidemics, with different gradients and peaks. These sub-epidemics vary geographically and in terms of their distribution among social or economic groups. In many countries in the poor world HIV spread first among drug users and commercial sex workers (CSWs). From there it moved into other groups: mobile populations, men who visited sex workers, and eventually into the broader population. One common feature in both the rich and poor world is that HIV spreads among people at the margins of society, the poor and dispossessed. (Examples of national and sub-national epidemics are discussed further in the case studies in Chapter 4.)

Incidence and prevalence

Incidence is the number of new infections which occur over a time period. The *incidence rate* is the number of infections per specified unit of population in a given time period. Rates can be per 1,000, per 10,000 or per million for rare diseases. The time may be per annum, but in the case of more rapidly moving infections it may be days or weeks. *Prevalence* is the absolute number of infected people in a population at a given time – it is a still photograph of current infections. The *prevalence rate* is the percentage of the population which exhibits the disease at a particular time (or averaged over a period of time). A numerical example and an illustration appear in Table 2.2 and Figure 2.6, respectively.

Data on incidence and prevalence are key statistics for tracking the course of the HIV epidemic. With HIV, prevalence rates are given as a percentage of a specific segment of the population. Commonly used groups are antenatal clinic attendees, adults aged between 15 and 65, blood donors, men with STDs, or the 'at risk' population – usually taken to mean 15- to 49-year-olds who are sexually active. Uniquely,

Table 2.2   Incidence and prevalence

Year	Population	Incidence (actual)	Incidence rate per 1000	Prevalence	Prevalence rate (%)
1	9,750	0	0	0	0
2	10,000	50	5	50	0.5
3	10,500	50	4.7	100	1.0
4	11,000	150	13.6	250	2.3
5	12,000	750	62.5	1,000	8.3

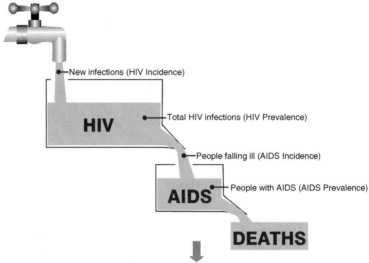

Note: The only point at which measurements are regularly made is HIV Prevalence

Figure 2.6   HIV/AIDS incidence and prevalence
Source: Whiteside and Sunter (2000)

HIV prevalence is given as a percentage rather than as a rate, as is the case for other diseases. Why this is the case is not clear; it may be because of the need to communicate figures simply, or because advocates find percentages most compelling.

Annual incidence is calculated by subtracting the previous year's prevalence from that of the current year. Because we don't know when people were actually infected – we only know the date on which their serostatus is ascertained – the data (incidence) which would be most helpful in measuring the impact of prevention efforts are simply not available. Moreover, high incidence may occur even when prevalence has levelled off, because those dying are being replaced by new infections.

Currently we have to use prevalence data to track how the epidemic is moving through a population, comparing one year with another. The aim of control and prevention measures is to reduce both prevalence and incidence. To achieve this the number of new infections produced by each existing infection must be reduced.

The reproductive rate

The gradient, final height and rate of decline of an epidemic curve is determined by the average number of secondary cases generated by one primary case in a susceptible population and the period over which this takes place. This is also known as 'the basic reproductive number' and is represented by the symbol R_0 (Anderson and May, 1992; Anderson, 1999). In order for an epidemic to be maintained, R_0 has to equal 1; in other words, each person who gets better or dies has to infect one other person. At this point the disease is endemic but stable. When $R_0 > 1$, each person infects more than one other person, the number of cases will rise. When $R_0 < 1$ then the epidemic will be disappearing. In South Africa in 2000 the R_0 for HIV was estimated at 5, while that of malaria was 100 (Whiteside and Sunter, 2000, p 10).

The percentage or number infected in a population depends on the degree of susceptibility of individuals in that population. This term is usually used in the narrow biomedical sense of transmission efficiency. 'Transmission efficiency is expressed as the probability that a contact will occur between infected and susceptible individuals multiplied by the likelihood that a contact will result in transmission' (Anderson, 1996, p 73). In this book we argue that susceptibility is far more than the result of biomedical events in the body; understanding and acting on this insight is fundamental both to reducing the rate of spread of the HIV/AIDS epidemic and to dealing with its long-term economic and social consequences.

Most epidemics are of relatively short duration. This is determined by the time from initial infection to the end (recovery or death) of the infectious period. Cholera epidemics may last only a few months in any one location. A measles epidemic with its typical two-week period from infection to illness will last between six months to a year. In the case of a disease where the gestation period is several years, the epidemic will last for decades. This is the case with HIV and it may be similar with nvCJD.

The HIV curve tells us where the epidemic has been. Projections tell us where it might go. HIV is not on its own important for understanding the social and economic impact of the epidemic. What is important is the AIDS curve (see Figure 2.5). If we are to consider impact we need to have an idea of the size of the potential AIDS epidemic which will hit a particular society.

How bad is the epidemic? How many people are infected and will die? How serious and global a crisis is it? These are all questions which are seldom posed in a precise way. Those who believe AIDS is a 'crisis' believe it is *the* major challenge facing most of the world. Thus 'Acquired immunodeficiency syndrome (AIDS) has become a major development crisis. It kills millions of adults in their prime' (General Assembly on HIV/AIDS, 2001). A memorandum issued on 2 June 1999 to World Bank staff and supporters announcing the new AIDS in Africa initiative (World Bank, *World Development Report*, 1998), stated: 'This fire is spreading. AIDS already accounts for 9% of adult deaths from infectious disease in the developing world. By 2020, that share will *quadruple* to more than 37%. The global death toll will soon surpass the worst epidemics of recorded history.'

Those who deny that there is an acute problem come in various shades: some say that there is no evidence of increased illness; others say that this can be explained by poverty, urbanisation or drug use. Even where the seriousness of the issue is recognised there is often debate over the exact figures. Effectively, people say: 'If you can't tell us exactly what is going on, why should we believe you at all?' This is a facet of denial processes which appears throughout the history of the epidemic.

Data sources

This section looks at how data are derived. We begin with AIDS case data and then go on to look at HIV. In Chapter 4 we establish the ways in which the epidemic trajectory differs from country to country, and how social, economic and cultural situations determine this. Here we provide a background to some of the difficulties in obtaining and interpreting such data.

Key data sources include governments, non-governmental organisations, academic establishments, and in some instances the private sector. Data are of variable quality but – *and this is important to note* – all data produced by all agencies originate from the countries themselves. Thus data reflect what is available in countries and what they choose to report. Epidemiologists and statisticians may make assumptions and extrapolate, but they are dependent on the information they are given.

Two main bodies collect and compile international data. UNAIDS produces estimates of AIDS cases, HIV prevalence in various groups, numbers of deaths and orphans. These data are collected and published annually in the *Report on the Global HIV/AIDS Epidemic*. Thus we are told that in 1999, 5.4 million people were newly infected, 2.8 million died and 34.3 million were living with HIV/AIDS. UNAIDS also produces country epidemiological factsheets.[7]

The second source of data is the United States Bureau of Census which collates official data and also data from many other published and 'grey literature' sources.[8] Staff of the Bureau can be seen at all conferences of note photographing posters, collecting papers and checking findings with people on site.

AIDS case data

In the early years of the epidemic, AIDS case data were the main source of information. Each year or month the 'body count' rose. This was most vividly demonstrated in Randy Shilts's documentation of the first few years of the epidemic, largely in the US (Shilts, 1987). As the 1980s unfolded, AIDS cases were reported from more and more countries across the world. Graphs were produced showing exponential increases in the numbers of cases and deaths. Unfortunately there was public confusion between HIV and AIDS, aided and abetted by press reports which failed to distinguish between infection and disease.

In the poor world reporting required that someone actually took the time and trouble to notify public authorities that they were seeing AIDS patients. The question was and still is: 'Do we have a clear picture of the number of AIDS cases or deaths?' The answer is 'No', and indeed we never did.

In most countries AIDS is not a notifiable disease, which means that medical staff are not legally required to report cases. Even if they do there are serious constraints to this process:

- reporting may be very slow. It takes time for data to flow into a central point and be collated
- data may be inaccurate because of unwillingness to report cases. This may be due to stigma associated with AIDS; to potential discrimination by medical insurance companies, not paying for treatment of AIDS related conditions, and by the life insurance industry excluding claims where the cause of death is given as AIDS
- the condition from which a person dies may not be recognised as being AIDS related. Instead the patient may be recorded as having, for example, TB or meningitis
- doctors may feel that it is pointless to report cases as there is no incentive, they are too busy or they get no feedback.

Many people in poor countries are not seen by the formal medical services. Figure 2.7 shows the numbers of 'filters' a report has to go

Person falls ill with AIDS	**AIDS case not recorded because:**
↓	
Is seen by formal medical service ➜	Person visits traditional healer/does not seek care
↓	
Is correctly diagnosed ➜	Is not correctly diagnosed or diagnosed with an opportunistic infection
↓	
Case recorded ➜	Case not recorded
↓	
Record sent to data collection point ➜	Report not forwarded/lost in post, etc.
↓	
Data collected and published ➜	Report lost/not published

Figure 2.7   The problems of AIDS case reporting

through before it becomes an official 'case'; in other words, before it is counted. The right-hand column shows the factors which can prevent this. Consider that somebody is dying in a small house, in a small village, several miles on foot from the nearest motorable road and many miles from the nearest all-weather road. There is a small clinic ten miles away but the medical orderly has not been paid for several months and has little in the way of drugs or equipment. The person's family has exhausted its resources and strength in caring for her. How is this person to become a 'case' recorded in the capital city some 300 or more kilometres away?

The fact is that no poor country has counted its AIDS cases. Indeed even in hospitals, many of which lack test kits, we cannot know how many AIDS cases there really are. What then is the value of AIDS case data? First, if they are collected consistently and in sufficient quantities, trends will be apparent. Second, they can give an indication of the scale of the problem. Finally, they can show where the epidemic is located by age, gender, mode of transmission and geographical area. Figure 2.8 illustrates the situation in Malawi in 1995. The first cluster

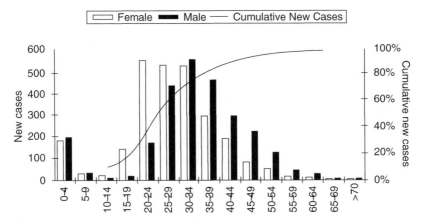

Figure 2.8 Malawi – age and gender profile of new AIDS cases 1995
Source: Loewenson and Whiteside (1997).

of cases is those resulting from mother-to-child transmission. The next is for young women, peaking in the 20–24 age group, and finally there is a cluster of male deaths in the 30–34 age group.

Most social and economic statistics have political ramifications. AIDS case data have always been 'political'. In the early years of the epidemic, countries were reluctant to admit to the existence of the disease because of what they felt its presence might suggest or imply about the morals and behaviour of their citizens, or what it might do to the tourist industry. This was the initial reaction in Kenya and Thailand.

Perhaps the most telling example of the politicisation of data was in Zimbabwe. The first report to the Global Programme on AIDS in Geneva was of several hundred cases in 1987. A few weeks later South Africa (then still under the apartheid regime) reported 120 cases. Within days the Zimbabwean government reduced its reported cases to 119 (*AIDS Analysis Africa*, 1990, p. 6).

The next potential data source is AIDS deaths. However, with few exceptions, there is no vital registration in poorer countries, and even where there is, information will not be collected on the cause of death by disease. Where death data are recorded information can be extracted (discussed in Chapter 6). But we must always remember that even if AIDS cases are accurately recorded at any given time, they reflect the HIV infections of five or more years earlier.

HIV data

HIV data tell us how many people are infected in a population, and are most frequently presented as prevalence. Ideally data would show exactly who in a population is infected and when they were infected. This would allow plans to be made for care and support of infected people and their families and human resource management. Deaths make families less able to provide for their members, the workforce less able to work, and increase demand for services such as health and welfare. Such data should also enable the epidemic to be tracked and the success (or failure) of interventions to be measured.

The ideal survey would cover an entire population. Every individual would give a blood or saliva sample for testing. Such a survey would furnish a point prevalence (the prevalence at that point in time). To track the epidemic, subsequent surveys would have to be carried out. This would be a logistical nightmare, would be costly and would raise ethical issues: do you compel people to take part? If people are identified then what do you do with them? As mentioned earlier, this type of survey has only been done in Cuba – an island with a population of 11.1 million.

Second best would be a population-based random survey which samples men and women across age groups to provide a representation of the situation in the whole population within certain calculable bounds of error. Such surveys have been done in a few places. They are expensive, require a lot of organisation, raise ethical issues and need to be repeated if they are to have value. In the past one of the major obstacles to population-based surveys was that the HIV test required blood. Taking blood is an invasive procedure to which many people will not consent. The development of saliva tests over the past few years has made population surveys much more viable.[9]

Presently available data are drawn mainly from samples of specific population sub-groups. These are then extrapolated to larger populations. UNAIDS notes that different types of epidemic require different types of surveillance:

> In largely heterosexually driven epidemics where there is evidence that men and women in the general population have become infected with HIV in significant numbers, HIV surveillance is based … on pregnant women attending antenatal clinics that have been selected as sentinel surveillance sites … the more regular the studies, the clearer the picture of current prevalence. Where data are not available for the current year, all available data points are plotted on

a curve, and an estimate for the current year is made according to what is known about the course of epidemics with predominantly heterosexual transmission. To account for differences in the spread of HIV, this is generally done separately for urban and for rural areas. (UNAIDS, 2000f, p. 116–18)

Many sub-Saharan African countries and a few in Asia and the Caribbean have conducted regular antenatal clinic HIV prevalence studies since the end of the 1980s. Antenatal clinic attenders provide a good sample because they are sexually active and adult. A major advantage is that blood is routinely taken from women attending these clinics for a number of standard tests and surveys can be repeated.

Box 2.2   Antenatal surveys

Antenatal HIV surveys are based on a sample of women attending antenatal clinics. A portion of the blood drawn for routine testing will be marked with the woman's age, the clinic's location and possibly some other social, economic or marital status data, and then sent for testing. This testing is called *anonymous* and *unlinked*. In other words, individual women cannot be identified as the source of a particular sample.

Such surveys should be done on a regular basis, either every year or every two years. In India they were initially done every six months to give rapid, consecutive results.

There are biases: younger women will be overrepresented as they are more sexually active and likely to fall pregnant; HIV positive women will be underrepresented as HIV infection reduces fertility.

An obvious drawback is that the survey is confined solely to women attending state antenatal clinics. It does not cover those women who either do not have access to state health care or who can afford to see private practitioners.

Population-based surveys were rare. However, where they have been done they show that in heterosexually driven epidemics the differences between these data and those from pregnant women are not great

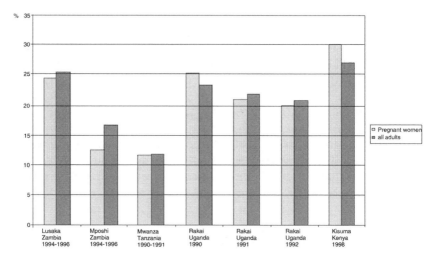

Figure 2.9   HIV prevalence rates among pregnant women and among all adults aged 15–49
Source: UNAIDS (2000F)

(Figure 2.9). Thus antenatal clinic data may be used cautiously as a proxy for the general population.

In most countries in Asia, South and Central America and Eastern Europe, the first manifestations of the disease, AIDS cases, were found in particular groups. These became subject to epidemiological surveillance. It was assumed that they represented high-risk behaviours. They included intravenous drug users; men who have sex with men, and sex workers and their clients. Here the methods for estimating HIV prevalence are different. What is needed is information on HIV prevalence in each group with high-risk behaviour, together with estimates of the size of each of these populations and the prospect of the epidemic bridging to the broader population. 'Since these behaviours are often socially unacceptable and sometimes illegal, information on both HIV prevalence levels and the size of the population affected can be much harder to come by. Consequently, uncertainties around these estimates may well be greater for countries where the epidemic is concentrated in specific groups' (UNAIDS, 2000f, pp. 116–18). A good example of the difficulties is countries where drug possession is a capital offence. In these circumstances it is particularly hard to track the epidemic in intravenous drug users.

UNAIDS presents data in its annual reports, but it is hedged with caveats. Estimates of new HIV infections and HIV related deaths are developed through 'simple back-calculation' procedures, which are based on the 'well-known natural course of HIV infection which determines the relationship between HIV incidence, prevalence and mortality' (UNAIDS, 2000f, pp. 116–18). Estimates for mother-to-child transmission (including breastfeeding) and HIV mortality in children are calculated from countries' age-specific fertility rates and documented region-specific rates of mother-to-child transmission.

Private sector companies and organisations are beginning to collect data for their own purposes. We know that in southern Africa insurance companies are gathering such information because they routinely test people before offering cover. These data are biased to those applying for policies and are often commercially sensitive, and so they tend not to be publicly available. For companies wishing to estimate how the epidemic is going to affect their workforce, the advent of saliva and urine tests mean surveys can be carried out more easily. These tests are non-invasive and relatively cheap. (In Chapter 10 we describe how, in consultation with the workers, this information was collected by one major employer in Botswana and how, if it is correctly and sensitively used, it can be valuable in designing company responses to the impact of the epidemic.)

Finally it is a routine procedure to test blood donations and these data can provide a picture of what is going on in what should be a low-risk group. Blood donors may be considered a low-risk group because organisations collecting blood try to exclude HIV positive people.

HIV data are also collected and constructed according to political social and other biases. The mere act of looking for HIV in one particular group has political and social significance. A national epidemic is the construct of a particular reporting system embedded in a specific polity which filters information into data; it is the signal which is modulated out of the background noise. The polity is a part of the modulating process. It defines and enables the reporting system, and may itself be an aspect of the relative susceptibility of societies. For example, a political system that insists on classifying HIV infections by 'race' would present one perspective. A system which refused to recognise the existence of male homosexuality or widespread intravenous drug use would present another filter; and a political system which could not afford to report accurately because there was no money for test kits would produce yet another slant.

Arguments about numbers may also be politically charged. This was apparent in the correspondence pages of the *South African Medical Journal* in 2000. Four independent researchers – Dorrington, Bradshaw, Bourne and Abdool Karim (Dorrington et al., 2000) – argued that the officially stated decline in HIV prevalence from 1998 to 1999 (from 22.8% to 22.4%) was incorrect. An examination of the 1999 results showed that prevalence fell only in Mpumalanga, a province with 7% of South Africa's population. Otherwise rates of infection showed little or no change in three provinces and rose in the remaining five. Dorrington et al. (2000) therefore concluded, using population weighted methods, that national prevalence should not have fallen; rather, a small increase was to be expected. Government officials and a respondent from the South African Medical Research Council (2000) argued that the data were accurate, and castigated Dorrington et al. for their pessimism, for their failure to approach the Department of Health before writing with 'whatever suggestions they might have', and for not 'joining in an active partnership against HIV/AIDS'.

Readers may think that this debate smacks of rearranging the deckchairs on the *Titanic*. The magnitude of the crisis is not debated, just the detail. However such a discussion points to the danger of debating figures rather than focusing on what they tell us about dealing with prevention and impact mitigation. It also shows the defensiveness of some governments (Dorrington et al., 2000).

The use of data

Data have three key functions: advocacy, prevention and prediction.

Advocacy requires people to see and understand the potential for the epidemic to develop and the impact it may have. The problem, clear from the preceding discussion, is that AIDS data are inadequate and outdated and HIV data do not show a visible epidemic.

Prevention remains the goal of all in the field of HIV/AIDS. HIV data give a picture of where the epidemic is located, the scale of the problem and who should be targeted for prevention interventions. They help in assessing if prevention activities are working. A decline in prevalence among younger women is seen as the first sign of hope. However this needs to be treated with caution, as it is not clear if the infections are averted or simply deferred. Women may be uninfected in their late teens because they do not have sex or because they use condoms. They become infected later, when they become sexually active or decide to have children.

Lack of incidence data also means that if the prevalence plateaus, we cannot be sure whether this is because people who die are being replaced with new infections. The turnover can be considerable. An apparently stable epidemic hides many deaths and new infections. The new generation of tests – both blood and saliva – may assist in providing incidence data which will help to show whether interventions are having any effect. But few give any consideration to the question of the impact of the disease. HIV infections become AIDS cases and AIDS deaths. AIDS cases need care, and AIDS deaths cut to the core of households and societies, leaving orphans and impoverishment.

Prediction tells us about the future course of the epidemic and its possible impacts. This is done through modelling. Here we use HIV data because AIDS case data have limited value. While it is useful to know the scale of the problem facing us in the present, what is most important in planning for impact is to know what will happen in the future. How many people will fall ill? How many orphans will there be? In order to look into the future the epidemic has to be projected through a process of modelling.

Mathematical models (which are translated into computer programmes) may be used to create projections of the course of the epidemic and its impacts, and more specifically estimate their magnitude.

HIV/AIDS projection models may be used for several different purposes, such as:

- projecting HIV prevalence and numbers
- projecting future AIDS cases, AIDS related deaths and orphans
- examining the demographic impact of AIDS and addressing questions regarding the impact of AIDS on population growth rates, the population age structure, numbers of orphans,[10] and life expectancy
- simulating different intervention strategies and comparing their strengths and weaknesses
- assessing the impact of the AIDS epidemic; for example, in terms of increased health expenditure and interactions with other diseases such as tuberculosis[11]
- Creating different scenarios which illustrate the effect of different assumptions on the projected outcome

All models depend on data, and the amount and type of data required will depend on the model used, the questions to be answered and the data to hand. This in turn will depend critically on whether a country is able to collect information about its epidemic. Does it have the technical, financial and political resources to do so? It is important to keep in mind that models are simply tools which may be used to guide decision making. Models are by definition a *representation* of an *aspect* of reality and they cannot possibly replicate the complexity of any real situation.

Conclusion

This chapter has described the basic science of HIV and the AIDS. It has explored the epidemiological instruments through which we 'know' or construct our knowledge about the aggregate effects of the disease.

At every point we see that data about the epidemic – including what it is, how it is defined, and how it is measured – are not neutral. Data are the outcomes of social, economic and cultural processes. Data are political: it may be that the governments do not want to admit that the epidemic exists; perhaps because they don't believe that their citizens 'behave in *these* ways', or that there are potential economic consequences. Admitting that there is an uncontrolled epidemic may also mean acknowledging that government policies have failed.

The form in which data appear depends on who is looking at information and how: doctors look among their patients, actuaries among those who form their client pool, anthropologists and sociologists in the particular group they are studying. Bias also arises from who is paying for the data – if you have an AIDS project it is not in your interest to show there is no AIDS!

Data are used to model the development and impact of the epidemic, but this, too, is not a neutral activity: models have assumptions and biases built into them according to the disciplines and beliefs of those who develop them and those who pay for them. Results will be interpreted differently according to the biases (explicit or implicit) of those who use them.

We have indicated the disease has implications far beyond the individual bodies that it destroys. It has social and economic causes and consequences. In Chapter 3 we consider why epidemics should differ so dramatically between societies.

Part II
Susceptibility

3
Epidemic Roots

Epidemic history and stigma

We may think of epidemics as unusual events, moments when disease organisms cross boundaries between habituated and non-habituated populations. We should rather consider an alternative view: that epidemics have their deepest foundations in 'normal' social and economic life. This is because pathways of infection are mapped on to social, cultural and economic relations between groups of human beings in ways that are sometimes simple, but more often not simple. As we all share the same world, but unequally, so we are differentially exposed to disease organisms, and for that matter to many non-infectious illnesses.

Particular infectious diseases are more likely to be present in some environments than in others. There is an image that 'tropical countries' are host to more infections than are temperate areas. The argument is that the humidity and high temperatures support larger, more varied populations of disease organisms. Some typically 'tropical' diseases continue to exist because of enduring poverty. Heat and humidity plus poor sanitation, crowded living conditions and polluted drinking water allow disease to thrive. We should not forget that typically 'tropical' diseases such as malaria and cholera were common until quite recently in temperate Europe and North America (Farmer, 1996). In the poorest countries, it is the wealthier, better-fed, better-housed and more leisured who are most likely to escape infectious disease.

Epidemics do not just happen. They are not random events. They have histories.[1] Histories always depend on how they are told, by whom and for what reason. Histories of infectious disease reflect the ways in which channels and paths of infection have been created as part of the material and cultural lives of societies. As we will see in Chapter 4, each 'national epidemic' is an artefact of all the sub-epidemics – by social group and by geographical area.

HIV/AIDS mixes sex, death, fear and disease in ways that can be interpreted to suit the prejudices and agendas of those controlling particular historical narratives in any specific time or place. Fear of infection all to easily translates into fear of the infected. The disease has been used to stigmatise various out-groups. 'Gay plague', women sex-workers, foreigners, 'those people living across the lake', 'those people who are black/Haitian/white/rich', 'harijans', 'tribals', 'non-Han Chinese' and so on. People have used all these labels, and many more, to identify 'those who are to be stigmatised'.

Stigmatisation is itself an important part of the history of any particular epidemic. It is a social process: a feature of social relations, reflecting the tension, conflict, silence, subterfuge and hypocrisy found in every human society and culture. While illness and death are the public facets of an epidemic disease like HIV/AIDS, these others are its private facets.

Illness and death expose to the public gaze areas of life of which people may be most ashamed and frightened. Some may be concerned because that gaze threatens existing patterns of power and interest. Hence the sometimes painful and embarrassing public discussion of sexuality, of sexual practices, of cross-caste liaisons, of child sexuality, of women's dependence on and therefore vulnerability to men. All these disturbing issues have been exposed to examination as the epidemic has progressed. The unusual numbers of illnesses and deaths in particular social groups makes it impossible to ignore the sexual origins of this disease. This violates social taboos, which in the absence of AIDS protect interests and avert the public gaze. When taboos are violated these webs of interest, power, privilege, dissimulation, collusion and, above all, institutionalised inequality are exposed and questioned.

In the richest countries, it is the poor who are more likely to endure bad health and also to be more exposed to infectious disease. The distribution of illness and disease tells of the distribution of poverty in the world. There is nothing original in saying this; the shame is that it continues to need repeating.

Global patterns of disease: past and present

Death and disease come in many shapes and forms. We all have to die someday. The question is what will kill us and when. In the rich world most people can expect to live to a ripe age and die of a non-communicable disease. These are the diseases of age and affluence. In the poor world the burden of communicable disease is much greater, people will live for a shorter time and their lower life expectancy will in part reflect their exposure to infectious disease and natural hazards.

The different burdens of disease are shown in Table 3.1. Communicable disease accounts for 21% of life years lost in Africa and under 10% in the rich world. In Eastern Europe and East Asia, over 16% of years lost are due to injury. Even more striking are the total life years lost – highest in Africa at 575 per 1,000 people, lowest in the rich world at a mere 117 per 1,000. This brings into focus the global inequity in health prospects and status. Broadly speaking, the vast majority of communicable diseases include those caused by bacteria and protozoa[2] – cholera, diarrhoeal diseases and tuberculosis – and those caused by viruses such as influenza, smallpox, measles and AIDS.

Infectious disease epidemics – causes and consequences

What causes infectious disease? Answer: a disease organism of course; a bacterium, a virus, or a prion.

What causes disease epidemics?

Box 3.1   Snakes, lice and witchcraft

'I knew a Zulu whose son was bitten by a snake and died. He said that his son had been killed by witchcraft. This did not mean that he didn't see that his son had been bitten by a snake, or that he didn't know that some snakes are poisonous while others are not, and that the bite of a poisonous snake may be fatal. When he said that his son was killed by witchcraft, he meant that a witch caused the snake to bite his son so that the son died ... every piece of good fortune involves two questions: the first is "how" did it occur, and the second is "why" it occurred at all ... Beliefs about witchcraft explain why particular persons at particular times and places suffer particular misfortunes ... witchcraft as a theory of causation is concerned with the singularity of misfortune ... A Pondo teacher in South Africa ... [asked] "It may be quite true that typhus is carried by lice, but who sent the infected louse? Why did it bite one man and not another?"' (Gluckman, 1955, p. 85)

Table 3.1 Life expectancy and life years[3] lost by world region

Area	Life expectancy at birth 1998	DALY[e] loss 1990 (%)			DALYs per 1000 population
		Communicable diseases[f]	Non-communicable diseases[g]	Injuries[h]	
World	66.9	45.8	42.2	11.9	259
Sub-Saharan Africa	48.9	71.3	19.4	9.3	575
Established market economies[a]	76.4	9.7	78.4	11.9	117
Eastern Europe and the CIS	68.9	8.6	74.8	16.6	168
Middle Eastern Crescent[b]	66	51	36	13	286
Latin America and the Caribbean	69.7	42.2	42.8	15	233
East Asia[c]	70.2	25.3	58	16.7	178
South Asia[d]	63.4	50.5	40.4	9.1	344

Notes: This table is compiled from two different data sources. This means geographical areas may not be directly comparable. The life expectancy data are taken from the 2000 UNDP *Human Development Report (HRDR)*, the DALYs data from the World Bank 1993, *World Development Report (WDR)*. The first four notes explain possible variations in coverage, the four remaining notes expand on the data.

a. OECD in *HDR*.

b. Arab states in *HDR*.

c. China in the *WDR*.

d. India in the *WDR*.

e. Disability Adjusted Life Years 1990 – a measure of the burden of disease.

f. Causes listed include TB, STDs and HIV, diarrhoea, vaccine preventable childhood infections, malaria, worm infections, respiratory infections, maternal causes, perinatal causes and 'other'.

g. Causes listed include cancer, nutritional deficiencies, neuropsychiatric disease, cerebrovascular disease, ischaemic heart disease, pulmonary obstruction and 'other'.

h. Causes include motor vehicle, intentional injury and 'other'.

This is a different order of question and there are many answers to it. These depend on your perspective and frame of reference. The question is also located within frameworks of cultural assumption – as shown by the stories of the snake and the louse. Looking at that particular anecdote from an 'African' perspective, we might ask, 'Well, why do Western "scientific" approaches relegate these concerns to a category called "probability", "chance" or "luck"?'

There are *risks* which are 'decision dependent', which can, in principle, be brought under control through rational decision. There are *dangers* which cannot be brought under control by, currently available, science, technology or political means (Beck, 2000a, p. 31). As we shall see, at present we put prevention of infection between individual bodies into the first category, placing the social and economic origins of susceptibility to infection into the latter, because they are too difficult to understand. That is not very different from saying 'That's witchcraft!'

Risks and dangers

There is an element of political and ethical will which makes us determine some things as explicable and thus tractable and others as inexplicable and intractable. We all too easily place large social and economic problems into the category of those things which are too big and complex to deal with because they are 'social' and intractable. It is hard to give causal answers to such questions and searching for explanations may be symptomatic of a misplaced faith in the power of science. Some things are puzzles with rational 'solutions'; others are problems, dilemmas and conundrums which have neither a single nor necessarily any solution. How we think between these two categories will alter through history. At present, the root causes of disease epidemics and many other issues of public policy fall into the second category of the intractable.

Today we are much more aware of the length of some of the complex causal chains which affect our lives. Increasing consensus about global warming and climatic change have pressed that awareness upon us all. It seems that we are also apparently more likely to create such long-term effects because of the scale on which science and technology can now operate. A genetic modification here, deforestation here, a change in feed for cattle, and some years down the line there are multiple dangers. We engage intellectually and practically with the very large and the very small but less so with the long-term relationships between these two scales. We now recognise more easily that each engagement with the micro- or macroscopic realm may have major large-scale and long-wave implications. Genetic engineering is a case in point, microscopic scale and potentially macroscopic impact. Nowhere are the long chain relationships between the microscopic and the macroscopic worlds more evident than in the origins of the HIV/AIDS epidemic and its social and economic consequences.

The implication is that we must carefully reconsider two other issues: responsibility and the relation between the 'public' and 'private' spheres. If we recognise that an action now has very long-term ramifications then we may face a new definition of 'responsibility'. If we recognise that a 'private' action (for example, by a company) may have considerable 'public' – even global – effects, then we may have to reconsider what we mean by the terms 'public' and 'private' – terms which are absolutely fundamental to the nature of 'Western' societies which have tended to elevate the importance of the 'private' sphere at the expense of the 'public'. For example, we may have to think again about the 'privacy' claimed by companies when they say that they will not justify or explain publicly the costs of research and development of new drugs for reasons of commercial privacy. Recognising these questions has important implications for how we think about welfare and public health.

Such concerns may seem distant from those which opened the chapter. They are not. When we examine the thinking behind responses to the AIDS epidemic, we discover that it is the consequence of long-wave processes, remote 'causes' and remote 'effects'. Our ability to understand its complexity is better now than it has ever been. We can understand the HIV/AIDS epidemic in ways that were not possible for previous epidemics. These insights have challenging implications for what can be done to stem an epidemic, when, where and by whom. What you think you can and *ought* to do depends on how far back in time you push the ideas of 'cause' and responsibility. This poses the related question of what you take to be the parameters of the epidemic. Is it just the physical illness or is it also its remote origins in social and economic processes and the stream of social and economic results flowing from that illness? The longer the recognised wave amplitude of the event which you 'know' and 'recognise', the more likelihood that responsibility can and might be allocated at the level of public policy.

The idea that an epidemic is a chance event, an unfortunate agglomeration of probabilities, a concatenation of causes, is in part a result of a 'research funding policy driven by the "atomistic" or "medical" fallacy which holds that understanding at the individual level automatically provides understanding at other scales or between scales' (Wallace and Wallace, 1995, p. 333). Scientific thought and method has many strengths. But because its method is often to cut a problem into manageable pieces, it also has the great and distorting weakness of atomising, anatomising and dissecting (often literally so) the object to be examined. This loses sight of the complex systems of which the object is a part. This is the case with an HIV/AIDS epidemic.

An atomistic, individualised perspective does not sit easily with a consideration of the causes and consequences of the HIV/AIDS epidemic. If an epidemic is not mere chance but *susceptibility* which is tied to the economic and social character of a society, its intergroup relations, balances of power, lines of stress and fracture, then it follows that the social and economic *impacts* of an epidemic are not chance events either. This is because *vulnerability* to the effects of excess morbidity and mortality is not equally distributed. In the same way that the poor are more vulnerable to the effects of flooding because their homes are more likely to be on marginal land, so they are also more vulnerable to the effects of raised levels of illness and death. They have fewer resources of all kinds with which to weather the storms. Such questions are considered in detail in Part III of this book. In this chapter and the next we concentrate on questions of *susceptibility* – those features of a society which make it more or less likely that an infectious disease will attain epidemic proportions.

Determinants of the HIV/AIDS epidemic – differing perspectives

Figure 3.1 shows the clinical-medical view of factors which may be considered relevant for explaining why people become infected with HIV.

The twentieth century saw many radical transformations of medicine. Among the more spectacular were vaccination, antibiotics, the discovery

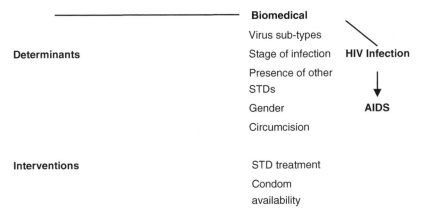

Figure 3.1 HIV epidemic – determinants and responses: a medical view

of DNA and consequent understanding of genetic code. There were also regrettable developments; the transition of the control of medicine from practitioners to the laboratory being one. Of great importance in the present context, was the division in 1916 in the US between 'medicine concerned with the health of the individual and one concerned with the health of populations' (Horton, 2000, p. 46; Garrett, 2000, chapters 4 and 6). The Rockefeller Foundation helped create schools of public health which were to be separate from schools of clinical medicine. This division of medicine into individual and public health resulted in a split in the perception of health and well-being which has not been repaired. One of the lessons of the HIV/AIDS epidemic is that this schism (White, 1991) must be repaired: it costs lives and causes suffering.

Once the divide had opened between individual health and public health, the creature which uncomfortably tried to span the divide was the epidemiologist. This discipline attracted followers who were part medical practitioners, part statisticians and part public health experts. They were bound to fall between all possible stools. Epidemiologists offer associational analyses based on statistically expressed ecological understandings. But epidemiological accounts are inadequate to the task of understanding public health issues as they apply to HIV/AIDS. Epidemiology all too often falls into the 'science' of the medical rather than expanding into broader social science analyses required for more comprehensive understanding of an epidemic.

What we see represented in Figure 3.1 are the constituent elements of a modern, Western interpretation: the view that HIV/AIDS is a problem of the body alone. Because of that, it is a problem to be solved almost exclusively by medical science, clinical practices, epidemiological knowledge and behavioural interventions that affect the ways that bodies behave towards each other. And yet, as we shall see in Chapter 5, the ways that we think of our bodies and what they can do, the ways that bodies behave and above all the ways that they desire each other, are products of history, culture, society and economy.

The recent history of interventions in the HIV/AIDS epidemic shows the continuing dominance of the limited, clinical-medical take on how you deal with an epidemic of infectious sexually transmitted disease. This is particularly surprising because the late Jonathan Mann – and his associates and co-workers at the WHO/GPA and at the François-Xavier Bagnoud Center for Health and Human Rights – were firmly of the opinion that HIV/AIDS was not solely a clinical-medical problem but required a much broader perspective. This led them to translate the problem into a concern with the relation between HIV/AIDS, health and human rights. The approach was powerfully institutionalised in the establishment of the François-Xavier Bagnoud Center for Health and Human Rights and Chair in Health and Human Rights at Harvard University. It was further developed in many publications, notably Mann, Tarantola and Netter (1993) and Mann and Tarantola (1996).

These ideas had a major impact on the development of UNAIDS (the United Nations agency which is charged with confronting the epidemic globally) when it was founded in 1996. That organisation has endeavoured to include social and economic aspects of the epidemic in its work plan. Despite these efforts, until very recently the main focus of UNAIDS and all national and regional programmes to do with HIV/AIDS has been on the clinical-medical and behavioural levels. Little attention has been paid in country programmes, Ministries of Health and government policies to the broader factors which contribute to the development of social and economic environments – what we describe as *risk environments* – in which infectious disease can expand and develop rapidly into an epidemic.

Epidemic disease, and HIV/AIDS in particular, is indeed a disease of the body – but that is only the presenting symptom. The epidemic (note, the *epidemic* – not the illness) is more deeply seated. An HIV/AIDS epidemic reveals many of the fractures, stresses and strains in a society. HIV/AIDS is but a symptom of the way in which we organise our social and economic relations. Concern with clinical-medical issues and with individual behaviour change to the almost total exclusion of the structural and distributional factors which result in those behaviours, has had serious implications. In particular:

- the well-known and continuing link between poverty and disease has been obscured from view (for example, Wilkinson, 1986; Fox, 1989; Blaxter, 1990; Backlund et al., 1996)
- recognition that while immediate focus on prevention is a correct and conventional response, it is short-term; we have to recognise that existing structural inequalities have historical roots
- failure to recognise what should have been obvious, that a lentivirus would have long-term social and economic effects.

The development of the human rights discourse has been important for the protection of some. But its placement at centre stage has much to do with the agendas of US politics and what is acceptable in the US policy discourse where social inequality and the distribution of income and wealth are by and large excluded from the political agenda. While human rights issues are indeed vital in relation to many aspect of this epidemic, they must always be considered in relation to structural questions of distribution. Human rights discourse translates issues into questions of legal process, inevitably focusing on legal persons (which may be individuals or collective bodies), their rights, obligation and capabilities for action. In the end this is a way of thinking and acting which is individualistic, emphasising the individual rights and responsibilities of legal actors. An epidemic is *par excellence* a *collective* event. While individuals do have responsibility for their actions, that responsibility has always to be considered in a context of what individuals can do given the structures of inequality and the histories within which they live their lives. Human rights and structures of inequality must both be taken into account in attempts to confront the epidemic.

Behavioural interventions – a necessary but limited response

The Global Programme on AIDS (GPA) was the World Health Organisation's response to the epidemic in the 1980s and 1990s. It was medically and epidemiologically driven and adopted a short term and conceptually limited fire-fighting perspective based on experience of other more explosive and shorter-wave infectious disease outbreaks (Garrett, 1995). The WHO adopted a series of 'Short Term Programmes' and 'Medium Term Programmes' in a laudable effort to contain the spread of the epidemic. These packages were all more or less the same as they were manufactured and exported from Geneva to the countries of Africa, Asia and Latin America. They were developed from *a priori* thinking about how to deal with an epidemic disease and met the criteria of (a) urgent need to react to an emergency, and (b) economy of scale. They also represented the best experience and thinking of the talented team in the GPA.

Box 3.2   The Knowledge, Attitude and Practice approach

Critics of the KAP approach have warned of the limitations of reducing sexuality to a series of isolated and quantifiable items of behaviour (e.g. whether people use condoms or not; how many sexual partners a person has per month). They argue that sexuality consists not of isolated items of behaviour, but of a complex of actions, emotions and relationships 'whereby living bodies are incorporated into social relations (Kippax and Crawford, 1993, p. 257) and which are too complex to be apprehended using quantitative research alone' (Campbell, 1997, p. 274).

Because this is a sexually transmitted disease, the plans were also associated with a series of what were first called Knowledge, Attitude and Practice (KAP) studies, an approach developed as part of the population control movement. These studies were supposed to acquaint local programme managers working in any particular country with the details of the local sexual culture. Information from such studies would enable them to tweak the general programmes designed in Geneva to fit the local situation. With these adjustments, national AIDS Control Programmes would take account of what local people and communities *Knew*, of their *Attitudes*, and of what *Practices* they had in sexual behaviours. It was soon recognised that what really mattered was what people's bodies got up to, so a *B* for *Behaviour* was added to evolve KAPB studies. The resulting programmes were firmly based on the tradition of individual psychology and on two main theories: the Health Belief Model and the Theory of Reasoned Action and Planned Behaviour.

The health belief model was developed in the 1950s and explains behavioural decisions by reference to individual knowledge, beliefs and attitudes (Salt et al., 1990; Montano, 1986; Janz and Becker, 1984). The theory of reasoned action assumes human beings are rational and key behaviours are under individual control. The key idea here is 'intention' – what people intend to do and how they rationally go about achieving their goals (Azjen and Fishbein, 1980; Azjen, 1985). Programmes that were rooted in this perspective retained a restricted view of sexuality, reflecting the rather simple perspectives of experimental psychology rather than taking account of the complex realities of human sexuality and its social and cultural nature.

However, adding Behaviour to the equation of what made for an epidemic of a sexually transmitted disease was a marked improvement. It moved the focus of concern away from the body to the mind. This was not only an improved conceptual approach, it also indicated further possible interventions and areas of engagement with the disease. Figure 3.2 shows this additional understanding and the resulting interventions.

In the late 1980s and early 1990s, the WHO/GPA saw that AIDS was not a problem limited to the clinic or the hospital ward. They could hardly think otherwise. Many of the main figures in the organisation (notably Jonathan Mann) had worked with the US-financed Project SIDA in Kinshasa Zaire in the early 1980s where the ever-present poverty and instability pointed firmly to the connection between poverty and the spread of the disease. But there was a large gap

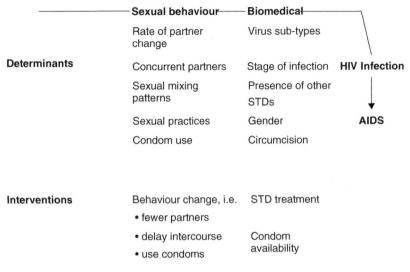

Figure 3.2   HIV epidemic – deteminants and responses: sexual behaviour

between the insight and the practice when Mann took over the WHO/GPA in Geneva. Institutional inertia was hard to resist and directed policy and action firmly into the clinical-medical framework.

The biological goal of any programme aimed at tackling an epidemic disease is to reduce the rate of transmission by intervening in the process of disease communication from one individual to another. In the case of sexually transmitted disease, this means a focus on the 'core transmitters' (see Box 3.3). These people are the 'superspreaders' (Anderson and May, 1992, p. 228). With diseases such as gonorrhoea, the optimal control strategy is contact tracing. Each sexual contact of a diagnosed person is traced so that in principle each infector and infectee in a sexual network is identified, counselled and treated. Thus is the disease outbreak contained or, ideally, wiped out. Such strategies require considerable financial and logistic resources; they are also dependent upon the availability and possibility of treatment. In the case of HIV/AIDS, none or very few of these conditions apply. There was until recently no treatment on offer and the finance and logistics for contact tracing were in any case unavailable in the poor countries and communities where the majority of infections were occurring.

The whole story of how epidemics come into existence, who has the highest likelihood of being infected and therefore who is most

---

Box 3.3   The core group concept

The idea of the core group is based on the notion that some segments of a population are more likely than others to transmit infections sexually. In the late 1970s James Yorke and Herbert Hethcote modelled this idea. They argued that a relatively small group of people – which could be defined in terms of their characteristics, geographic, socio-demographic, behavioural – were responsible for the maintenance of gonorrhoea at endemic levels in US society. They argued that within such a group, an infected individual generated one or more new infections (see Chapter 2 for discussion of R_0). They concluded that in the absence of such core groups the infection would not be sustained or propagated in a population. Yorke and Hethcote concluded that core groups were definable, relatively stable and in fact quite small. The implications for control were clear – get to the core groups and prevent the disease from breaking out from them. A major problem with gonorrhoea is that, particularly among women, there may be asymptomatic carriers. With a lentivirus such as HIV, this problem, as we have seen, is much greater.[4]

---

exposed, is indicated by the boxed columns in Figure 3.3. These are the areas where policy is likely to require a long-term perspective and where it is most likely to run into the problem that people throw up their hands and say that it is all too complicated or impossible. Their response is to stick to the easier, familiar and pragmatic interventions that can be done with individuals.

The everyday politics of competition for limited resources, and between competing ends, mean that long-term goals are sacrificed (or not dealt with because they are too complex) in favour of short-term, more pressing and more easily achieved ends. In this competition, public goods such as public health are likely to be sacrificed for private benefits on the altar of power. Governments have their eye on the next election/political crisis/threatened *coup d'état*/debt crisis rather than on the longer term, and on individual rather than public goods.

Yet it is longer-term policy perspectives and commitments to fund public goods which are necessary. The origins of an HIV/AIDS epidemic are historical and structural and its effects appear over the very long-term. Such long-term and very large-scale questions are contentious,

Determinants	Distal determinants		Proximal determinants	
	Macro environment	**Micro environment**	**Behaviour**	**Biology**
	Wealth	Mobility	Rate of partner change	Virus sub-types
	Income distribution	Urbanisation	Prevalence of concurrent partners	Stage of infection
	Culture	Access to health care	Sexual mixing patterns	Presence of other STDs
	Religion	Levels of violence	Sexual practices and condom use	Gender
	Governance	Women's rights and status	Breast feeding	Circumcision
Interventions	Social policy – redistribution	Social Policy Economic Policy	Behaviour change communication	STD treatment
	Legal Reform – Human Rights Taxation Debt relief	Legal Reform Employment legislation	Condom promotion and marketing Voluntary counselling and testing	Blood safety Anti-retroviral therapy during pregnancy
	Terms of Trade		IVDU harm reduction	Vaccines and microbicides (when developed)

Figure 3.3   The whole story
Source: Barnett et al. (2000).

closely tied to difference, wealth, income and distribution. These are areas where group and individual interests and positions are threatened. While clinical treatment and behaviour change may easily be categorised as purely technical, the 'broader issues' raised by distribution and difference are more contentious and obviously political. These issues touch on many global problems: the international distribution of wealth and poverty, debt, trading relationships and employment legislation.

Socio-economic and macro-level interventions

Of course, interventions at the biomedical and behavioural levels are vital. This is undeniable. But there is little in the armoury. There is no vaccine. Multi-drug therapy prolongs life but is expensive, requires sophisticated medical backup, and will not be available to the huge numbers of people who are infected worldwide. Prices may be falling but in many countries infrastructure will be the constraint.

Box 3.4   Behaviour change

'[T]here are remarkably few policy success stories on a national scale. Thailand is the clearest case: after an intense national campaign to raise condom use in commercial sex, the condom use rate for brothel-based sex workers reached more than 90%, STD cases declined precipitously, and HIV prevalence among army conscripts dropped by more than half. Infection rates among pregnant women have since declined, although are still high at 1–2%, and these accomplishments seem mostly sustained throughout the East Asian financial crisis. In Uganda, HIV prevalence has declined among pregnant women and young people who are delaying sexual activity. However, it is difficult to attribute either of these outcomes to public policy. The decline in prevalence may be due to heightened mortality among HIV-positive individuals or the natural evolution of human behaviour faced with a generation of high mortality associated with sexual behaviour.' (Ainsworth and Teokul, 2000)

Condoms are problematic, not least because they require male compliance. The development of microbicides (chemical substances that kill viruses and bacteria and can be used vaginally) which would offer greater female control over matters of sexual health has been inexplicably neglected. No safe preparation has been developed. Treating other STDs reduces rates of HIV transmission but there are questions as to the sustainability and cost of such programmes. Behaviour change interventions do work as long as they are maintained. This has been seen in the US and Western gay male communities, Thai brothels, and among intravenous drug users and with needle exchange programmes in the UK and the Netherlands. But these interventions are aimed at core transmitters. In epidemics in Africa and elsewhere such strategies will not be adequate because these epidemics are generalised rather than concentrated in core transmitter groups.

Experience from gay male communities in the US and Western Europe, and heterosexual communities in Uganda, suggests widespread behaviour change occurs in response to large increases in mortality, at which point the HIV epidemic may be nearing its peak. It is also possible that such large-scale behaviour changes require very special circumstances, circumstances which are closely related to some of the key issues raised in this chapter – the nature of society and the expectations of the future which it is possible for people to have.

Societies confronting generalised epidemics, or where the epidemic is already generalised, should contemplate interventions that do not usually receive sufficient consideration. These are at the social, cultural and economic levels, described as macro environment and micro environment in Figure 3.3.

Two kinds of macro-level intervention are required. The first will confront social and economic factors increasing *susceptibility* to infection. This is prevention through effective and broad ranging public health programmes and social and economic policies which reduce income inequality and improve governance. Here people feel that they are living in a society that offers security to them and their children. The second must engage with the social and economic impacts of death and illness, and how some population groups are particularly hard hit because they are especially *vulnerable* to impact. These interventions are complex and closely connected to wider issues of social and economic welfare policy and public health.

Three concepts are important in developing these ideas: *risk environment*, *susceptibility* and *vulnerability*. Below we explore the related concepts of *risk environment* and *susceptibility*. In Chapters 6–12 we examine the concept of *vulnerability* to the medium- and long-term impacts of the epidemic.

Risk environment

In epidemiology, the concept of 'risk' is used in a strictly statistical sense. Thus:

> the degree of increased risk associated with a specific behaviour or other factor is measured as the relative risk or relative odds of infection comparing those with the factor to those without the factor. (Brookmeyer and Gail, 1994, p. 23)

This can be expressed mathematically and produces the concept of a 'risk group'. A 'risk group' is defined as all those individuals belonging to the set with the characteristic that is associated with increased relative risk or relative odds. They are 'core' or 'super-transmitters'. If, for example, a study shows that commercial sex workers, lorry drivers or people with a high level of education who travel a lot (to note three commonly cited groups) have markedly higher levels of infection than the general population, these may be described *statistically* as 'risk groups'. The description is merely a statement of the relative probability of finding infected individuals in this group as contrasted with another group.

However, in popular perception the notion of a risk group presents problems. In the case of human disease, especially fatal sexually transmitted infections, the precise statistical concept of a risk group used in specialised technical discussions within professional journals and conferences, is all too easily translated into another, less precise, vernacular use of the same term. When this happens, 'risk' is no longer the observed characteristic which raises the odds of being infected, but rather the 'risk' which 'they' (those who possess an observed characteristic – Haitian, sex worker, African, gay man – but may not be infected) pose to 'us' the uninfected. This has occurred with HIV/AIDS. Specialised and precise epidemiological language has been translated into everyday and less precise language, becoming connected to ideas and emotions such as those of blame and stigma.

This is an important point. Sexual intercourse (of whatever variety: oral, anal, vaginal) is not intrinsically a 'risky' (in the popular sense) behaviour, beyond the obvious risks of conception in the case of the heterosexual variety. However, when a deadly disease appears *and* the social and economic environment is such as to facilitate rapid and/or frequent partner change, then that environment may be described as a *risk environment* and the act of sexual intercourse becomes a *risk behaviour*. *The riskiness of the behaviour is a characteristic of the environment rather than of the individuals or the particular practices.*

Risk environments: an example from the US

There is a picture of American big cities as 'hollowed out'. The wealthy and the businesses which they support have fled to the suburbs leaving at best a townscape of closed retail outlets and low-quality housing, at worst a burned-out core inhabited by people who are all or some of the following: immigrants, the poor, the sick, AIDS patients and HIV infected people, substance abusers, the criminal, the mentally ill. This is a risk environment.

Wallace and his co-researchers try to understand how this has come to pass (Wallace, 1991a, 1991b, 1993; Wallace and Fullilove, 1991; Wallace and Wallace, 1990, 1995; Wallace et al., 1994). They suggest that in

New York it is in part the result of political decisions to withdraw services from inner-city areas and in particular of decisions to withdraw fire services. In areas of decrepit housing stock with many poor people, the result of these policies was urban burn-out followed by out-migration. This was in the 1970s and the concurrent social results were frequent family moves accompanied by breakdown of social support networks. In such neighbourhoods, people already faced many kinds of stress associated with ethnic discrimination (most of these people were/are black and Hispanic), low education, unemployment and poverty. As the momentum of out-migration built up and residential patterns became unstable, so social networks became over stretched, and support – what we might now call 'social capital' – became less available. Stress broke the links between people: the result was 'urban meltdown'.

Many of the processes identified in such milieux are similar to or apparently the same as those which can be observed in Africa and elsewhere. They have particular implications for the ways in which 'maleness' is expressed, constructed and experienced in different places and its role in epidemic development.

The argument is that such meltdown adversely affected communal controls on behaviour. It interfered with people's pursuit of economic opportunity and made the adequate socialisation of young people difficult. At the same time, survival in this kind of environment elicited cultural expressions that exaggerated risk behaviours such as drug use, crime and violence (Wallace et al., 1996). In a noisy place you have to shout, and in such a disrupted environment there is a lot of noise – actual noise, such as 'ghetto blasters', but also the push and shove of people making out and the noise of risky competition to survive under conditions of stress. In a social and cultural space where there is little organisation, high uncertainty and a harsh daily struggle to survive, shouting becomes the norm. Only this is not just oral shouting, it is many other kinds of elaborate 'noisy behaviour' which will protect and/or permit an individual to overcome challenges and be seen to occupy territory.

We shall see in Chapter 4 that there are parallels here with the ways in which male identity is constructed in communities far away from New York. Similarly exaggerated maleness also appears in Africa (Bujra, 2000a, 2000b). And not only there. Groups of young Thai men make collective visits to brothels (Soonthorndhada, 2000); Indian male lorry drivers insist that driving makes them 'hot' and that this heat must be frequently 'cooled' by sex with a woman or a boy.[5] These are examples of exaggerated masculinity associated with risk and uncertainty.

Junior status, exaggerated masculinity and poverty: an aspect of susceptibility

In US cities the meltdown environment affects socialisation by removing social and cultural control during childhood and adolescence. By reducing educational attainment and employment prospects, it prolongs the period preceding that in which adult behaviour is possible or expected (Wallace 1993, pp. 892–3): it is difficult to be a social adult when you cannot enter an adult social role. The result is the 'youth' problem. The 'problem' is paralleled in many parts of Africa where 'youth' is a distinct social category that can extend from 13 to 30 years old. In some cases this 'youth' status is associated with cultural definitions of age and its relative worth and is formally recognised by age grading and initiation in many African societies. In these societies, the roles of junior and senior members are clearly delineated and rites of passage mark transitions from one status to another.

In other cases, the longevity of junior status may have to do with the circumstances of migrant labour where a young man's identity is split between an urban place where he can earn and a rural place where he lacks a recognised social position. Or it may be associated with orphaning – perhaps as a result of AIDS – and interrupted education and socialisation. In either case, there is a tendency for the development and reproduction of exaggerated forms of masculinity, associated with expectations of frequent sexual partner change (Campbell, 1997; Bujra, 2000a).

Box 3.5   Zulu age grading

Age grading was practised during the reign of Shaka. His groupings of similar aged males was designed as a military strategy.[6]

Groups of males and females born in a two-year period were bonded together. The male age groupings were the bases of the regiments for their clans during warfare. Shaka reorganised these clan age bands as he formed one nation – the Zulu Nation. Males of similar ages (regardless of clan) where drafted into regiments or *amaButó*. Similarly, girls were formed in *amaButó*, each with their own name and the special purpose of providing wives for the opposite male *amaButó*. Of particular significance was that men were not allowed to have sexual intercourse until married, and were not allowed to marry until the king gave his permission. The male control thereby defined female sexuality. (Bryant, 1949, pp. 490–7)

In parts of Africa, and not uniquely there, wider cultural roots may reinforce this expression of male sexual identity. Some observers (Caldwell et al., 1989) suggest that many African systems for regulating sexuality and defining ancestry and descent place a very high premium on fertility and a low value on long-term bonds between sexual partners.[7] In discussion with the authors, a Rwandan man expressed this view in 2001 when he said: 'In the US and Europe, gay men have sex for pleasure; in Africa we have sex to make children and to people the land; after genocide we have to have more children if we are to survive and fill the land once again.' Such a view – even if true of some African societies and cultures – should not be taken as suggesting that there is anything unique or peculiar about 'Africa' (a continent which is as varied and heterogeneous as any other). Further, this is most certainly not an argument about 'African morality', 'African sexual drive', 'Africans as a race' or any other such reductionist and racist positions. It is part of a broader argument about the peculiarity of the 'Eurasian system' of kinship and marriage. It suggests that we should look critically and objectively at the 'Eurasian' system and consider the possibility

> that there is a distinct and internally coherent African system embracing sexuality, marriage, and much else, and that it is no more right or wrong, progressive or unprogressive than the Western system or ... Eurasian society. (Caldwell et al., 1989, p. 187)

We have argued that 'risk' is not an attribute of individuals or groups. It reflects the environments in which people live their lives. These environments are shaped by their particular histories. We have seen that expressions of sexual identity may be associated with social and perhaps physical survival in risk environments. Life lived in a risk environment affects who you are, who you become, how you earn your living and what you (and others) do with your body. But none of this is about 'culture' driving decisions against the grain of what is rational. People who inhabit a risk environment make decisions that are rational for them in their circumstances. However it is the case that in a risk environment, people may be compelled to take risks that are against their long-term interests because they have little hope for the long term.

Susceptibility

In a risk environment, individual, group and general social predisposition to virus transmission is increased. This we describe as *susceptibility*. Susceptibility refers to any set of factors determining the rate at which the epidemic is propagated. Over time an environment can change. Factors that contribute to increased or decreased susceptibility may at first sight seem to have little to do with disease. However, many of them have considerable importance for the environment within which an infectious disease is transmitted.

Box 3.6   Sexual favours and women's access to education in Nigeria and elsewhere

'THERE IS NO ROMANCE WITHOUT FINANCE'
(*Nigerian adage from River State*)

'Women students may be more susceptible to infection than some other groups in certain circumstances. A study in Nigeria suggested that a woman may end up having sex with three people at once to make her way through university – her teacher (to ensure good marks), a "sugar daddy" (to pay her fees and living expenses) and her boyfriend' (Edet, 1997, p. 42).

'Dr. Bayo's findings on Campus girls "campus night crawling" is similar to findings made in Uganda's Makerere University study. The study found that in spite of the very high (98–100%) level of AIDS awareness and knowledge, the girls engaged in risky sexual behaviour – e.g sex with older "rich" men (at times just pretenders); and for the boy, since they can't afford "standards" (money, gifts, etc. to girls) they either prey on college girls or prostitutes in the nearby slums surrounding the University. Actually the dynamic socio-sexual behaviour going on in Makerere Campus has put most Campus girls beyond the reach of most Campus boys! One night stand is a common practice in the University. In fact some studies have indicated that CSWers for the mid and high income bracket customers are mostly campus girls, although they deny it! Interestingly, after affairs with the "Sugar Daddies", they fall back on their Campus colleagues for fun sex; and during the holidays, they return to the one in the "village" (at minimum 3 partners). As a result, AIDS has taken its toll on the University, from students to the academic and support staffs!'[8]

They may be infrastructural: for example, the development of a road which makes contact easier between previously inaccessible areas. Similarly, aspects of the natural environment may have bearing on susceptibility. A natural environmental factor might include a drought which resulted in unusual population movements and mixing. Other very important constituents of susceptibility are economic, for example, increased inequality of income distribution; or social – the operation of labour and associated housing markets in urban areas. People will go to great lengths to find education, employment and housing. Sometimes those lengths may include provision of sexual favours. Thus, differential income, status and social standing may determine livelihood choices and ultimately sexual networks.

The idea of susceptibility reveals aspects of situations, circumstances, organisations and processes as they contribute to the increased or decreased 'riskiness' of an environment within which disease may be transmitted. The relative 'riskiness' of an environment will enhance or diminish the ease with which disease is transmitted. This variability may occur at a number of levels, from the physiological (abrasions during dry sex) to the macro-economic: financial stress which makes life tough, livelihoods more difficult and makes some people necessarily less risk averse in their sexual behaviour.

Susceptibility may be thought of at various levels. An entire 'society' or country may be considered susceptible because its population is constantly on the move – through national or international migration, civil unrest or environmental events. A household may be susceptible because one of its members is a migrant worker.

Susceptibility is an ecological notion. It can be used to describe environments at any level, from damage to the epithelial cells of the reproductive tract as a result of a sexual practice, to a fall in the value of a country's currency that limits public expenditure on STI treatment. It describes features of institutions and organisations. The people working in a government ministry, a hospital or a manufacturing enterprise may each have an increased susceptibility to infection for many reasons. The ministry of education may post married couples among its teaching staff to different areas of the country. A hospital may not have sufficient rubber gloves for its health care staff. An enterprise may insist on short-term, seasonal contracts with its labourers, resulting in its main workforce being migrants for part of the year.

Local epidemic; global networks

Local epidemics take on particular forms, reflecting different levels and types of susceptibility. The example of the enterprise and its contracts with its workers is revealing. It tells us something about the relation between local epidemics and globalisation. One of the ways that multinational enterprises reduce and control costs is by subcontracting, outsourcing and directly employing as few people as possible. Local subcontractors are always in competition among themselves for contracts with the multinationals. This is what 'efficiency' and 'competition' mean in practice. These contractors too must cut costs as far as possible. When a local employer takes on migrant labour at minimum wages and for short-term contracts, these migrant workers may well take HIV/AIDS infection back to their home area many hundreds of kilometres away. The resulting 'local' epidemic has its origins far away. This is because of the risk environment that members of the community encounter in their place of employment. That environment may be determined by decisions taken in boardrooms in Zurich, London or Tokyo. The chains of infectious causation from one individual to another are determined and created as an intrinsic part of the production relations associated with globalisation.

There are also cultural aspects of susceptibility. The construction and reconstruction of what and whom we desire and how. Sex has many variations of meaning and significance. Sex is a deeply private activity in almost all societies. But it is learned, coded and interpreted in many different ways and carefully controlled and disciplined in all societies through the manipulation of symbol, metaphor and ritual.

Globalisation increasingly replaces local perspectives. In a world of globalised markets, diversity and cultural discreteness are destroyed. They are replaced by the brand images, usually of objects but also of forms of sexuality, whose branding is linked to film actors, musical performers, fashion houses, sports stars and their products and marketing support organisations. In this process, systems of sexual symbolism and transaction which were once embedded in local webs of obligation and commitment are replaced by increasingly unidimensional, market-mediated versions of what is, inevitably, a limited range of physical actions. The value – wherein lies the constructed desire – has been replaced by the price, an approximation to a common medium of sexual experience. The porn image emphasises price and structure over symbol and metaphor. Sex has always had a 'price' of some kind in most societies throughout history. Globalisation and consequent standardisation and demystification now mean that its intimacies are increasingly delinked from local cultural and social systems. Globalisation increases susceptibility through destruction of local values and norms, replacing these by new constructions of desire.[9]

Susceptibility: a conceptual approach to explaining and predicting the epidemic

There have been a number of attempts to explain different epidemics by developing indices or statistical correlations. They have been of limited use.[10] The problem is that some of the richer, more developed African countries, such as Botswana and South Africa, have serious epidemics while other countries, despite economic and development determinants pointing to the potential for an AIDS epidemic, do not. Examples of two countries where dramatic epidemics might be expected are the Philippines and Sri Lanka. The first has very unequal distribution of income, high levels of overseas labour migration and a reputation for a relaxed attitude to sexual commerce: surprisingly, it has extremely low HIV seroprevalence. Sri Lanka has massive amounts of overseas labour migration, skewed distribution of income and has been in a state of civil war for many years. The indicators developed to date do not allow us to understand why these countries, with what might be considered ideal circumstances for the development of a generalised epidemic, do not have such epidemics. Below we develop a perspective which may begin to tell us something of why epidemics can vary so markedly between societies.

Social cohesion and inequality

The hypothesis is that the shape of the epidemic curve, how many people are infected and how rapidly the infection spreads will be determined by two key variables:

- the degree of social cohesion in society
- the overall level of wealth.

Social order, social cohesion and HIV/AIDS

Each society has regulations about where, when and with whom sex is possible, and also about what constitutes 'sex' and 'sexual intercourse' (former US President Bill Clinton, in 1999, for example). There appears to be some relationship between the degree of order in a society and the variability of patterns of sexual mixing between groups. In times of rapid change and even more in times of political uncertainty or disruption, these mixing patterns are more likely to become 'disassortive' (Anderson and May, 1992, pp. 290–7). In other words, people are likely to find sexual partners from groups outside of their 'usual' networks than would be the case in 'normal' times and with greater frequency. In periods of rapid economic change where livelihoods are uncertain either because of growth or decline, people's livelihood strategies may facilitate faster change of sexual partners within and between diverse groups. Thus social order and attendant social cohesion play an important part in regulation of patterns of sexual mixing in populations. As we have seen in the case of risk environments in some American cities, and as we shall see in Chapter 5 in relation to Africa, the existence of a risk environment reflects the breakdown of social order and cohesion.

Internationally, expansion of markets, increased speed of communications, fluidity of relationships, their short duration and rapid change, are all characteristics associated with globalisation. As noted, activities in one part of the globe have rapid consequences for others. We have seen this in relation to the competition for investment among subcontractors of large multinational corporations. Resultant poor working and living conditions and job insecurity may and often do have implications for sexual networking.

With regard to social order and cohesion, there is a continuum from authoritarian societies where most aspects of life are regulated and prescribed with attendant sanctions for violation, to those where social order depends on the free play of the market, representative political organs, voluntary commitments by individuals and groups. No existing society falls at either of these extremes.

Directed social action and social control of individual behaviours may be rooted in either authoritarianism or voluntary commitments within civil society and the domestic sphere. Regardless of its origin, the possibility of directed and controlled behaviour reflects the cohesiveness of society and its ability to act collectively. Many argue that the authoritarian route is less constant, requiring frequent reinforcement, whereas the 'representative' route (viewed in the Western tradition as democracy) is more enduring as its sources of authority are widely dispersed and, at least nominally, based on principles of consent.

Social control through authority

Social control and discipline may derive from the exercise of centralised and homogenising authority over people. This may take the form of religious control, as in the case of some devout communities where there is little distinction between the public and private spheres and where 'private' behaviour of all kinds, including sexual behaviour, is very closely regulated. Similarly, the application of a particular political ideology may have the same effect. This was so in the Soviet Union where it was impossible to travel without permission, to book a hotel room without authority, and where, in most aspects of life, individual 'private' behaviour was subject to state surveillance. For example, people suffering from sexually transmitted infections were subject to close state supervision. An extreme form of authoritarian control of sexual behaviour existed in apartheid South Africa and in Nazi Germany. In each of these, legislation proscribed some sexual mixing.[11] Control may also be less crude but nevertheless effective, as where an initially military regime (such as that in Uganda) or an inter-mittently militarised civilian regime (like that in Thailand) exercises close control over its citizens. In Uganda, the establishment of a chain of administrative and political councils extending down to and includ-ing the parish level introduced a communication channel directly from the centre to the household. In Thailand, the 100% condom campaign in brothels was introduced at a moment when a military government was in power. This gave added authority to the edicts of a government that potently combined the symbolism of religion, monarchy, state and nation.

Social capital, consent and action

Social capital is the stuff of social cohesion in non-authoritarian soci-eties. Social cohesion can be thought of in terms of investment and storage of wealth and resources on a parallel with money capital. The idea of social capital has been explored at great length in social sciences (Mauss, 1925; Bourdieu, 1980, 1986; Bourdieu and Wacquant, 1992; Coleman 1987, 1988, 1990; Putnam et al., 1993; Fine, 1999; Harriss and De Renzio, 1997; Putzel, 1997). It exists in the traditions of most peoples where, for example, gift-giving and the ceremonials of birth, death and marriage form reciprocal ties and linkages between individuals and groups. The underlying concept is simple and familiar: you do something for me and I owe you. The favour, gift or work is to be reciprocated at some, usually unspecified, time in the future; the idea of reciprocation is central to the principle of social capital. Build up enough and you can draw it down in large quantities, and as it is often symbolic you don't even have to draw it down explicitly. Social capital is the foundation of social cohesion. It requires constant tending and reinforcement, and we shall return to this in the dis-cussion of impact and impact mitigation (Part III) where we describe the work that maintains social capital as *socially reproductive labour*.

There are two points to make about the concepts of social capital and social cohesion. First, while they have been seen as positive and desirable, this is not necessarily the case. Social capital can have a dark side (Portes and Sensenbrenner, 1993; Portes and Landolt, 1996; Fine, 1999). Your socially cohesive group may exclude mine, even hate it. Indeed, exclusion of my group may be a vital part of your group's legitimating beliefs. Second, emphasis on personal ties, the intimacies of religion, kinship, caste, region, ethnicity, craft, may militate against effective involvement and engagement at the level of the state, the large enterprise, the multinational company. Emphasis on the local, the neighbourhood and community may in fact disempower people and exclude them from access to higher levels of social, political and economic organisation.

Social cohesion is likely to work both ways:

- as an expression of people's underlying social confidence
- as a social environment which will feed back to increase people's sense of confidence and trust in others (Wilkinson, 1996, p. 10).

Despite its limitations and ideological content, the idea of social cohesion does tell us something useful about the nature of social and economic susceptibility to communicable diseases which are sexually transmitted.

The idea of social cohesion was explored as a way of explaining differences in political and economic developments in northern and southern Italy. Robert Putnam and his collaborators used this concept in a comparative study of different regions of Italy (Putnam et al., 1993). They suggest that the regional economic and political differences can be explained by variations in social capital endowments between communities. Many politicians and thinkers in the post-Cold War world have seen ideological and theoretical advantage in the idea of social capital. It moves away from notions of social class to a broader and less determinist perspective. This allows for competing and complex affiliations, and points to a social and political world of fluid alliance and shifting association. Such ideas were in keeping with the conservative political and social milieu of the 1980s and 1990s and with the 'Washington Consensus'.

Social cohesion built on social capital reduces individual or small social group risk by spreading it among more people and enabling directed action by large units. In a highly socially cohesive society or sub-group, individuals find some insurance for the future and are able to mobilise resources in pursuit of joint goals to avoid or control risk. There is safety in numbers and linkages and there is more safety when people can have expectations of the future because their plans and projects are more likely to be realised.

Box 3.7   The Washington Consensus

The Washington Consensus is the name given to a set of economic prescriptions constructed around a package of policy instruments which were viewed by the International Monetary Fund (IMF) and the World Bank, both based in Washington, DC, and subscribed to by the US Treasury, as necessary to basic economic reform. These prescriptive policies appear as structural adjustment programmes (SAPs).

The recommended macro-economic measures, the conditional ties that attach to loans from the IMF, are as follows:

- fiscal discipline: limiting budget deficits and entailing cuts in spending which means cuts in social spending (health, education, welfare)
- financial liberalisation: interest rates being determined by the market
- privatisation of state enterprises
- trade liberalisation: declining tariffs and opening economies to foreign competition
- foreign direct investment: no barriers
- the management of exchange rates: exchange rate stability

Additional policy measures include the deregulation of labour markets, a change in public expenditure priorities away from subsidies, and tax reform in broadening the tax base and cutting marginal tax rates. These policies constitute the lending framework of the IMF and are the Enhanced Structural Adjustment Facility.

With the centrality of privatisation and trade liberalisation in these policy recommendations, the Washington Consensus is clearly aimed at facilitating the globalisation of capitalism.

Wealth and income

Wealth and income are relatively unproblematic concepts. Wealth generally equates with health; income is a partial proxy for wealth. However, income distribution may be unequal. In this respect Wilkinson's recent work on health and inequality is important (Wilkinson, 1996). It reminds us of the relationship between general health, socio-economic inequality and the degree of social support available in a society. There is, however, no need to introduce inequality in addition to wealth and social cohesion as variables. Societies with low social cohesion and high wealth appear to have high Gini coefficients, indicating income inequality.

This hypothesis is supported by the view that

> trust and civic co-operation are stronger in countries:
> * with property and contract rights effectively protected by formal institutions;
> * with higher and more equal incomes;
> * and with populations less polarised by class, education and ethnicity. (Feldman and Assaf, 1999, p. 33)

If income distribution is a reasonable but inevitably fuzzy proxy representing underlying inequalities in economic, educational and other forms of material and symbolic capital then, as Wilkinson suggests:

> Because these processes of social differentiation feed on ... inequalities and destroy social cohesion, the extent to which we have an integrated and harmonious society with high levels of social involvement, or at the other extreme a society that is divided, dominated by status, prejudice and social exclusion ... gives rise to aggressive subgroups antagonistic to the rest of society, and the stigmatisation of the most disadvantaged ... closely related to the extent of income inequality. (Wilkinson, 1996, pp. 171–2)

Social cohesion and wealth combined

Combining social cohesion and wealth gives four 'types' of society:

* Type 1: high social cohesion and high wealth – many societies of the rich world
* Type 2: high social cohesion and low wealth – some societies with strong religious cultures or good governance
* Type 3: low social cohesion and low wealth – countries experiencing civil war or economic collapse, such as Uganda in the early 1980s
* Type 4: low social cohesion and high wealth – societies in transition, such as South Africa, where wealth is very unequally distributed.

These are summarised in the matrix in Figure 3.4.

There are few studies of the relationship between HIV/AIDS infection and social and economic inequality. The World Bank's 1997 study of

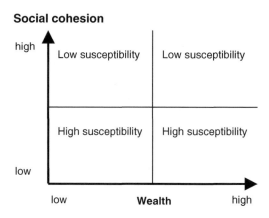

Social cohesion

Figure 3.4   Social cohesion, wealth and susceptibility

72 countries showed that high urban adults rates of HIV infection were associated with low national income and unequal distribution of income (World Bank, 1997a). The relationship between wealth and HIV infection at the national level is apparent in Figure 3.5, although the considerable scatter of points around the regression line in the graph indicates the effect of other variables.

If social cohesion and wealth are indeed major influences on the gradient and peak of the epidemic, then logically there will be four different epidemic curves as, shown in Figure 3.6.

Curve 1 describes the epidemic in a society with high levels of social cohesion and high income; a low peak and slow decline follow a slow growth with low endemic prevalence. Curve 2 is a society with high levels of social cohesion and low income. Here we might expect to see levels of infection kept in check by socially defined behaviour. A slow growth in prevalence will characterise this society. Curve 3 is a society with low levels of social cohesion and low income and the epidemic may take time to gain momentum, but once it does so the curve will be exponential and the level of infection may remain high. The final curve, number 4, is a society with low levels of social cohesion and high income; here the curve will show a sharp increase in prevalence followed, hopefully, by a sharp decline. Although the society is susceptible to infection in the early stages, wealth means it has the capacity to respond.

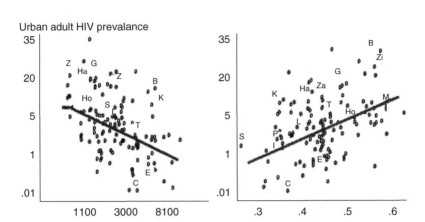

Key: B = Botswana, C = China, E = Egypt, G = Guyana, Ha = Haiti, Ho = Honduras, I = India, K = Republic of Korea, L = Laos, M = Malawi, P = Pakistan, S = Spain, T = Thailand, Za = Zambia, Zi = Zimbabwe.

Figure 3.5   GNP per capita, income inequality and urban adult HIV infection, 72 developing countries
Source: <http://www.worldbank.org/aids-econ/confront/present/lima/sld009.htm>

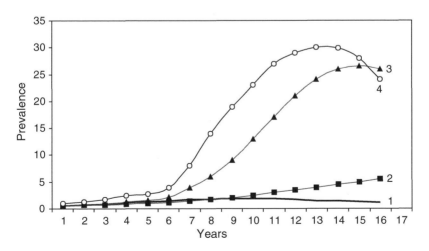

Figure 3.6   Epidemic shape: social cohesion and inequality

A number of further points must be made about this paradigm:

- Societies that are wealthy in aggregate but lack social cohesion often exhibit inequality in the distribution of wealth
- Societies can and do change. Social cohesion may break down or build up and countries may experience economic growth or decline. The cases of Uganda and Ukraine are germane. Construction of cohesion in Uganda, as evidenced through grassroots government and NGO activity, may have been crucial in turning the epidemic round. In Ukraine social cohesion is breaking down as, along with other countries in the region, it makes a halting and difficult 'transition' from centralised state control to 'free market' capitalism
- The paradigm shows that growth alone is not a panacea. Economic and social development with social justice is also necessary. This means addressing issues of equality, human rights and the construction of 'civil society'. HIV/AIDS interventions that ignore these issues will not be effective or sustainable in the long term
- There is a clear justification for interventions at the socio-economic and macro level, and governments have a substantial responsibility in this area.

Relative susceptibility: the differing shapes of HIV/AIDS epidemics

Chapter 2 showed how HIV/AIDS epidemics can be described and some of the problems of assembling and using data. A *'national epidemic'* is an artefact. As represented by the curves in Figure 3.6, it reflects choices made by those describing the epidemic. It is a function of the reporting systems which produce the data. A national epidemic is of course made up of sub-epidemics. Different epidemics curves – within countries and between countries – vary in gradient and peak according to the conditions in different countries and their constituent populations.

Conclusion

This chapter has argued that a generalised HIV/AIDS epidemic does not just happen. There are social, economic and cultural reasons why such events occur. We referred to these predisposing conditions as elements in the relative susceptibility of societies or parts of societies to generalised epidemic. In particular we described the way that some circumstances and historical junctures present as risk environments where sexual relations of any kind carry an unusual or raised risk of sexual disease transmission.

It is increasingly clear that health in richer, 'developed' societies is related to social factors which may be described by the term 'social cohesion'. Where marked income inequality and low social cohesion march together, ill health and ill-being are the result.[12] The causal links in this observation are being explored. However, given that the main killers in rich societies are 'lifestyle' diseases and not infectious diseases, the hypothesis is that there are social and psychological pathways which are brought into play by the 'hidden injuries of class' (Sennet and Cobb, 1973). For degenerative diseases characteristic of most rich countries, health, social cohesion and income are tied together through the nexus of people's concerns about their relative status and the effects that these concerns have on their levels of anxiety (Wilkinson, 1999a, 1999b).

By contrast, an infectious disease is an event that requires some communication between bodies, however tenuous, by breath, body wastes, touch, or by transmission via an intermediate host. Human communication takes many forms, verbal, non-verbal, physical and symbolic. It is subject to a wide range of rules and differing codes of regulation. These forms of regulation can be seen as valves that prevent or facilitate the flow of disease organisms between human hosts. Abrupt or continuing rapid changes in the social, political and economic life of a society or of a part of a society will inevitably produce cultural change, physical or social mobility, breakdown of control, or all of these. In this chapter we have shown how the 'causes' of an epidemic have to be located in relation to such social and economic events. In certain circumstances risk environments develop and these increase susceptibility. The implications of these findings are that interventions to confront a long-wave epidemic event such as HIV/AIDS cannot be limited only to the treatment of individual bodies or to pleas for behavioural change. HIV/AIDS teaches us the necessity for a much broader engagement with all aspects of public policy which affect human well-being.

In the next chapter we examine some national epidemics and suggest some of the ways that macro-economic and social processes in those societies may, in part, explain the differences between their respective epidemics.

4
Cases

While the precise routes to a risk environment may differ, the outcomes are similar. There are as many national epidemics as there are countries. There are also different sub-national epidemics. These sub-epidemics differ depending on the stage of the epidemic and the particular history and circumstances of the risk environment.

It is surprising that different epidemics have not for the most part been categorised across countries according to types or levels. Multilateral agencies producing global data routinely classify countries with regard to other features, but they do not do so for AIDS. For example, the World Bank characterises countries by income level and geographical area, and the UNDP has four classifications.[1]

In 1997, the World Bank classified national epidemics into three categories: nascent, concentrated or generalised (World Bank, 1997a, p. 87). They are differentiated as:

- *Nascent.* HIV is less than 5% in all known sub-populations which are presumed to practise high-risk behaviour
- *Concentrated.* HIV prevalence is above 5% in *one or more* sub-populations presumed to practise high-risk behaviour; but among women attending urban antenatal clinics it is still below 5%.
- *Generalised.* HIV has spread far beyond the original sub-populations with high-risk behaviour, which are now heavily infected. Prevalence among women attending urban antenatal clinics is 5% or more.

This categorisation is useful but limited. It does not say anything about how epidemics might develop or what social and economic processes are driving them: the epidemic dynamic. It is important to know why the epidemic has spread in certain ways in some countries and not in others, and to have some idea of its future trajectory. If we know what is driving it then we will have a clearer idea of how to prevent its spread. Moving from descriptive to dynamic categorisation of epidemics points to public policy interventions beyond existing prevention programmes and links HIV/AIDS control to wider problems of public health and public policy. This is the advantage of the concept of susceptibility and why understanding the plausible relationship between seroprevalence, social cohesion and wealth becomes important. Here we look at a number of different epidemics. The countries we consider are those for which we have data and in which we have worked. This is an inevitable bias: no attempt has been made at random selection of cases. These case studies provide evidence that the epidemic is driven by more than biomedical and behavioural factors. Culture, society and economics all play a role in determining the course of the epidemic. In Table 4.1 countries are organised in terms of social cohesion and wealth.

Our first category is countries which can be characterised as societies with high social cohesion and high wealth – the UK is our case study. Second are countries providing examples of high social cohesion and low wealth – those societies with strong religious cultures or good governance or integrating ideologies: we draw on data from the Philippines, India and Senegal. Third are countries with low social cohesion and low wealth – countries experiencing civil war or economic collapse, such as Uganda in the early 1980s, or possibly the current situation in Eastern Europe. Fourth are countries with low social cohesion and high wealth; South Africa and Botswana provide examples.

Table 4.1 The case studies[2]

Determinants		Example(s)	Notes
High social cohesion	High wealth	UK	
High social cohesion	Low wealth	Philippines, India, Senegal	India provides two sub-case studies
Low social cohesion	Low wealth	Uganda, Ukraine	The situation in both these countries is dynamic
Low social cohesion	High wealth	South Africa, Botswana	

High social cohesion, high wealth: the UK

The epidemic in the UK (population approximately 58 million) is small. The first AIDS cases were diagnosed in the early 1980s and by 1983 totalled 51.[3] By the end of 1998, 16,007 people had been diagnosed as having progressed to AIDS, of whom 12,701 had died (Public Health Laboratory Service [PHLS], 2000). It is estimated that there are around 30,000 HIV positive adults in the population, of whom one-third are currently undiagnosed. In the last two years there have been more infections as a result of sex between men and women than from sex between men. Data released in 2001 showed that the number of newly diagnosed cases was higher than in any year since testing became available in 1985.

The largest numbers of diagnosed AIDS cases (69%) are in men who have sex with men. The introduction of anti-retrovirals provided free of charge by the National Health Service means that as a proportion of the total AIDS cases this group has been getting smaller since 1995. The next group of AIDS cases (12%) consists of people from abroad – particularly from Africa – and UK residents who have lived or visited abroad. The third largest group is injecting drug users (6%).

Medical practitioners' voluntary reports are the main source of data about AIDS cases in the UK. It is believed that a very high percentage of actual cases are identified. One of the main reasons is that people who suspect they might be infected have a real incentive to know their status. Public medical services offer a range of free care up to and including anti-retroviral therapies.

HIV data come from a variety of sources, including STD clinics, unlinked antenatal testing and delivery-room blood-spot testing. Seroprevalence rates for men and women are low. The rates in London are highest. The greatest number of infections is in homosexual/bisexual men. In 1997, 9% of gay men attending STD clinics in London were HIV positive, while among IVDUs attending clinics the rate was 3.9% and among heterosexual men it was 0.8%. By comparison, the general prevalence derived from sentinel surveillance was 0.8%. The figures for women were consistently lower than for men; women IV drug users had a prevalence of 1.5% and maternity room blood-spot counts indicated 0.2%. Most areas outside London had lower rates of prevalence (all data from PHLS, 2000).

The total number of infected people has increased slowly but steadily, but the proportions in each of the infection categories have altered. Thus the shape of the UK's epidemic may be described as initially concentrated among men who have sex with men, with smaller heterosexual and IVDU incidence. In the early years, the men-to-men statistics were probably associated with the gay sexual politics of the late 1970s and early 1980s. There appears to have been very high rates of partner change and sexual experimentation, although in the UK this did not often take the form reported during the same period in the US (Shilts, 1987). In the gay male community the number of new infections has stabilised in the range of 1,000–1,600 per year since 1986.

Among drug users who share injecting equipment, the epidemic has been localised in relatively poor and immobile people in a few urban centres, notably Edinburgh, Glasgow and London. Increased injecting drug use was a feature of many societies in the 1980s. With the economic recession of the 1980s it was often associated with urban social deprivation and marginalisation. The IVDU situation has been contained by interventions such as needle exchange schemes and the education of intravenous drug users about the dangers of infection and how to clean equipment.

The male–female incidence has consisted predominantly of people who appear to have contracted HIV abroad;[4] either people who have come to live in the UK from an area of high HIV prevalence, particularly Africa, or people who contracted the infection abroad (*AIDS/HIV Quarterly Surveillance Tables,* 1997).

Why was the UK epidemic contained so successfully for so long? The general health status of the UK population was high in the late 1970s and early 1980s, despite clear gradients in the distribution of health and illness on lines of socio-economic class. At this time the public health care system was under financial pressure, and the entire society was undergoing a radical process of economic and social restructuring. However, surveillance and treatment of sexually transmitted infections remained effective and well-resourced, with no cost to the client. High levels of confidentiality were maintained and there was an effective system of contact tracing.

In the gay male community, a predominantly young group of men possibly with higher than average levels of disposable income, there was growing consciousness and action associated with the politicisation of questions of sexual choice and orientation. Some sexual lifestyles were associated with high risks of contracting the common sexually transmitted diseases. These infections were treated and, apart from the appearance of drug resistant strains, there was a degree of equilibrium between organisms and hosts. After three decades of free universal health care, these men's health status was high, providing a bulwark against the effects of frequent infection. The potential for an epidemic in this group was confronted by effective mobilisation and an energetic self-help response. Messages about safer sexual behaviour and the diagnosis and treatment of HIV and AIDS were effectively transmitted and acted on.

The UK thus exhibited a low level of general societal susceptibility to disease transmission. Increasing income and wealth disparities in the 1980s and early 1990s do not appear to have had any noticeable effect on the diagnosis and treatment of STIs. Widespread and often free availability of condoms kept HIV rates in the heterosexual population low. Female commercial sex workers, a potential bridge population, adopted condoms or other safer sexual practices and seem to have had sufficient bargaining power to negotiate the terms of their trade. Seroprevalence rates among female sex workers remain at low levels.[5]

We may summarise the situation in the UK during that period. At the biomedical level the population was not very susceptible, as a result of mainly free and universal medical provision, especially the satisfactory treatment of STIs. There was a clear government response to the need for public education; and condoms were, and are, easily available, either without cost from general practitioners and other health facilities, or at low cost from many retail outlets including dispensing machines in dance clubs, pubs and other public places. Among the gay male population there was a high level of self-generated response. The IVDU epidemic has been the subject of a number of imaginative needle exchange schemes, funded and organised by central and local government together with the non-government sector. It was among this group, who may fund their drug use by commercial sex work, that an important bridge to the general population could have developed but has not.

In the years 1999 and 2000, a rise has been reported in heterosexual transmission and for the first time the numbers of new infections via this route have exceeded those among gay men. It should also be noted that with anti-retroviral treatments people survive longer. Paradoxically, availability of this treatment option means the pool of infected people becomes larger.

High social cohesion, low wealth: the Philippines and India

The Philippines

The Philippines has extremely low HIV prevalence. This may seem contrary to some outside perceptions of a country of easy sexuality and a flourishing commercial sex trade. The population is mobile and comparatively poor. Together, these features should facilitate the spread of HIV. However the data show that the epidemic is under control – it has been described as 'low and slow'.

In 1993, GPA expert James Chin estimated that there would be about 100,000 infections (HIV and AIDS) in 2000. In 1998, epidemiologists, including Chin, met and agreed that there would be about 38,000 infections in 2000. In May 2000, a further consensus meeting reduced this estimate to 13,000 infections (Health Action Information Network et al., 2000).

This assessment has been borne out by the numbers of recorded AIDS cases and HIV infections to date. The first AIDS cases were reported in 1984. The annual number of cases is shown in Figure 4.1. To date this has never exceeded 60 cases per year (UNAIDS, 2000e). By the end of 1999 only 441 AIDS cases had been recorded (Philippines National AIDS Council, 2000). The number of people who have tested HIV positive is very small, 1,325, and this includes all those recorded as having become ill with AIDS. The largest category of infections is among homosexual and bisexual men, as shown in Figure 4.2.

The Philippines Department of Health has taken a pragmatic view of surveillance. Numbers are currently so small in a population of 76 million that it does not make sense to carry out sentinel surveillance. Instead there is a programme of 'risk group surveillance' at ten sites where particular populations are tested: sex workers, injecting drug users and men who have sex with men. All these sites have reported prevalence rates of more than 1% for these groups

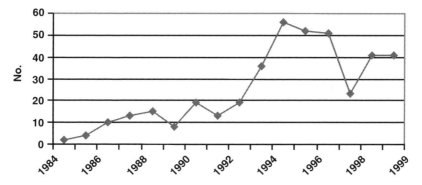

Figure 4.1   AIDS Cases, Philippines 1984–99
Source: UNAIDS (2000e)

1	Heterosexual
2	Homosexual
3	Bisexual
4	Perinatal
5	Other
6	No exposure reported

Figure 4.2   Philippines: reported modes of transmission
Source: Philipines National AIDS Council (2000)

(Philippines National AIDS Council, 2000, p. 12). The Department of Health claims that by monitoring specific populations it has established an early warning system able to pick up any increase in HIV prevalence. In the Philippines lack of HIV data does not reflect inability to collect the information, rather it demonstrates a logical decision about resource allocation.

Why has the epidemic remained low and slow? The concepts of susceptibility and vulnerability have been applied in the Philippines, (National Economic and Development Authority, 2000). The authors of the National Economic Development Authority's Report claim that the following factors are slowing the epidemic.

- The country is an archipelago detached from the Asian mainland. The lack of land borders has helped to reduce the spread of the disease
- Most Filipino men are circumcised
- The society is sexually conservative which includes late sexual debut and low rates of extramarital sex and resort to CSWs
- Low rates of injecting drug use
- The Church is a powerful moral force in Filipino society
- Literacy rates are high, at over 90%
- There have been multisectoral awareness and information campaigns involving government, NGOs, academics and the wider community, as well as people living with HIV/AIDS
- The NGO sector is strong and vocal, and an important part of a political system where popular mobilisation and street protests have been able to change governments relatively peacefully.

In addition it is significant that HIV/AIDS interventions have taken place in a supportive environment. In 1998 the legislature passed the AIDS Prevention and Control Act (RA 8504). This prohibited compulsory testing for HIV and emphasised human rights, and it provided that individuals with HIV should have basic health and social services, that there should be accredited HIV testing centres, and that HIV/AIDS education should be integrated into schools at all levels.

Filipino informants say that the moral authority of the Church, the vibrancy of the NGO community and the strength of family discipline all contribute to social cohesion in the face of large-scale public corruption and political uncertainty. Will this change? The Department of Health asks if the epidemic will remain 'low and slow'. It carries out 'Risk analysis ... to look at how our susceptibilities and vulnerabilities might change, for the worse' (National Economic and Development Authority, 2000, p. 24). Issues identified are: increased population mobility, including militarisation, especially in Mindanao; sexual conservatism which can result in unwillingness to discuss sex and promote condom use; low and incorrect condom use; lacerating sexual practices such as insertion of bolitas (small metal balls) into the penis; gender inequity; and invisibility of the epidemic.

Surveillance reports suggest that the country does not have a problem. Given that current surveillance methods monitor groups where the epidemic will appear first, any increase in HIV prevalence will rapidly be apparent. The Philippines will probably maintain a low and slow epidemic. The country may be poor but it seems that there is a certain level of social cohesion which ensures sexual discipline despite sometimes chaotic appearances at the level of formal political life.

India

How many people are infected in India? In the late 1990s, UNAIDS stated that India had the largest number of HIV positive people in the world. This was hotly challenged by the Indian authorities. Following extensive consultation, the government's National AIDS Control Organisation (NACO) estimated that as of mid-1998 there were between 2.3 and 3.5 million infections (NACO, 1998). The UNAIDS estimate at the end of 1999 was 3.7 million (UNAIDS, 2000f).

As of February 2001, only 19,115 AIDS cases had been reported nationally (Table 4.2). These figures are considered to be a fraction of the actual AIDS cases in a country with a population of over 1 billion.

Table 4.2   AIDS case surveillance in India (as of February 2001)

AIDS cases in India	Cumulative	This month
Males	14680	893
Females	4435	225
Total	19115	1118

Risk/transmission categories

	No. of cases	%
Sexual	15839	82.86
Perinatal transmission	336	1.76
Blood and blood products	784	4.10
Intravenous drug users	815	4.26
Others (not specified)	1341	7.02
Total	19115	100.00

Age group	Male	Female	Total
0–14	459	265	724
15–29	5767	2167	7934
30–44	7141	1586	8727
> 45 yrs	1356	374	1730
Total	14723	4392	19115

Source: Adapted from NACO (2001).

Table 4.2 shows that most infections are sexually transmitted. Other important features of the epidemic as reflected in the table are: the sizeable 'blood and blood products' category, previously due to the practice of paid blood donations, now supposedly addressed through legislation;[6] and the size of the 'Others (not specified)' group, which is the third largest 'risk category' – about which little appears to be known.

The HIV data from India are problematic. Until 1998, the National AIDS Control Organisation reported all tests carried out, no matter why they were done. These included testing for clinical reasons, at blood banks, as part of small serosurveys, and tests ordered by the authorities for different reasons. There may have been double count-ing of HIV positive people who were tested more than once and/or in different localities. The situation was set to improve with the introduction of standard antenatal clinic attender surveys. However, several years' worth of results will be required before a clear picture of the epidemic in India is available. These data are not as yet publicly available, and indeed the March 2001 NACO website stated that:

Data on HIV Sero Surveillance has been withdrawn
The update on sero surveillance data collected from various surveillance centres have been withdrawn because of gross under-reporting of HIV infections. Further, based on scientifically valid HIV sentinel surveillance in place in 232 sentinel sites in the country, which provides insight on total disease burden in the country from time to time, the sero surveillance data has limited value.

We take this to mean that as of 2001, the Government of India has very little idea of the extent of the epidemic in the world's second most populous country. The sparse data we do have show that numbers of infections are rising and only three states out of 32 report no AIDS cases, which is more likely to reflect limitations of the reporting system than the epidemiological reality.

There are many distinct epidemics in India. In Maharashtra, it is concentrated in urban centres among women commercial sex workers and their clients and now spreading into the general population. In Manipur and the north-east of the country, the epidemic is centred in IVDUs but is also, according to recent reports, spreading beyond this group.

Given difficulties with data and the diversity of India, it is unrealistic to speak of a 'national' epidemic. We will look at the situation in two very different states, Rajasthan and Manipur.

Rajasthan[7]

A cumulative total of 263 AIDS cases was recorded as of February 2001 (NACO, 2001). HIV data are hard to come by. According to the Indian National AIDS Control Organisation, 347 HIV positive test results had been recorded as of 1998 (NACO, 1998, p. 20).

Table 4.3 India: seropositivity and rates per 1,000 screened samples and total reported cumulative AIDS cases 1993–97,[8] 1998

	Sept 1993	*March 1994*	*March 1995*	*Dec 1995*	*April 1996*	*July 1996*	*Jan 1997*	*1998*
Seropositivity rate	6.98	7.32	7.28	7.79	8.07	15.97	17.0	22.7
Reported AIDS cases	459	713	1094	2109	2574	2639	3183	5204

The state has a population of over 44 million people. Overall this is one of the driest areas of India with frequent droughts. Of the population, 12% are 'tribal' peoples, nearly double the national average. They are among the very poorest in India and their livelihood strategy exposes them to potential infection. Poor people's income potential in this part of India is probably constrained less by access to land itself – although than can be a problem – but rather by access to irrigation. Unable to provide for themselves and their households from their land – a situation often exacerbated by drought – both men and women enter various forms of labouring work. This may be daily, and may involve travel to nearby towns or more distant migration to other states. Rajasthani people travel to neighbouring Gujarat to work on the commercial cotton plantations for months at a time.[9] They also travel to other countries including the Gulf states.

Raised levels of STI prevalence, close urban/rural relations, marked income and wealth inequalities, complex interethnic relations and identities, gender inequality, heavy dependence upon long-distance lorry transport, and labour migration all contribute to the creation of a risk environment. In such circumstances social and economic conditions facilitate rapid transmission of infection once bridging has occurred between high prevalence urban sub-populations and the general population. For the moment, available data do not show that this has yet occurred in Rajasthan.

Manipur [10]

The same dearth of data applies in Manipur, but here the dynamic of the epidemic is different.

Manipur has 0.2% of India's population (about 2 million people) but over 7% of the total number of reported HIV infections in the country (NACO, 1998, p. 20). Manipur's first AIDS case was identified in 1990 in an intravenous drug user. There are few time series data, but the HIV epidemic has been tracked among drug users in Imphal, Manipur's capital. In 1994, 85.6% of IVDUs tested in Imphal were infected. This had fallen slightly to 69.8% in 1998, the last year for which we have information (NACO, 1998, p. 29). In 1999, Imphal also recorded 2.3% of pregnant women infected at one site (UNAIDS, 2000b, p. 12). The largest concentration of infections among IVDUs in India is in Manipur. In 1990, 95% of those who were reported to be HIV positive were IVDUs. By 1997 this had dropped to 75%, indicating that infection has spread into the wider population.

Manipur is currently experiencing an epidemic among young urban men. There are factors peculiar to this state that increase susceptibility. It is geographically isolated and culturally distinct from much of the rest of India. It became part of the Indian union only in 1949, after a brief period of independence following the departure of the British. Some suggest that the main reason for its incorporation into the union was as a buffer zone against Chinese encroachment towards Assamese oil reserves. The relationship between Manipur and India was, and has to a degree remained, colonial. The area was starved of investment until it achieved statehood in 1972. However, since then it has seen little in the way of development. This lack of economic activity combines with disrupted livelihoods and central government neglect to create high levels of youth unemployment. This, in turn, drives intravenous drug use.

Proximity to Burma (with which it shares a long border) and the Golden Triangle are additional factors. Indeed, nowadays, the main drug-smuggling routes pass through Manipur and some of them have entrepots in Imphal and in Moreh. Dissident sources[11] in the area suggest that these activities exist with at least tacit and perhaps active co-operation from politicians, state officials, and local civil servants as well as elements in the security forces. Many of these people are outsiders and see assignment to Manipur as an opportunity to make money to supplement their salaries. Activists suggest that, ironically, it was sometimes the relatively wealthy sons of these officials who were among the first IVDUs. With increasing urbanisation, the decay of the extended family and household system, few if any significant local industries and little sign of development, the situation is not going to change – except that the disease is now spreading from the IVDU community to the general population of the state. However, for the time being, this epidemic is geographically localised and separate from the rest of India.

Some conclusions about the 'Indian' epidemic

Any discussion of relative susceptibility in India must take account of the enormous diversity of the country. The situation in Rajasthan suggests a high level of susceptibility associated with population movement between rural and urban areas, and in particular medium- and long-term labour migration. Levels of rural and urban poverty and marked income and wealth inequality indicate that many population sub-groups are likely to pursue livelihood strategies which expose them to infection. 'Tribal' women have a reputation for participating in sex work on some of the transport routes. Poor households will be vulnerable to the impact of excess death and illness, and health systems will certainly be affected. Manipur's isolation suggests its epidemic is unlikely to contribute markedly to generalisation of the *Indian* epidemic. However, considered regionally, in relation to adjoining areas of Burma, the Manipur epidemic may generalise. National boundaries may disguise such epidemics and thus the region may be susceptible precisely because the populations at risk extend over an area where boundaries adjoin and where both official and illicit traders are active.

Given the data constraints, it is impossible to know the size of the Indian epidemic or whether it has become generalised. It appears to be socially and geographically limited to certain groups and areas. However it would be unsurprising if a few states did not already have generalised epidemics. And in any case, as knowledge of an 'epidemic' is the outcome of political and social processes (see Chapter 3) it is likely that the scale of the Indian epidemic may have escaped the notice of the Indian government. Indeed this is borne out by discussions with NGO workers and community activists, all of whom feel that HIV/AIDS is present to a larger degree than officially acknowledged. Particular features of Indian life prevent the issue from being addressed. In India – although not uniquely so – the politics of AIDS policy is tightly tied to the political and cultural processes whereby this complex nation is constructed (Corbridge and Harriss, 2000). For the moment it is unlikely that the Indian state will be able to come to grips with an epidemic so bound up with areas of taboo such as gender, caste, ethnicity, masculinity and money. The politics of these in the maintenance of 'India' will take precedence.

Low social cohesion, low wealth: the Ukraine and Uganda

The Ukraine[12]

Prior to the breakup of the Soviet Union, Eastern European authorities congratulated themselves on escaping the AIDS epidemic, and the data supported this view. Draconian control of sexually transmitted infections and sexual behaviours, and state provision of health and social services meant that HIV/AIDS had been kept at bay.

In the Ukraine up to 1994 the few positive tests had been associated with foreigners. Since then both an AIDS and an HIV epidemic have appeared and the situation is now considered to be generalised.

By the end of 1997 only 419 AIDS cases had been reported in the Ukraine (see Table 4.4).

Table 4.4 Ukraine: cumulative AIDS cases by age, sex and transmission category reported to end 1997

Mode of transmission	Male	Female	Total No.	Total %
Adult:				
Homo/bisexual men	20	–	20	5
IVDUs	209	68	277	66
Blood transfusion	1	3	4	1
Heterosexual	47	34	81	19
Undetermined/other	15	7	22	6
Children:	NA	NA	15	4
Total	292	112	419	100*

* Totals do not add up to 100 due to rounding.
Source: Barnett et al. (2000b).

The official procedure for recording an AIDS case in the Ukraine was complex. Each case had to be fully investigated and diagnosed. Only then could the confirmed case reports be sent to the central authority and thus enter the official statistics. Only three specialised HIV clinical centres could diagnose and report AIDS. They became increasingly overstretched as the epidemic gained momentum and resources became scarcer. These early data show that the majority of cases were adult and male and the main form of transmission was intravenous drug use.

During the initial period of the epidemic (from 1987 to 1994 – spanning the Soviet and post-Soviet periods) there was mass HIV testing. Over 39 million[13] (39,226,986) tests were carried out. These were performed on all blood donors, pregnant women, sexual partners of HIV positive persons, social and professional contacts of HIV positive people, hospitalised patients, military personnel, people who were abroad for more than three months, 'promiscuous persons' (sic), patients with STIs, prisoners, men who had sex with men, and drug addicts. The test was compulsory: if the authorities decided you would be tested then you were tested! Civil liberties and human rights were not considered. The system derived from the Soviet tradition of public health. The public health justification was that people who were infected represented a 'danger', the authorities needed to contain this danger and to do this they needed to know who was infected. Of the 39 million tests only 398 were positive, and the majority of these (215) were foreigners (see Table 4.5).

In 1994, large-scale testing of populations seen by the authorities as 'at risk' was scaled down, but it was not replaced by sentinel surveillance:

Table 4.5   Ukraine HIV positivity by transmission category 1987–94, 1995, 1996

Transmission group	1987 to 1994		1995		1996*
	No.	*%*	*No.*	*%*	*No.*
Foreigners	215	54	9	0.6	22
Ukrainians	183	46	1480	99.4	5400
Of whom homo/bisexual men	25	6.3	2	0.1	
IVDUs	3	0.8	1021	68.6	
Blood transfusion	5	1.3	0	0	
Heterosexual	103	25.5	304	20.4	
Nosocomial	10	2.5	0	0	
Perinatal	8	2	8	0.5	
Breast milk	2	0.5	0	0	
Undetermined	27	6.8	145	9.7	
Total HIV positive identified	398		1489		5422

* Breakdown by transmission group was not available when the table was prepared.
Source: Hamers, 1997, Table 2.

instead, people who are identified by the authorities as 'commercial sex workers' and/or 'intravenous drug users' can be subjected to a compulsory test, as can people who show 'epidemiological signs'. There is continued screening of blood donors and pregnant women, although testing of the latter group has declined markedly in the past few years. The number of tests fell from 'close to 2 million in 1992 to 300 000 in 1996' (Hamers, 1997, p. 11) (see Table 4.6). This situation remained essentially the same in 2001 (Ukraine Government, Ministry of Health, 2000).

HIV data confirm what the AIDS case data suggested – that prior to 1994 there were sporadic infections, mainly among non-Ukrainians. Since 1994 the vast majority of those infected have been Ukrainian. The male:female ratio is uneven, with more males than females infected (4,130 to 1,270 in 1996). The majority (more than 70%) of new cases are among IVDUs.

There are additional data on some groups; in particular IVDUs, the group where spread of HIV has been most rapid. In 1996, 51,681 drug users were registered with the Narcology Dispensaries of the Ministry of Health and 63,450 with the police. These are estimated to represent about 10% of the national total of drug users.

Drug use in the Ukraine is predominantly intravenous (85% of drug users inject). The drug of choice is locally made *kompot* which is sometimes taken using shared equipment or even mixed in the blood of fellow users. So the risk of infection is increased. Evidence suggests that

Table 4.6 HIV tests, positive results and rates: blood donors and pregnant women, Ukraine

	1987–94			1995			1996			1997 to June		
	Tests	HIV positive	HIV positive per 1000	Tests	HIV positive	HIV positive per 1000	Tests	HIV positive	HIV positive per 1000	Tests	HIV positive	HIV positive per 1000
Blood donors	14885029	12	0	1624488	34	0	1408077	398	0.03	877567	518	0.06
Pregnant women	9943576	12	0	373044	8	0	351855	181	0.05	212553	187	0.09

Source: Data provided by Dr Yuri Kruglov.

drug use can be found at some level throughout the Ukraine. In the late 1990s, drug dealers were targeting the smaller urban centres and even the rural areas as larger markets became saturated.

In summary, the limited data indicate that the HIV epidemic now poses a serious problem in the Ukraine. Indeed, very recent research (Balakireva et al., 2001) indicates that an optimistic projection of numbers of people HIV positive by 2010 might be just under half a million, while a pessimistic projection would be around 1.5 million. These data are probably indicative of the situation in many other parts of the former Soviet Union. From sporadic occurrences among foreigners, infection has spread rapidly among the intravenous drug using population, and increases are being observed among pregnant women and blood donors. This means that HIV has now spread into the general population.

There are distinct dangers. The Ukraine is a society in transition and at the moment most of the changes in quality of life and economic development are negative. The breakup of the Soviet Union had acute social, political and economic implications for the newly independent Ukraine. The Soviet system was highly centralised and controlled via four main mechanisms: the party, the internal security apparatuses, the official trade unions, and the administration. Entitlements to social, economic and cultural goods were largely administered within this structure. The economy was integrated on a union-wide basis, with the Ukraine specialising in heavy industry. Of production, 75% was associated with capital goods and military requirements, and only 25% with consumer goods. Since independence, there has been a period of acute economic decline. Unemployment and underemployment (characterised by short- and part-time working) have become widespread. In 1995–96 around 18% of the workforce were on unpaid or partly paid leave while 5.6% were on short-time working (*Ukraine Statistical Annual*, 1995). Women make up a greater proportion of the registered unemployed than men. In some cases, this crisis of employment is geographically concentrated. Around Donetsk and Lugansk – areas of heavy industry once tied to the USSR's arms establishment – entire communities have seen the virtual disappearance of their economic base.

The sudden and dramatic collapse of the USSR's integrated economy and service infrastructure has meant that many people survive only by entering the 'shadow economy'. This is of course unregulated, unaccounted and often involves activities which are on the borderline of legality. Substantial sections of the Ukrainian population are poor (World Bank, 1996) and are having to work extremely hard to survive:

mean household expenditure on food is around 57% of total income. This is a risk environment with high susceptibility to infection. The situation is made worse by political uncertainty (Nahaylo, 2000) and uncertainty about national identity (Kuzio et al., 2000).

Uganda

The first cases of AIDS were documented from Rakai District of southwest Uganda in 1982. 1988 saw clinically defined cases throughout the country. The main mode of transmission is heterosexual intercourse. Current estimates are that 820,000 people are living with HIV/AIDS in Uganda (UNAIDS, 2000f). AIDS is responsible for up to 12% of annual deaths and has surpassed malaria and other conditions as the leading cause of deaths among individuals aged 15–49 (National AIDS Commission, 2000). There is no requirement to report AIDS cases, but UNAIDS estimates that 110,000 people died of AIDS in 1999 alone (UNAIDS, 2000f).

HIV surveillance is carried out using sentinel surveillance of antenatal clinic attenders at public health facilities. The current national seroprevalence figure for adults is 9.51% with much higher figures in some areas. The national and some regional data are shown in Figures 4.3 and 4.4.

A sample sero-survey was undertaken in 1988 in all parts of the country accessible in the then-prevailing security situation. This excluded some northern areas. The results showed that the epidemic was already generalised. Some areas and age cohorts exhibited rates of infection as high as 35%. As Figs 4.3 and 4.4 show, the prevalence rate had stabilised and begun to decline in most sites. Incidence rates are

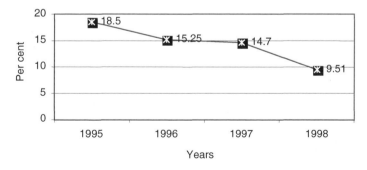

Figure 4.3   Uganda: national prevalence of HIV
Source: Uganda AIDS Commission <http://www.aidsuganda.org>

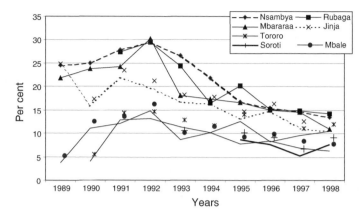

Figure 4.4   Uganda: Seroprevalence rates among antenatal clinic attenders
Source: AIDS Control progamme/ Ministry of Health <http://www.aidsuganda.org>

also declining (Okiror et al., 1997; Kilian et al., 1999; Stoneburner and Low-Beer, 2000).

The reasons for Uganda experiencing such a large epidemic are considered in more detail in Chapter 5, but we can summarise them here. During the period 1970–86 there was a breakdown in political order and economic collapse. This made people poor and removed any sense of security and continuity. The need to survive in such conditions created a group of risk takers who were placed in an environment that made them sexual risk takers. Women, already disempowered, were further socially, economically and politically disadvantaged by these changes. The result was that exchanging sex for food or goods or protection become more necessary for their survival in these unstable times. Deterioration of health and education exacerbated the environment for disease to spread. People did not have access to treatment for STIs and other diseases. Uganda was very susceptible to the rapid spread of HIV.

The 'shape' of the Ugandan epidemic may be summarised as radiating from specific centres (Kampala, Rakai District and the main communications routes from the African east coast to the centre of the continent) along communication routes into the general population.

Uganda's 'success' in confronting the epidemic owes much to the government's initial frankness in dealing with it on the international stage and to President Museveni's strategy of 'selling' HIV/AIDS as one of the areas needing foreign assistance.

Low social cohesion, high wealth: Botswana and South Africa

Wealth and social cohesion are relative terms. Nowhere in Africa is this illustrated more starkly than in Botswana and South Africa. These two 'wealthy' African countries have the highest levels of adult prevalence (35.8% of adults are believed to be infected in Botswana), and the largest number of infected people of any country, 4.2 million in South Africa. They are respectively the second and third wealthiest countries on the continent. Botswana has an annual per capita income of $3,240, second only to Gabon at $3,350 and ahead of South Africa ($3,160). No other African country comes close to these three.

We can ignore AIDS case data. They are not collected. However both countries have good-quality HIV sentinel data, mainly from annual surveys of antenatal clinics.

The first HIV prevalence survey in South Africa was in 1990 by the then Department of National Health. Since then an annual anonymous unlinked survey has been done each year in the month of October among state antenatal clinic attenders. The results are accurate and comparable year on year, and province on province there is a national protocol for the study. The samples are large: in 2000 a total of 16,607 specimens were tested from 400 sites. There is good coverage, 80% of all pregnant women attend public sector antenatal clinics. The survey is not representative of all social groups. An estimated 90.2% of African women attend the state clinics. Other ethnic groups and more wealthy African women (the middle- and upper-class groups) are underrepresented. The clinics cover a mixture of urban and rural sites.

The results are shown by province in Table 4.7 and Figure 4.5. Data are available only for some provinces and for national level prevalence prior to 1994. This is because until then South Africa was divided into 'white' areas and black 'homelands'. The 'homelands' were excluded from earlier surveys, as they were not considered to be part of South Africa under the apartheid regime. They were reincorporated when the new government acceded to power in 1994, at which point the provincial boundaries were redrawn.

National prevalence increased steadily up to 1998 when it appeared to level off briefly. The upward trend was resumed in 2000. Only three provinces had rates below 20% in that year. The provincial variation shows the following:

- In some provinces the epidemic is apparently stabilising but at high levels of infection

118

Table 4.7 Provincial breakdown of HIV prevalence rate in women attending antenatal clinics in South Africa (%)

Province	1990	1991	1992	1993	1994	1995	1996	1997	1998	1999	2000
W. Cape					1.2	1.7	3.1	6.3	5.2	7.1	8.7
E. Cape					4.5	6.0	8.1	12.6	15.9	18.0	20.2
N. Cape					1.8	5.3	6.5	8.6	9.9	10.1	11.2
Free State	0.6	1.6	2.9	4.1	9.2	11.0	17.5	20	22.8	27.9	27.9
KZ-Natal	1.6	2.9	4.8	9.6	14.4	18.2	19.9	26.9	32.5	32.5	36.2
Gauteng					6.4	12.0	15.5	17.1	22.5	23.9	29.4
Mpumalanga					12.2	16.2	15.8	22.6	30	27.3	29.7
Northern					3.0	4.9	8.0	8.2	11.5	11.4	13.2
North-West					6.7	8.3	25.1	18.1	21.3	23.0	22.9
National	0.8	1.4	2.4	4.3	7.6	10.4	14.2	17	22.8	22.4	24.5

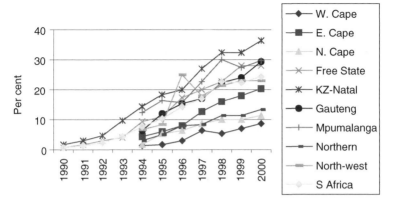

Figure 4.5 South Africa: HIV prevalence among antenatal clinic attenders

- The national epidemic is made up of sub-epidemics. A comparison of the Northern and Western Cape with KwaZulu-Natal and Mpumalanga shows this clearly
- Differences in prevalence mean different responses are needed. In the Western Cape prevention can still work and hold prevalence down. In the high-prevalence provinces prevention should remain a priority, but the impact of the inevitable cases of AIDS will soon be felt and has to be planned for.

The situation is similar in Botswana. The surveys follow the same procedures as in South Africa. Sentinel surveillance has been carried out in antenatal clinics since 1992. Gaborone and Francistown are sampled annually whereas other sites are only sampled every other year. The resulting data have been used to produce national estimates, as shown in Figure 4.6.

Table 4.8 shows HIV prevalence by site. We can see that prevalence is generally higher in urban areas than in rural, and in the northern part of the country than in the south. This pattern is consistent with an epidemic that has spread from the northern border and is now concentrated in urban areas where population density is highest.

Data are also available by age for South Africa and Botswana. This is shown in Figures 4.7 and 4.8 for South Africa and sites in Botswana, respectively. What seems to be happening is that declines in the under-20s age group are matched by increased prevalence in the 20–24 age cohort. This implies that infections are being delayed rather than prevented.

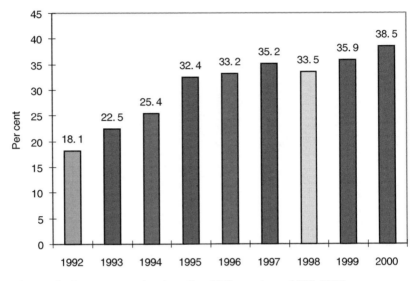

Figure 4.6   Botswana: national median HIV prevalence 1992–2000

Table 4.8   Annual HIV prevalence, Botswana (%)

Sites	1992	1993	1994	1995	1996	1997	1998	1999	2000
Francistown	23.7	34.2	29.7	39.6	43.1	42.9	43.0	42.7	44.4
Gaborone	14.9	19.2	27.8	28.7	31.4	34.0	39.1	37.1	36.2
Ghantsi		9.5		18.9			22.3		26.4
Kanye (Southern)			16.0		21.8		24.67		40.7
Molepolole (Kweneng East)		13.7		18.9			37.2		30.4
Selebi Phikwe			27.0		33.1		49.89		50.3
Tutume			23.1		30.0		37.45		35.4

These two countries are important case studies. They have dramatic epidemics that can be described with good-quality data. We simply do not know what is happening in many other countries where war and disorganisation mean that data are not collected and any that exist certainly cannot be relied on.

What possible explanations are there for such dramatic epidemics? Why is there such a high degree of susceptibility in these two count-

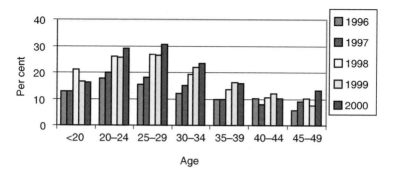

Figure 4.7   South Africa: age-specific HIV prevalence 1996–2000

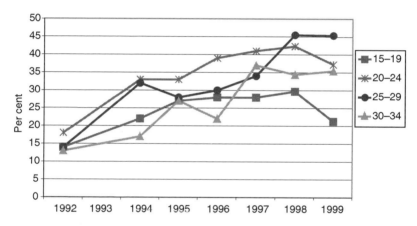

Figure 4.8   HIV prevalence by age group in Gaborone, Botswana
Source: National AIDS Coordinating Agency (NACA), Botswana (2000)

ries? It is evident that national wealth alone is not a defence against such an epidemic. These questions are considered with regard to South Africa in the next chapter. What of Botswana?

Botswana is one of the fastest-growing economies in the world and is in the UN's upper-middle-income category. It has also done well in terms of human development. The adult literacy rate is 75%; and 96% of primary school-age children are in school. The country has a well-developed, decentralised, primary health care system. Before HIV/AIDS life expectancy was 60.3 years and infant mortality 61 per 1,000 live births.

Until recently the population of this semi-arid country depended on subsistence agriculture and pastoralism. Economic growth has led to rapid urbanisation. Of the estimated 1,496,000 people, 729,000, or 48%, live in urban areas. This figure has increased from 18% in 1981. The population has been growing rapidly: 3.48% per year between 1981 and 1991. Until 1991 employment opportunities increased but growth has now slowed. The 1991 census found that the unemployment rate was 14%. Unemployment has risen since then. The estimated unemployment rate in 1994 was 21% and it is higher among women than men – 22% compared to 14% in urban areas. It is also higher among young people, the rate in the 20–24-year age group was 36% (Goverment of Botswana/UNDP, 1998, p. 22). Despite rapid economic growth, income distribution is highly skewed. The Gini coefficient in 1993/94 was 0.54%, close to South Africa's Gini coeffecient. The richest 20% of the population receive 59% of the income; the poorest 40% receive only 12% of total income (Goverment of Botswana/UNDP, 1998, p. 20).

Traditionally the Batswana were a mobile population, moving between their villages, the lands, where crops were grown, and the 'cattle post', remote grazing areas around which cattle are kept. The urban areas now provide a fourth destination, and the development of a good all-weather road network has greatly assisted population mobility. Botswana is also a corridor for transport of goods from South Africa to Zambia, the Democratic Republic of the Congo, Angola and Malawi, as well as from Namibia to its eastern neighbours.

While the country is politically stable, socially it is in flux. Between 1971 and 1996, the proportion of ever-married women fell steadily from 63% to 39%. The percentage of teenage pregnancies has remained constant at about 15% of teenagers. Rapid economic growth, an expanding transport network, population mobility, urbanisation, cross-border trade and inequality are all characteristics of a risk environment. The population of Botswana is highly susceptible to HIV infection and the data are good enough for us to be certain that the epidemic is now generalised and very serious indeed.

What these case studies show

These case studies illustrate the creation of risk environments in a range of different settings. They show how:

- susceptibility varies from society to society, and within societies
- common features of risk environments can appear in very different social, economic and cultural settings

- variations in a country's resource base and political milieu may enhance or detract from that country's ability to describe and be conscious of its epidemic
- a country may change in terms of its social cohesion and wealth distribution and thus change the trajectory of its epidemic – as in the cases of Uganda and Ukraine.

As the epidemic unfolds it seems that the scale and consequences will be worst in Africa. While we are not certain what will happen in Eastern Europe and Asia, initial evidence suggests that their epidemics will not be as serious and, perhaps more important, the impact will not be as devastating. Why is this the case? We believe the answer to the relative size and rapid of spread of HIV lies in the concepts of susceptibility and risk environment. The devastation will be greater in Africa because it is poorer, both financially and in human resource terms. In the next chapter we explain why Africa is a special case.

5
Why Africa?

At the beginning of the nineteenth century, Africa's income levels were roughly one-third of those of Europe. Since then, the continent has fallen behind the rest of the world (World Bank, 2000a, p. 1). Sub-Saharan Africa accounts for 32 of the UN's 40 'least developed' member countries. Its foreign debt has trebled from US$84.1 billion in 1982 to US$235.4 billion (World Bank, 1997a, p. 202).

At independence in the 1960s many African countries were richer than their Asian counterparts. A wealth of natural resources held out promise for future trade, growth and development (World Bank, 2000a, p. 18). However as Tables 5.1 and 5.2 show, this promise was not met.

The World Bank notes that 'The region's total income is not much more than Belgium's, and is divided among 48 countries with a median GDP of just over $2 billion – about the output of a town of 60,000 in a rich country' (World Bank, 2000a, p. 7). Africa is in danger of becoming a marginalised backwater of global society, occasionally

Table 5.1   Global economic trends

	Africa excluding South Africa	Africa	South Asia	East Asia	Latin America
Economic indicators[1]					
1970 per capita income	525	546	239	157	1216
1997 per capita income	336	525	449	715	1890
1970 investment per capita	80	130	48	37	367
1997 investment per capita	73	92	105	252	504

[1] In 1987 US dollars.

124

Table 5.2 Development indicators

	Sub-Saharan Africa	South Asia	East Asia	Latin America and Caribbean
Life Expectancy				
1970–75	45.0	50.1	63.2	61.1
1995–2000	48.9	62.7	70	69.5
Under 5 mortality per 1000				
1970	226	206	118	123
1998	172	106	46	39
Food security and nutrition				
Change in daily per capita				
supply of calories 1970–97 (no.)	–34	364	856	324
Change in daily per capita				
supply of protein 1970–97 (%)	–4.1	12.7	59.7	13.1

Source: UNDP, *Human Development Report* 2000, pp. 189, 240.

controlled by 'peacekeeping' activities when regional disorder threatens to affect the wider world (Duffield, 1996; Hoogvelt, 2001). The HIV epidemic is a result of these processes of decay and will push the people of Africa into further marginalisation and poverty.

Africa bears the major burden of the epidemic. Of the estimated 34.3 million people living with HIV/AIDS in 1999, 24.5 million or 71.4% were in sub-Saharan Africa; of the 2.8 million deaths in 1999, 2.2 million were Africans; and of 13.2 million orphans generated by the epidemic 12.1 million are in Africa (UNAIDS, 2000f, p. 124).

Until recently it appeared that west Africa had escaped the worst of the epidemic affecting the rest of Africa. Here, HIV-2, a form of the virus that is less aggressive, has a longer lifecycle and therefore does not kill so rapidly, was dominant. This is no longer the case and HIV-2 is now being displaced by HIV-1. In addition the degree to which the epidemic had spread in this region may have been disguised by poor data, particularly in the most populous country, Nigeria (124 million people in 1999). The return to civilian government here has meant that in spite of continuing civil unrest, HIV/AIDS is receiving more attention. It is now known that general seroprevalence in the Nigerian population is rising rapidly and currently stands at just over 5% (UNAIDS, 2000f). Poor data and regional unrest in Liberia and Sierra Leone mean those epidemics have been for the most part unobserved and unreported.

Seroprevalence rates have been lower in west Africa than elsewhere on the continent. The reasons for the differences in rates of epidemic development as between west Africa and the rest of sub-Saharan Africa remain unclear. The most rigorous study to date (Buve et al., 1999) compared rates of sexual partner change and sexual behaviour in four cities: two in east Africa with high seroprevalence and two in west Africa with lower (but not inconsiderable) levels of infection. The study did not look at social and economic characteristics of the study populations and thus cannot directly answer the kinds of question posed in this book. The main findings were that high levels of STIs, particularly genital herpes, and low levels of male circumcision were strongly associated with high rates of HIV prevalence. This finding points to ways in which some significant cultural practices, particularly male circumcision, may affect the overall relationship between inequality, poverty and infection. High levels of STIs are likely to be related both to absence of male circumcision and of adequate reproductive health care. Thus, the epidemic may take off in west Africa as it has elsewhere on the continent. But its rate of spread may be mitigated by the frequency of male circumcision.

In this chapter we look at different areas of the continent to show how their histories have contributed to elevated susceptibility to an HIV/AIDS epidemic. We will see that although there are some marked similarities between these examples there are also dissimilarities. What this illustrates is that the general concept of susceptibility has many different forms and manifestations.

Explanation of what has happened in Africa requires a broad historical sweep and risks simplification. Here we outline the main forms and processes which can be observed. This demands consideration of very long-term historical and geographical trends including the landlocked nature of much of Africa, the great historical movements of peoples across the continent, its sparse population, and the slave trade. In addition, there are more recent events, including failure – and in some cases disintegration – of post-colonial states in parts of the continent; an enormous debt burden; heavy dependence upon primary products, and failure to industrialise.

Geography and early history

Geography is not destiny, but it certainly plays a role! Jared Diamond's book, *Guns, Germs and Steel* (1999), suggests that differing continental forms and whether they have their widest orientation running north–south or east–west have important implications. In particular, latitudinal width meant that, in Eurasia, early agricultural innovations could be moved within the same climatic belt rather than across climatic belts. This was significant for Africa where north or south movement involved crossing agro-climatic belts. This limited the transferability of agricultural systems and thus development and the growth of population (Diamond, 1998, pp. 186–7). This may be one reason why Africa's peoples have always been sparsely distributed across its vast landmass.

This theory of geographical determinism is supported by Bloom and Sachs's (1998) analysis looking at Africa's recent economic growth. They conclude that geographical factors – most notably the adverse ratio between coastline and landmass – and the sparse distribution of population lower Africa's growth potential by just under 1% as compared with other major world regions. Low population density has additional effects: it makes the provision of infrastructure and services expensive, and means that it is more difficult to integrate populations into meaningful political units and to link both internal and external economic activities through markets.

This situation is made worse by disease. Ill health as a result of infectious disease is more common in Africa than anywhere else in the world (Feachem and Jamison, 1991). While nutritional deficiencies also play a role, these are themselves linked to disease. Thus, chigger, sleeping sickness, TB, various STIs, bilharzia and above all malaria have contributed to the burden on Africans across the continent and the centuries (Hartwig and Patterson, 1978). Of the world's total malaria cases, 80% are found in Africa. According to the World Bank, this accounted for 11% of the continent's disease burden and cost many African countries more than 1% of their annual GDP (World Bank, 2000a). While onchocerciasis affects 18 million people in the world, 99% of these live in Africa. Such infections are both caused by and cause poverty. Ill health reduces production and saps energy. Intermittent or chronic ill health is 'normal' in many poor societies and this is particularly the case in Africa. Thus, as fifteenth-century European capitalism was expanding, in Africa it encountered a region which was already geographically and demographically challenged. Contact with Europe exacerbated those challenges.

On the other side of the Atlantic, the European encounter with the Americas was associated with the destruction of the indigenous populations. This created a huge demand for labour on the newly established sugar plantations. European merchant adventurers turned to the western coast of Africa, from today's Senegal to Angola, to meet this demand. Their activities extended far inland and collided with an area of internal population movement troubled by many local wars (Oliver, 1991, p. 125). The pattern was mirrored, albeit on a smaller scale, on the east coast where Arab traders were making similar forays into the hinterland to meet demand for slaves around the Indian Ocean. From both west and east coasts, the slave trade extended disruption through African intermediaries far into the heart of the continent. These early contacts created the conditions for a long history of *sustained* disruption and dislocation that opened the way for the spread of HIV/AIDS in the twentieth century. Centuries of population movement associated with extended periods of unrest and warfare created a continent-wide risk environment.

Our argument is that epidemics in Africa are the product of histories that have made many of that continent's societies 'unhealthy'. The African HIV/AIDS epidemic has to be seen against this broad sweep of African history. To understand AIDS in Africa today we have to go back and consider events in the last century; in the nineteenth century, the period of the so-called 'scramble for Africa'; and before that to the slave trade. An examination of Africa's history is necessary for other reasons: considered over the long term it is symbolic of the truly exceptional nature of what has happened to the peoples of Africa and to the African continent. Recognition of these historical developments, plus long periods of consistently adverse terms of trade, must inform any understanding of contemporary Africa.

We must balance this view with the knowledge that external pressures did not impinge upon an unspoiled Africa. External forces and their effects do not adequately explain the subsequent and more recent history of Africa. Africa's problems are not solely the result of what came from outside. There are and have been sufficient Africans in positions of advantage and access willing to participate in the spoliation of their own continent. Perhaps above all, recent decades have seen the failure of post-independence states to achieve legitimacy in the eyes of their citizens.

An abnormal normality

Since the sixteenth century, there has been little in the way of 'normality' in many regions of Africa, if that means periods of relative social peace and material security. Formal colonialism, which at best provided civil security, predictable legal systems and some degree of stability, lasted barely 60 or 70 years for those parts of Africa which, from the mid-1950s onwards, were to become 'nations'. Four decades after independence, colonial rule has faded from memory: most Africans are now two or more generations distant from colonial times. In any case, that colonial stability was at the surface. For much of the period there was simmering opposition to foreign rule. Outright rebellion was not infrequent.

For the last five centuries Africa has not experienced normality, at least not by the standards of the rest of the world. In Africa there has been an 'abnormal normality'. This is the foundation for the disorder, inequality, exploitation and poverty in which an epidemic such as HIV/AIDS could grow and thrive. Aspects of this dislocation as they are manifest today have been exacerbated by external shocks and internal social conflicts, by poor economic management and unusual levels of inequality. We shall examine some of these factors briefly.

Most African countries have small populations for their area. Their economies remain heavily dependent on primary commodity exports (World Bank, 2000a, p. 8). If this were not a sufficient handicap, Africa's share in world trade has fallen dramatically since the 1960s, and the continent now accounts for less than 2% of the total (World Bank, 2000a, p. 9).

The countries of Africa are by and large artificial constructs, reflecting nineteenth-century competition between imperial powers. The result has been borders that contain accidental agglomerations of peoples, traditions and languages. The outcome has been perennial crises of state legitimacy from independence in the 1960s and 1970s up to the present. With the Cold War as a background factor, the military coup became the standard mechanism for change of government throughout the period 1970–90. Many countries had at least one coup or attempted coup during that period.

'Africa has perhaps the world's highest income inequality' (World Bank, 2000a, p. 92). On conventional measures, Africa is second to Latin America (see Table 5.3); but when consumption rather than income is used to measure inequality, Africa comes first (World Bank, 2000a, p. 92). Furthermore, Africa's inequality differs from that of other regions. Rural inequality is almost as high as urban inequality, 20% of the population accounting for 6% of consumption in each sector. In addition, inequality in Africa is high despite the low average income (World Bank, 2000a, p. 93; Ali and Elbadawi, 1999).

HIV/AIDS epidemics are related to income inequality and absence of social cohesion. Dislocation, inequality, civil unrest, population mobility, radical changes in community beliefs and standards have been

Table 5.3   World income inequality by region (%)

Region	Gini coefficient	Share of top 20% of population	Share of middle	Share of bottom 20% of population
Africa	45	50.6	34.4	5.2
East Asia and Pacific	38.1	44.3	37.5	6.8
South Asia	31.9	39.9	38.4	8.8
Latin America	49.3	52.9	33.8	4.5
Industrial countries	33.8	39.8	41.8	6.3

Note: Data for Africa calculated on a consumption basis. Adjustment to an income basis (as used for the other regions) would involve raising the Gini coefficient by 6 percentage points, making Africa's Gini coefficient 51%.
Source: Deininger and Squire (1996), cited in World Bank (2000), p. 93.

constant motifs in the story of HIV and AIDS in Africa (Setel, 1996; Caldwell et al., 1989; Kaburu Bauni, 1990). Dislocation has been linked to radical movements of population. It is associated with urbanisation (Konde-Lule, 1994), and the continuing and longstanding interaction between urban and rural areas (Schoepf, 1988, 1991, 1992, 1993). HIV/AIDS adds to that continuing dislocation. Many countries in Africa are experiencing the loss of generations of people in their prime and truncation of individual life horizons, as life expectancy becomes briefer. The effects will reverberate through the decades and centuries to come.

Here we examine aspects of African history as that history impinges upon the development of social, economic and environmental settings – risk environments, as described in Chapter 3 – where a sexually transmitted disease such as HIV/AIDS can spread rapidly and dramatically.

The following brief historical reviews are offered because:

- Uganda is a country where there was a complete economic and political collapse with subsequent regeneration. Here the epidemic has been acute and may now have reached its peak. Uganda's history shows development of an extreme susceptibility
- Tanzania is following an epidemic trajectory similar to that in Uganda with a different, less violent history
- Congo illustrates the long-term issues which underlie susceptibility; and
- South Africa is a society where history has seen the development of high levels of legally entrenched susceptibility.

In each case we see how risk environments have developed and the ways in which they are similar to and differ from each other. We examine the effects of national histories and their impact on specific groups and geographical areas in Uganda and Tanzania. The Congolese and South African studies epitomise general trends: they are examples illustrating processes seen throughout the continent.

Uganda: risk environment, susceptibility, division and contradictions

Development of a risk environment and increased susceptibility in Uganda has much to do with the growth of ethnic, regional and class differences as 'Ugandan' society came into existence from the late nineteenth century to the middle of the twentieth century. While many other societies have such marked divisions, in Uganda these divisions became lines of conflict that tore a recently established polity to pieces. There the development of the epidemic since the late 1970s and the reconstruction of the society in the period since 1986 have gone together. The epicentre of the epidemic was Buganda in the south of the country, an independent African state until the late nineteenth century.

The colonial history of Buganda revolves around the cultivation of two major cash crops – cotton and coffee. The opening of the Uganda railway in 1902 linked Mombasa on the Indian Ocean to Kampala and reduced the cost of transporting commodities produced in the African interior. When they arrived in Buganda, the British encountered a centralised, 'feudal' state with an effective ruling class. In 1900 this ruling class was co-opted by means of a land tenure reform which converted feudal tenure into individual tenure. All the power holders of Buganda, from the king down to the lowliest parish chief, were allocated parcels of land. Thus, Buganda was converted from a feudal system to a society of landlords and tenants in which landlords were able to establish their economic, political and social domination. Cotton production was the foundation of this system. Buganda chiefs organised their people to produce cotton and coffee and also drew adjoining peoples into the production process (Isaacman and Roberts, 1995, p. 27).

Cotton production ensured that the newly acquired territories were self-financing and guaranteed cheap raw materials for the declining Lancashire cotton industry. The British aimed to keep Africans in the rural areas, producing cotton. They were discouraged from entering into trade. Instead trade (and ultimately ginning) was put into the hands of Asians imported as labourers and settlers. These people were simultaneously a link between the British and the people of Uganda, and a barrier to the development of an indigenous Ugandan trading class. As a 'foreign' stratum, it was assumed that the Asians would be loyal to the British and that their main interest would remain in import and export rather than in the internal development of the country. By 1938, these 'Asians', imported by the British, controlled cotton ginning, wholesale trade and commerce (Mamdani, 1975, pp. 32–3). Africans remained in the agricultural sector, but in an agricultural sector which was undergoing rapid change.

Land tenure reform facilitated the development of a wealthy Ganda peasant class. Society was divided into the traditional aristocracy, an economic class of independent smallholders and rural entrepreneurs, labourers – both local and ethnically related people who had migrated from the Belgian territory of Ruanda-Urundi (present-day Rwanda and Burundi) and the Asian ginnery owners, traders and merchants. Nationalist movements in the late 1940s organised political opposition to this status quo. The 1950s saw a succession of violent incidents and boycotts aimed at 'Asians', and by the 1960s the language of political protest had become a racial one – 'Africans' against 'Asians'. This was to have very dramatic results in the next decade.

In the colonial period Buganda retained a degree of autonomy within the structure of the British Protectorate. In the period leading up to Ugandan independence there were pressures for secession. The years after independence in 1962 were characterised by continuing struggles between the central government in Entebbe/Kampala and Buganda.

By late 1960s, lines of violent division had emerged across Uganda between Africans and 'Asians' and between Buganda and the Government of Uganda. Dramatic falls in global cotton and coffee prices made the situation worse (Mamdani, 1975, pp. 48–9). The government's response to the crisis was a rash of fiscal measures. The power of state personnel increased and was exercised through patronage and pay-offs. This was not in the interests of the small class of African traders and merchants who saw themselves in competition with the 'Asian' petty traders who could often better afford the necessary bribes.

In 1969, the government made a distinction between Asian petty traders (who were encouraged to leave Uganda) and members of the larger Asian commercial class who were granted citizenship and thus encouraged to stay. This made it clear that 'the governing bureaucracy preferred an Asian to an African petty bourgeoisie. The latter was a political threat, the former was not' (Mamdani, 1975, pp. 52–3).

Another contradiction had appeared in Uganda's political and economic life, that between the governing class and the African petty bourgeoisie. The latter looked to the army for support. Milton Obote's government attempted to neutralise the army by isolating individuals seen as a threat. One of these was a senior officer called Idi Amin. Attempts at neutralisation through military reorganisation were ineffective, and Amin finally affected a coup against Milton Obote in 1971. The main supporters of his coup were the members of the African petty bourgeoisie who saw it as a way of defeating the state personnel and the Asians, both groups which frustrated their interest in moving from being petty bourgeoisie to grand bourgeoisie. Regionalism figured in the equation too. Amin received support from his ethnic homeland in the north of the country, a region which had always seen itself as relatively dispossessed compared with the more prosperous south.

The Amin period was characterised by economic mismanagement and terror. This is important for understanding the creation of a risk environment. The key was *magendo*, a LuGanda word which means the 'pilgrimage of greed'. *Magendo* developed as a system of illicit, semi-legal and illegal distribution after Amin had finally expelled all the Asians and destroyed existing systems of distribution. Amin's economic policies froze agricultural prices and drew large quantities of cash crops into the black market. Here lay the roots of *magendo*. This was of particular importance in Buganda which supplied the food needs of the major towns of Kampala and Jinja. In addition, the *mafuta mingi*, the 'fat ones' – the operators in the illicit economy – also began to move into transport. The essence of the *magendo* economy was smuggling of coffee, paraffin, sugar and gold out of the country, of vehicle spares and other necessaries into the country, and of food within the country. Transport was essential and was a good if risky investment. Illicit markets, secretive transport and the human interactions that tied such a system together were a risk environment *par excellence* and fertile ground for the development of an epidemic of HIV/AIDS. The profits from this trade were invested in housing, commercial buildings and land (Rothschild and Harbeson, 1981; Bond and Vincent, 1990), and no doubt in paying off helpful government officials. The exciting, risky and often deadly atmosphere of these times has been graphically described as follows:

> The basic supply-route from the port of Mombasa, through Nairobi to Uganda, ran like a great artery of corruption from western Kenya

to Kampala, on north to the Sudan, on west and south to Rwanda, Burundi and Zaire. Long stretches have been beaten to pieces as hundreds of trailer-trucks pound continuously up and down the roads. The tough drivers and crews, who are paid overtime and danger money, changed their Kenyan shillings at the border. They are often delayed for days, drinking in the bars, eating in the hotels ... sleeping in the brothels which line the route. From this main artery corrupting tentacles of the black market with its illicit deals and violent transactions penetrate into the Uganda countryside, pulling into its stream the desperate, the opportunistic, and the down-and-out. (Southall, 1980, p. 632)

Buganda, and within it Rakai District, the focal point of Uganda's HIV/AIDS epidemic, is adjacent to the lorry route from Mombasa in Kenya to Bujumbura in Burundi. It fronts Lake Victoria and has many casting-off points for nighttime journeys to Kenya and Tanzania. When Amin was overthrown in 1979 by the Tanzanian army, the invading army passed though here. The invasion was itself significant for the development of the epidemic and has been closely described by Hooper (1999, pp. 42–3, 767–72).

The troops moved through this area which had already seen regional disruption, particularly influx of refugees from the 1959 outbreak of ethnic conflict in neighbouring Ruanda-Burundi. Between 1959 and 1964 some 200,000 WaTutsi had fled the country to seek safety in Congo, Tanganyika, Uganda (President Museveni's mother was part of this exodus) and Burundi (where, while ethnically similar, power was in the hands of the WaHutu). There is no clinical or laboratory-based evidence to support the hypothesis that this seeded the epidemic, but Hooper (1999) assembles a series of anecdotes which suggest that some of these people may have been HIV positive and later developed AIDS. Many of the refugees on both sides of the Uganda–Tanzania border were moved to an area near the Kagera River.

In 1979 Amin's regime was overthrown by a combined Tanzanian and Ugandan invasion from the south into Uganda, across the Kagera River and into Rakai District. For operational reasons, the invading army spent several months in the area astride the border during 1979–80. The first reports of AIDS were from this area of the country in 1982 (Serwadda et al., 1985; Carswell, 1986; Musagara et al., 1989; Hooper, 1999, p. 37).

Under the rule of Dr Milton Obote, the leader installed by the Tanzanians, decay of the state structure continued. This regime did not allow 'normality' to reappear in people's lives. The illicit economy continued to thrive as a vital part of people's survival strategies. In 1986, Yoweri Museveni defeated and expelled Milton Obote and took office as president of Uganda. His government rapidly established a higher level of civil and political order in most of the country. However, Uganda remained a troubled society for the next decade and armed opposition groups remain active in parts of the country. In addition, Uganda's army is prominently involved in the Great African War in the Congo between forces from Uganda, Zimbabwe, Angola, Namibia and Rwanda, as well as various Congolese factions and warlords. All of this contributes to even greater population movement across this huge region spanning many millions of square kilometres in Central Africa.

Rakai District – the first visible African epidemic

In 1989 and 1990 local people told how AIDS had made its way into the lakeside communities in Rakai from Tanzania during the late 1970s and early 1980s. Conditions here created an environment that raised the potential for effective transmission of a sexually transmitted infection. These were all associated with the illicit trade and survival in times of extreme disruption. Conditions included high mean rates of sexual partner change, high mixing of partners across geographical areas, large numbers of concurrent partnerships, and geographical mobility. Gender relations, rooted in local tradition and disrupted by disorder, increased the levels of individual and social susceptibility to the disease.

Survival strategies in times of hardship created demand for the provision of food, lodging and sex at truck-stop townships, border towns and the smuggling villages on Lake Victoria. It was men who benefited most from this volatile and lucrative trade, though some women took part. In an interview in 1989, one respondent remembered these times and said: 'People had money and could exchange it into any currency. Young men dropped out of school to earn the easy money. Women joined in because it was much safer for them than for men.' The *magendo* economy of the 1970s and early 1980s inflated men's cash incomes compared to those of most women. This increased women's insecurity and dependence. Already unequal gender relations were thrown into further imbalance, an imbalance that inevitably took on a sexual complexion.

During the Amin period, the existence of illicit economic activity had a serious destabilising effect on the already unequal balance between men and women. This was reinforced by a male ideology which here, as in many other societies, evaluates male status in relation to other men at least partly in terms of sexual conquest and the procreation of children.

In a community with fairly relaxed sexual attitudes – at least when judged by the *public* standards of many other cultures (Kyewalyanga, 1976, pp. 155, 208) – younger women responded in a number of ways. Some became prostitutes, selling sexual services in return for cash. Others became 'kept women', in stable non-resident relationships where a visiting man gave gifts to help with household requirements. Yet others entered into various types of marriage. In brief, women gained access to economic resources, often, but not uniquely, through sexual relationships with men.

The distribution of these types of relationship varied from place to place. Along the main transport routes from the lakeside, 'kept women' and prostitution were to be found. It is likely that opportunities for the more casual types of sexual relationships increased in the 1970s and perhaps encouraged greater mixing between different groups. In such circumstances, the rate of partner change can be assumed to be fairly rapid. In the remoter villages, more traditional relationships based on beer brewing, drinking and sex were the norm. But it was not until the disease had been introduced by travelling men, often of a higher educational status or with cash to spend, that these traditional networks took the infection further into the rural areas.

Thus *magendo*, the position of women, warfare and civil unrest combined to make Rakai into a risk environment. The rate of change in Rakai District, Buganda and Uganda over the past century has been so rapid as to meet the definition of 'abnormal normality'. The following comment by a woman in Uganda in 1989 provides a chilling summary of a woman's life in a risk environment: 'During times of war soldiers took money and sometimes killed men, but always took money and sex from women.'[1]

This survey of Uganda, and particularly of Buganda, shows how change and fluidity in social, economic and political relationships create circumstances where HIV could lodge and spread rapidly. Susceptibility takes many forms. In this case it is rooted in changes in structures of power, between ethnic groups, classes, genders and political actors. In contrast, in Tanzania and specifically among the people of Mount Kilimanjaro, its roots lie in changes in self and societal perception.

Tanzania – 'development', population movement and susceptibility

The first cases of AIDS in Tanzania were reported in the north west of the country, in Kagera region, across the border from Rakai, in 1982

(Government of Tanzania, Ministry of Health, 1992). The people share cultural and social features with their neighbours. It was the area through which the invading army passed on its way from Tanzania to assist in the overthrow of Idi Amin.

Tanzania is a risk environment where rapid change is associated with what is often described as 'development'. This case study focuses on the area around Mount Kilimanjaro and shows how integration of the locality into a system of global relationships affected livelihoods, demography, and people's minds. The result was that people began to inhabit new niches of risk with increased susceptibility to infection.

Slaves and disorder

Before the advent of formal colonisation, the coast and interior of this part of Africa had undergone dramatic changes and disruption. Modern Tanzania consists of two parts, the mainland and the islands of Zanzibar and Pemba. It was on these two islands that the main east African slave trade was established. By the middle of the nineteenth century, when European 'explorers' began to make their way into the African interior, they were following a well-trodden path – well-trodden by thousands of slaves, traders in ivory and other goods (Hall, 1996, p. 436). Peoples of the African interior, such as the Nyamwezi, the Ngoni and the legendary King Kazembe, were happy to trade with distant partners. By the mid-eighteenth century the Sultan of Zanzibar was responsible together with his merchants for the enslavement of 30,000 people from the interior per year. In addition he had an estimated 12,000 slaves working on the 5,000 acres of his personal clove plantations (Hall, 1996, p. 446).

Cotton, coffee and colonialism

What is now the United Republic of Tanzania was allocated to Germany as part of the 'scramble' in the 1880s and was passed to Britain at the end of the First World War. The 30 years after initial German colonisation saw a series of events which disrupted the human settlement patterns in the region: rinderpest destroyed cattle and smallpox killed people.[2] Famine appeared in the 1890s, the result of disruption of agricultural systems as the area was 'subdued' and tsetse fly populations increased. Cotton was a feature of this episode of colonisation – Germany needed assured sources to be able to compete in the world textile market. People of the area fought hard against the enforced cultivation and there was considerable social disruption. Indeed, the two decades from the 1880s onwards were a period of outright conflict and sometimes bribery of local elites culminating in the Maji-Maji war (1905–07). This uprising began as a revolt against forced cotton production. German military forces operated over a wide area (Kjekshus, 1996, pp. 148–9) and required food and labour. This had adverse effects on local communities as did labour recruitment for railway construction and other major infrastructural undertakings (Kjekshus, 1996, p. 156). Coffee cultivation was introduced after the initial drive to cultivate cotton. This was to be the transforming product in the area around Mount Kilimanjaro.

The Chagga of Kilimanjaro

Among the Chagga, the introduction of coffee, the development of markets, migration and changes in land use resulted in fundamental transformations both of livelihoods and personhoods (Setel, 1999a). It is not that such changes have not happened elsewhere: they have; but here we have information on the ways that risk environments, susceptibility and the personal sphere are interrelated.

Settlement and the subsequent population movements and dynamics of the Chagga on Mount Kilimanjaro were the result of a number of processes, some internal to Africa and some resulting from Africa's contact with the world beyond. These included:

- the pressure of the continuing historic great Bantu migration from the north – still active after 2,000 years
- the introduction and spread of cattle disease associated with this migration
- the slave trade along the east coast
- a population increase leading to a quest for fertile land under pressure from succeeding waves of migration from the north.[3]

Between 1,000 and 1,500 metres above sea level, the slopes of Mount Kilimanjaro are green and fertile. In the nineteenth century new migrants, people who became known as the 'Chagga', settled here. These migrants prospered and multiplied. The introduction of coffee made land valuable. Population growth and land shortage – there was a total of only 1,300 square kilometres of suitable land at the critical altitude – meant subdivision, exclusion and eventual out-migration of large numbers of people. Chagga land was hemmed in by adjacent grants to European enterprises which made competition for land more pressing. By the late 1930s, supposedly rural Kilimanjaro 'seemed something like an emergent sprawling city, with many areas approaching urban population densities and possessing a concentration of churches, schools, clinics and shops more typical of towns' (Setel 1999a, p. 68).

The people had developed a complex livelihood system dependent on a portfolio of crops cultivated across a range of altitudes. Their farming, ways of thinking about age, power, gender and inheritance were/are tied together in their concept of the *kihamba* – the homestead. In Setel's words:

> The formal organization of each *kihamba* not only provided a cultural map of linked productive and reproductive relations, but it also charted a model of the ideal gendered and generational life course. The unborn, the living, and the dead were all co-resident there. In the fertile soil beneath the banana plants lay buried the bones of the ancestors and the umbilical cords of their male issue. The *kihamba* represented prosperity, proliferation, and supremacy of an ordered succession of the generations beneath the umbrella of the patriclan. (Setel, 1999a, p. 32)

The problems with this apparently integrated and idyllic life were that it was no more integrated or problem-free than any other mode of human existence. Sons risked parental displeasure and disinheritance if they disobeyed fathers; women were subject to the will of men. The *kihamba* system, apparently stable, integrated and controlling, could only exist and reproduce itself from generation to generation as long as people remained on the mountain. But, as the population grew, young men and women began to leave the mountain to seek their fortunes. Setel points out that this migration was not only a transition in place; it was and is a transition in personhood. Not only among the Chagga, but also for most people, time, location and person are intimately tied. it is this 'tying together' which enables people to act, to express their capabilities, to define and redefine the world; in short to find their way and to know what to do and how to do it.

The reordering of desire

In the twentieth century, the land crisis drove many Chagga off the mountain and into new ways of life – schools, churches, clinics and coffee farms. These changes meant that people began to 'think about themselves as men and women in ways which had no place in the lives of their grandparents' (Jeater, 1993, p. 227, quoted in Setel, 1999a, p. 49). Social and economic change is often also ecological change.

New patterns of settlement, new livelihoods, new neighbours, new relationships – all of these are accompanied by a reordering of the bacterial and viral world which we inhabit and which inhabits us. A new personhood, new experiences, new options – new temptations! The world of the *kihamba* regulated people's lives, including their sexuality, through routine and ritual. Everything was tied to the social, economic and cultural reproduction of that way of life. Rearrangement of people's lives also reordered desire and exposure to disease, particularly sexually transmitted infection.

Desire was limited by *kihamba* life. Among the Chagga, there exists the story and the concept of *tamaa* – a deeply felt urge with negative connotations which, when excessive, becomes synonymous with bad moral character. This bad moral character was/is revealed through the misallocation of an individual's productive and reproductive energies and resources (Setel, 1999a, p. 59). People's move from the *kihamba* to the world below the mountain involved a release of desire. One of Setel's informants told him that 'many people thought *tamaa* was inseparable from the development process, a product of the colonial encounter and the mixing of cultures in postcolonial society' (Setel, 1999a, p. 60). This dangerous allure of the new was nicely summarised by one person who perhaps idealised the past when he reflected:

> 'Life was simple one to two hundred years ago. In the past, our grand-fathers … had fruits, animals … they didn't have *tamaa*. *Tamaa* did not exist. *Tamaa* entered our society when foreigners came; when Europeans brought material goods that weren't known here – things like shoes, tables, cloths, plates, bowls, coats, boots, forks, knives, blankets, mattresses, beds, cars, lamps, metal sheeting, pressure lamps, flat irons. (*Tamaa*) is always based in something you have seen. After all, you can't desire a 'Benz (Mercedes-Benz car) if you've never seen one.' (Setel, 1999a, p. 60; slightly edited from the original)

This thing, *tamaa,* was not just or even mainly about sex. It was about being removed from the *kihamba* way of life, with its close regulation, into a world of anxious predilection to acquire something better (Setel, 1999a, p. 62). This desire – which had its origins in a period of economic growth when coffee cultivators were prosperous – was exacerbated in the succeeding period of economic decline during the 1970s, with its 'Acquired Income Deficiency Syndrome' (Setel, 1999a, chapter 5). Rapid change, population growth, economic growth, economic decline all made their contribution to creation of risk environments.

It became more profitable for the new landowners to hire labour and for their sons to go elsewhere – in the best circumstances to education and a government job, in the worst circumstances to urban unemployment. By 1957 the Chagga had become a migrant group throughout Tanzania (Setel, 1999a, p. 68). The vagaries of the world coffee market in the 1960s and 1970s soon meant that incomes on the mountain were less assured. The solution was even more migration. People moved out of the area to seek work, education and experience and returned periodically to marry, visit, celebrate a rite of passage or inherit some land. At first the migrants were almost exclusively men, but by the 1950s they were joined by women, many of whom made their own independent living arrangements. In Moshi town, near Kilimanjaro, there was a surfeit of men, matched by a contrasting deficit on the mountain. The scene was set for the appearance of HIV/AIDS. The sizeable migrant male population often had wives back 'home' on the mountain protecting inherited land by occupation but living unfulfilled 'partial' lives. These women said of their menfolk: 'Even when they're here, it's like they're not here' (Martina, quoted in Setel, 1999a, p. 74). Migrant husbands in town; semi-deserted wives on the mountain; HIV/AIDS – a situation tragically encapsulating in one storyline the lethal combination of social, personal, environmental and economic change, developing risk environments and disease niches.

The endgame was as follows:

> Paradoxically, the *kihamba* regime itself contained many elements that contributed to the emergence of demographic and economic conditions of risky sex and disordered domesticity. The sexual values of the nineteenth century, which appear never to have been associated with a stable social order, changed even more rapidly in the face of a developmental process about which the Chagga felt increasingly ambivalent. Coffee wealth, education, and the embracing of colonial institutions and Christianity brought the Chagga prosperity. Yet the demographic consequences of migration, social mobility, and spousal separation caused many to call into question the cultural and practical ramifications of development. The production of persons through the ordered domestic sexuality of the *kihamba* regime was a thing of the past for many Chagga in the 1990s. What replaced it was a sense of loosened control over sexuality, over the terms and conditions under which sex took place, how relationships formed and ended, and the timing of the birth of children. (Setel, 1999a, p. 145)

In contrast to what happened in Uganda, these people's lives were not in recent years disrupted and made desperate by conflict and mis-government. In fact for many decades they were doing all right. What happened among the Chagga was a process to be found in many parts of the world – 'development'. Here internal and external factors worked together to produce redistributed risk and novel niches for infection among individuals. It is important to note that not very much of the substance of these events was actually about sexuality: rather, it was about disease transmission and the conditions of human life which create channels, niches and pathways for the more or less effective transmission of a virus. The reordering of desire was a part of these other changes.

The Democratic Republic of Congo: violence, corruption, war and risk environment[4]

Few populations on earth have been abused to the same degree as those of the Democratic Republic of Congo (DRC). Because of the degree of disruption and disorder in the country we have few hard facts about the extent of what must be a major epidemic of HIV/AIDS. This is a risk environment *par excellence* where population movement and violence have been combined for long periods.

Known until recently as Zaire, this huge, sparsely populated country of around 50 million people is larger than Western Europe (2,345,410 square kilometres against under 2,000,000 square kilometres). It is now the site of the first Great African War. Forces from many adjoining countries (and the Congo has nine international borders) and more distant Namibia, Zambia, Zimbabwe and even Chad (<www.reliefweb.int/IRIN>), contend either directly or through proxies for control of territory, population and, above all, natural resources – particularly diamonds.

The whole of the DRC has long been tied into a complex network of mainly illegal trading:

> Northeastern Zaire is part of a regional area extending eastwards to the ports of the Indian Ocean and north to the Sudan, but only as far west as Kisangani. Shaba is tied to Zambia and South Africa and its trade in smuggled imports penetrates to Kasai and Kivu. Lower Zaire forms a regional trading area with the Democratic Republic of the Congo [Congo-Brazzaville] and Angola, including Cabinda. Beyond all these regions, trading ties for some commodities extend

much further afield: to Europe, South and West Africa, India, and the Far East. (MacGaffey, 1991, p. 23)

Unrecorded trade across the DRC's southern, eastern and north-eastern borders links these regions more closely to neighbouring countries than to the DRC. Today that trade includes arms from Ukraine and Kosovo in exchange for diamonds.

An extreme abnormality

Little is normal about Congo. The slave trade was followed by grotesque exploitation under the personal rule of King Leopold of the Belgians from 1885. The Government of Belgium took control of the state in 1908 and continued to exploit the country's human and natural resources. Independence in 1960 saw a rapid transition to the brutal dictatorship of Mobutu Sese Seku, supported during the Cold War by the US and France.

Early contact with Europe

The first recorded European contact with this part of Africa was in 1482. The Manikongo, a king elected from among his peers, ran his kingdom with an elaborate bureaucracy and a degree of decentralisation. This society had such large numbers of slaves that a sixteenth-century Portuguese observer opined that the slaves outnumbered the free (Oliver, 1991, p. 122). These were people taken as captives in war as well as offenders against the law of the state or people who had been given as part of dowry payments (Hochschild, 1999, p. 9). Some were domestic slaves, some were plantation slaves, and some no doubt were sexual slaves. There were also many slaves whose social and economic conditions differed little from that of those of the free. Progressive manumission of slaves meant that more unmanumitted slaves had to be acquired to enable the hard and unforgiving tasks to be done. Internal African demand soon linked with external demand from European traders.

The trade had considerable effects over the next 300 years. From Central Africa, 5 million people were extracted (Keim, 1995, p. 116). Of these, more men than women were taken and they did not last long on the sugar and tobacco plantations of Brazil and later the Caribbean and North America. Their constant replenishment demanded expanded capture. The effects of this harvest went deep into the social and economic life of the continent until the nineteenth century.

The scramble for Africa and King Leopold of the Belgians

In the 1880s the states of Western Europe competed for territory and resources in Africa. They wanted raw materials to feed their burgeoning industries and sought markets for the products of those same factories. This was the scramble for Africa and King Leopold of the Belgians decided that he wanted a piece. By dint of careful personal diplomacy he achieved something remarkable. At a meeting in Berlin in 1884, while the European powers divided Africa between them, King Leopold gained *personal* control over the Congo. This Congo 'Free State' was his chattel and was 'free' only in the sense that it was free of control or oversight by any authority other than King Leopold.

By the turn of the twentieth century, rubber determined the fate of millions of people in Congo. Leopold had gone deeply into debt to pursue his ambition: it was now payback time. Wild rubber was the main source of revenue for the Congo Free State.

Collecting wild rubber required that people go deep into the forest. Collecting agents were paid by the weight of rubber they delivered, and the people who collected it were suborned by the most terrible means. Women and children were corralled and sold back to their menfolk when the rubber was delivered (Hochschild, 1999, p. 161). 'The entire system was militarized' (Hochschild, 1999, p. 163); whipping and mutilation were widely used to force rubber collection.

Perhaps 10 million people died as a result of depredations during the so-called 'Free State' (Hochschild, 1999, p. 297). After the slave trade and King Leopold even the most resilient societies and economies would have been staggering. But more was to follow. The Belgian state took over administration of this huge country and did little that was different. In 1960 the Republic of Congo, ill-prepared with few trained administrators, teachers or specialists, received its independence.

Patrice Lumumba, the leader of the independence movement and the country's first prime minister, was perceived as a communist sympathiser, a threat to US strategic mineral interests. Zaire was the world's largest cobalt exporter – at one time producing 90% of the cobalt used in the US aerospace industry. Western governments and the Belgian Union Minière destabilised the country by encouraging secession of the mineral-rich province of Katanga. Lumumba opposed these moves to dismember the newly independent country and was killed by members of Mobutu's army with the possible collusion of the CIA within a few years of independence.

The patrimonial state – kleptocracy in action

For the next 30 years Mobutu Seke Sesu held sway, until the fall of the Berlin Wall made protection of his corrupt regime no longer necessary. The Congo certainly did not 'develop' during Mobutu's regime. Instead its already poor infrastructure rotted further, its human resources remained sparse, and the few qualified people fled. This huge country is replete with mineral and other natural resources yet its per capita income has never risen above sheer poverty in the whole 'independence' period. 'The ruling class in Zaire has effectively "privatised" the public bureaucracy and converted it into an instrument for self-enrichment from independence until now' (Gould, 1980, p. xiii). A violent history; constant unrest since independence; a state corrupt to the core (Williams, 1972): it is hardly surprising that conditions were in place for an epidemic of HIV/AIDS. In addition, gender relations are regulated by retrogressive legislation. Formal regulations require that a woman have her husband's permission to take out a trading licence or open a bank account, and any contribution on his part to her enterprise ensures that he controls her earnings (MacGaffey, 1991, p. 34). Taken together, we once again have important constituents of a risk environment.

In view of this history, it is inevitable that data on the state of the epidemic are inadequate and old. UNAIDS reports (a) that mean adult seroprevalence was 5.07% as of the end of 1999, and (b) that collection of data from outside the capital, Kinshasa, was 'infrequent' (UNAIDS, 2000a). However, a small indication of the true situation in the country may come from the single observation that in Lubumbashi 9% of antenatal clinic women tested were HIV positive in 1999 (UNAIDS, 2000a). The likelihood is that rates are in fact much higher than this.

Another turn of the screw

The troubled history of the Congo, now the Democratic Republic of the Congo, can now be brought up to date. Mobutu was overthrown by an invading army lead by Laurent Kabila in 1997. Within four years Kabila had been assassinated and succeeded by his son. Most of the country is not controlled by Kinshasa and a multi-country war is waging across the Congo. Many armies are fighting this war. We know that socio-economic instability and war hasten the spread of HIV. Military forces have higher levels of infection than civilian populations and those in the Congo have exceptionally high levels of infection. Estimated prevalence in the Angolan and Congolese armies is 40–60%; that of the Tanzanian forces is between 15–30%, while it may be as high as 80% in the Zimbabwean army (Mills, 2000).

How many new infections will be spawned? How many recombinant forms of the virus will appear as a result of this latest episode of disorder? It may seem inappropriate to consider the question of social and economic impact of HIV/AIDS in such circumstances. What is there for it to impact on? But we should. Here is a vast region with multiple problems: state instability, extreme poverty, war, population dislocation. Each of these will exacerbate and be amplified by the epidemic. Questions of 'development', whatever that might mean in such circumstances, cannot be broached without taking into consideration the additional challenges posed by HIV/AIDS. For example, it is estimated that there are already almost half a million AIDS orphans in the Democratic Republic of Congo (UNAIDS, 2000f). Their present care and future tenuous participation in the life of their communities must be high on the agenda as an impact.

And why and how does the disease spread in Zaire (now Democratic Republic of Congo) in 'normal' times? Listen to the story of Mama Tabala, aged 35, and her husband, who live in Kinshasa. Once a taxi driver but now unemployed, Monsieur Tabala drinks. Mama Tabala looks after their child and two others who are their wards. They are poor. When Monsieur Tabala has money he buys food for himself. Mama Tabala meets all the household expenses by herself. When her nephew who lives with them became sick she was so pressed for cash to buy food and medicine that

> she took several sexual partners. Other women in the neighbourhood criticised her for this ... One, who is more realistic, said: 'Look, you who criticize Mama Tabala, your husbands contribute to the budget, but hers doesn't help at all. There she is, attractive and well-built, still young. She has to feed the family, pay the rent, and clothe everyone. What else can she do? If only there were not that terrible disease that kills, that doesn't let anyone escape.' (Schoepf and Engundu, 1991, p. 143)

South Africa – institutionalised and legalised inequality: reaping the whirlwind

The HIV/AIDS epidemic began to spread through South and southern Africa in the late 1980s. The 1990s saw an explosion in HIV prevalence and the already extremely high rates continue to rise. Adult HIV prevalence was estimated at 19.94% at the end of 1999. South Africa's peculiar history has made it fertile ground for the spread of HIV.

South Africa's history has been exploitative and bloody, but there are important differences from the preceding cases:

- the system was based on 'racial' discrimination and after 1948 this was institutionalised and legalised
- the past 200 years have been characterised by mobile populations and a breakdown in social structures
- South Africa has high levels of urbanisation and a large white minority.

In contrast to the other countries we have considered, this was a settler society with strong and enduring links to the intellectual and political worlds of Europe and North America. The settlers shared a vision of 'civilisation' which distanced them from the rest of the population and by means of which they legitimised their dominance.

The country's written history begins with Portuguese mariners' tentative steps to explore the coast in search of a sea route to the Indies. Bartolomeu Dias first rounded the continent's south coast in 1488. For the next two centuries there was little European settlement, for the most part confined to the coast. These people earned their living by supplying ships plying the profitable trading routes to Asia. The Dutch established their major centre of settlement at the Cape and its immediate environs. The Portuguese had a number of small forts on the Mozambican coast.

Cape Town was effectively a company town, owned, run and governed by the Dutch East India Company. This had important long-term implications for the development of the region. First, the early settlers were company employees; indeed, non-company men were discouraged. Thus it was an unattractive location for free immigration. Second, relations between the settlers and the native inhabitants were fraught and exploitative but the local population was not so easily disposed of as in the Americas. Third, there was little attempt to expand beyond the initial settlement and development was discouraged.

In the late eighteenth century the Cape was fought over during the Napoleonic Wars. In 1814 Britain was confirmed as the new master of the colony. It was of strategic importance to the entire British imperial project, a vital point on the route to India prior to the construction of the Suez Canal.

What followed was to set the pattern for the next 150 years. Dutch farmers moved into the interior of this vast and sparsely populated continent away from what they perceived as restrictive British rule.

White and black populations were brought into prolonged contact and conflict for the first time. The Boers were moving into territory devastated by the *mfecane* or *difaqane* translated as the crushing and clubbing. This was a reign of terror, war and violence that stemmed from the establishment of the Zulu nation under Shaka – an endpoint of the historic Bantu migration from the north to the south of the continent, mentioned above. These 'tribes' (many of them in formation, decline or transition) cannonading across the sub-continent resulted in a degree of depopulation and destabilisation.

By the mid-1800s southern Africa was a farming/subsistence society. Its cores were the British-controlled Cape Province and the colony of Natal. To the interior were the Boer republics that became the Orange Free State and the Transvaal. On the periphery were autonomous African states, most with a complement of missionaries who were committed to protecting the interests of 'their' natives. Some black people at the Cape were protected by laws which accorded them certain rights. However, for most Europeans, the black population was seen as either providers of labour or rural people living Arcadian lives who could be safely ignored. When the blacks protested, sometimes violently, because they were losing land or their rights were being infringed, Arcadia was transformed into 'savagery'.

In 1867 diamonds were discovered on the borders of the Orange Free State. This was to transform the history of the entire sub-continent. By mid-1870 the town of Kimberly had been established and, by British sleight of hand, the official border between the Cape and the Free State had developed a kink that put the diamond fields in the Cape. By 1872 the diamond fields had a population of between 30,000 and 50,000 people, of whom 13,000 were European. Manual labour was provided largely by people from the interior, the majority of whom were Pedi from the Northern Transvaal, Tsonga from Mozambique and an organised contingent of Basutho. These were all volunteers and target workers; they worked for long enough to get money to buy specific items.

The black population did not consider that working for whites was necessarily worthwhile or desirable. This was most evident in Natal, where the major cash crop was sugar. Zulus, given a choice between working in the hot, sweaty, dirty cane fields or continuing their traditional lives saw no contest. The European solution to this problem was to import Indian labour, an addition to the population mix that was to become modern South Africa. The imperial Government of India insisted that a proportion of migrants be women, and the workers could stay in South Africa once their contract expired. If they chose to stay they were allocated land to the value of their return passage. Many stayed and a new, imported, community began to develop, particularly in Natal Province.

Diamonds are small and valuable. They can be easily concealed and there was a ready market for them no matter where they originated. Control of labour and its conditions was vital, both at work and after, if theft was to be avoided. Attempts to control black mine labour took two forms. From 1872 all employees were required to carry passes. In practice, whites did not bother to register and were seldom harassed by the authorities. Non-employee blacks had to carry certificates of Cape citizenship to avoid harassment – a pass to avoid a pass. The advantages of controlling the workforce soon became apparent to the European mine owners and managers. By 1885 the first compounds were in place, and within a short period black workers were living in compounds from the time they arrived to the time they left the mines. The conditions were crowded and unsanitary. The ultimate humiliation was that at the end of each contract, a worker would be confined in a room for a few days, naked and wearing a type of boxing glove. This was to ensure that workers did not swallow diamonds: their stools were examined for any that they might have managed to conceal.

The rich Witwatersrand goldfields were discovered in the Transvaal in 1886. The development of the mines meant that white immigration increased and the need for black labour expanded. Themes that were to dominate southern African history for the next 100 years can now be identified.

- White mastery was clear. Whether Afrikaner or British, the whites held economic and political power. There was a limited black franchise in the Cape but most whites resented this and even the most liberal saw universal black franchise as being at least 100 years away (ironically they were right, but for the wrong reasons).
- Conflict between the British and Afrikaners was inevitable. This erupted into war in 1880/81 when a brief skirmish resulted in the British forces being comprehensively trounced. The longer war of 1899–1902 (the 'Boer War') saw an eventual but expensive victory for the British. This led to the establishment of the Union of South Africa in 1910. Despite British military victory, Afrikaner interests soon gained political control.
- The English and the Afrikaners were in broad agreement about the position of black people. They were to have no political rights and

economic advancement was resented. They were a labour pool and legislation was geared to ensure that they were stripped of rights, forced to offer their labour and firmly controlled.

- The countries surrounding South Africa – with the exception of Zimbabwe – were placed in a core–periphery relationship. Botswana, Lesotho and Swaziland were British protectorates ruled through a policy of benign neglect. South-west Africa became a South African administered territory after its removal from German control in 1918. Mozambique was divided into company-controlled estates run for the benefit of South African capital. Zimbabwe mirrored South Africa on a smaller scale.

The legislative framework

Once pass laws and the exclusion of black people from the franchise had been established, the next step was to divide the land. The best land was allocated to the whites. What remained could not support the black population – they had to seek wage labour on white farms, in white-owned mines and industries. Proposing the Glen Grey Act in 1894, Cecil John Rhodes, the premier of the Cape and controller of the diamond industry, was open about the motives:

> It is our duty as a Government to remove these poor children [the Thembu] from [a] life of sloth and laziness, and give them some gentle stimulus to come forth and find out the dignity of labour. (quoted in Welsh, 2000, p. 309)

The first post-Union legislation to deal with 'the native problem' was the Natives' Land Act of 1913, which effected geographic separation between whites and blacks, seriously curtailing black land purchase and ownership outside the reserves. Other repressive legislation followed in the period leading to 1948. The Nationalist Party's accession to power in that year saw the refinement of the apartheid system.

Under apartheid the country was subjected to extreme social engineering, influenced by Nazi Germany and designed for the benefit of the minority white population. The state sought control through racial criteria governing:

- who could vote
- where people could live and own land
- what work people could do
- what education and health care they received

- who they could marry
- with whom they could have sex.

Migration

The stated policy of government was that:

> Bantu are only temporarily resident in European areas for as long as they offer their labour there. As soon as they become, for some reason or other, no longer fit for work or superfluous in the labour market they are expected to return to their country of origin. (South African Government, 1967)

South Africa's black population was forced into crowded, impoverished homelands which led further to the breakdown of traditional cultural structures and livelihoods. Adults, mainly men, migrated to urban areas to work in white-owned factories and mines and live in single-sex hostels. The law now prevented them from bringing their families to town. This created a culture of urban and rural wives and of sexual liaisons spanning the continuum from 'town wife' to 'prostitute'. Many children were cared for by adults other than their parents, which resulted in family breakups. Health services were limited and many diseases, including STIs, went untreated.

At the peak of this system in 1985, 1,833,636 South Africans were classed as 'migrants' (Whiteside, 1986), that is, they were not regarded as resident in the areas where they worked. Of these, 771,397 came from the 'independent homelands' of Transkei, Bophutatswana, Venda and Ciskei; and 1,062,239 from the 'self-governing' homelands of Lebowa, Gazankulu, Qwa Qwa, KwaZulu, KwaNdebele and KaNgwane.[5]

However South Africa's economic influence extended far beyond the country's borders. It was (and is) the richest country in the region, which meant that it drew in labour from as far away as Malawi and Angola. And this labour was needed. Despite the apartheid system there was not enough indigenous labour. In 1985, 27,814 Batswana, 139,827 Basotho, 30,144 Malawians, 68,665 Mozambicans and 22,255 Swazi were employed officially as migrants in South Africa. In addition there were many illegal migrants, mainly employed in the agricultural sector. The number of legal migrants continues to fall (as shown in Table 5.4) and the number of illegals continues to rise. No one knows quite how many illegal migrants there are today in South Africa. It is certain though that South Africa and Botswana are still the honeypot for most Africans, the place where streets are paved with gold. And

Table 5.4   Trends in employment of foreign migrants in the South African mining industry

Country of origin	1984	1989	1994	1998
Lesotho	75787	98085	84700	60450
Botswana	18599	15229	10837	7752
Swaziland	12152	16555	14829	10336
Mozambique	42294	44015	44044	51913

Source: Whiteside and Sunter (2000), p. 63 (data from Employment Bureau of *Report and Financial Statements*, various years).

today they come from as far away as west and east Africa. Hausa and Swahili are now widely heard on the streets of Johannesburg, Durban and Cape Town. In such conditions, the construction and reconstruction of sexualities occurs. For men who are migrants, whose fathers and even grandfathers were migrant labourers, the exaggerated masculinity referred to elsewhere resulted in a particular construction of risk taking: promiscuous sexuality (Campbell, 1997; Bujra, 2000a).

Conflict and change

The South African black population was not acquiescent. In the 1950s the African National Congress (ANC) realised that negotiation with the Nationalist government would get nowhere and the white opposition would never represent African interests. Armed opposition was the only way forward and this began in the early 1960s. For the first 20 years it was inefficient and badly organised. South Africa was seen as a bastion against communism and received explicit and more important tacit support from the West.

By the 1980s internal opposition and international approbation most effectively expressed through sanctions and boycotts began to influence the government and it was clear that there would have to be change. In February 1990, all political parties were unbanned; the leadership, including Nelson Mandela, was released from prison and the white government began to negotiate itself out of power. In May 1994 the ANC won the first election based on a universal franchise and took power.

The legacy

The AIDS epidemic reflects the history of this region. Migration and mobility have created patterns of sexual behaviour and mixing which are perfect for the spread of sexually transmitted disease. Indeed we note that the migrant-sending countries have higher rates of HIV prevalence than South Africa itself. South Africa is the crucible for HIV transmission in the region. Labour comes into an area of high sero-prevalence, where working and living conditions encourage sexual mixing. Infected men return to their home communities where 'local' epidemics are established. In the periphery there are neither the resources nor the ability to establish AIDS control programmes. In the longer term it is these communities that bear the cost of increased illness and deaths.

Then there is inequality. In 1993 in South Africa, the richest 10% of the population received 47.3% of the income, whereas the poorest 40% of the people had only a 9.1% share. Land inequalities mean that 71% of the rural population – mainly black – lived on 14% of the land, while the balance of farmland was owned by only 67,000 farmers, almost all white (Whiteside and Sunter, 2000). The same situation pertains in Zimbabwe, although here the 'land reform' means that the major landowners are black cronies of the leadership. There are also regional inequalities: in 1998, per capita income in Mozambique was US$210, in Lesotho US$570 – compared to South Africa's US$3,310.

Breakdown of family structure in the rural areas and townships, government policy toward its black population and the violence that accompanied the end of apartheid combined to create a widespread philosophy of fatalism. This perception that 'what will be, will be' in turn diminished individual worth, responsibility and accountability. The feeling is still prevalent and makes people live for today without valuing tomorrow. It can be summed up in a shrug of the shoulders and the response: 'If AIDS kills me in five years' time, so what?'

Conflict resulting from the cycle of oppression and resistance led to the widespread destruction and disruption of civil society. The ANC's political slogan of the late 1980s, 'Make the townships ungovernable', was to have far-reaching consequences. Society has been militarised. Armed forces proliferated, including the defence force, homeland armies, liberation movements, self-defence units and political militias, as well as shadowy groups of vigilantes and unofficial police and intelligence units. Apart from internal conflict, wars were being fought by South Africans in Angola, Mozambique and Namibia. Conflict between the armed wings of the political parties continued up to the 1994 election, and in KwaZulu-Natal continued beyond the election albeit at a much lower level. Conflict results in inability to absorb and act on messages contained in educational programmes about HIV. Military forces have higher levels of infection than the general population and are more likely to spread their infections.[6]

An astonishing fact that emerged from the Truth and Reconciliation Commission (TRC) was the use of HIV as a weapon. According to submissions made by two apartheid-era security officers, Willie Nortje and Andries van Heerden, speaking at the TRC in 1999, HIV positive *askaris* (former ANC operatives who had gone over to work for the apartheid state security forces) were used to spread the disease. These men, known to be HIV positive, were employed in 1990 in two Hillbrow hotels in Johannesburg with explicit instructions to infect sex workers (Roberts, 1999).

The ending of apartheid and election of the new government in 1994 resulted in relaxation of the draconian controls on society. But these were not replaced immediately by a strong civil society – hardly surprising, as this is something that has to be built over time rather than imposed. In addition, there was no immediate redistribution of resources or lessening of income inequality.

Crime and gang violence are now endemic in South Africa. As a consequence, rape and gang rape have become potent methods of spreading HIV. In 1998 a total of 54,310 sexual crimes were *officially* recorded. The true figure is no doubt very much higher (Institute of Security Studies, 1999). Rape has much higher odds of HIV transmission because of physical trauma; its frequency tells us something about the nature of gender relations in the South African communities.

Political changes have not meant prosperity for all South Africans. Unemployment has risen since 1994. Job shedding started in the late 1980s, largely due to sanctions. However it increased sharply after 1994 when South Africa joined the World Trade Organisation and import tariffs ceased. A million jobs, mostly unskilled, were lost between 1993 and 1997, offset against 60,000 skilled jobs gained. In South Africa about 35% of the labour force lacks formal employment and a far larger proportion lack the skills needed to participate in export industries.

Ironically, the economic autarky associated with apartheid protected South Africa against some global forces. Globalisation may have positive outcomes in countries where the labour force is able to obtain long-term employment and participate in the production of goods and services for export. Here export-led growth will increase employment opportunities and eventually raise household incomes. But in South Africa things are different. The labour force lacks skills, the strong union movement protects those in employment and Western countries have been less than generous with Favoured Nation status and preferential tariffs.

The upshot of global changes in the structure of demand for goods and services and competition has been to marginalise different components of the labour force in direct proportion to their skills and ability to find employment in sectors that are competitive in the global economy. (Tomlinson, 2000)

What applies in South Africa applies equally in the rest of southern Africa. With the exception of Botswana these countries are poorer than South Africa. They have less resilience and, in the case of Angola and Mozambique, have been victims of the view taken by powerful nations that wars are engagements best played away from home.

South African society and AIDS – the Carletonville study

We have an insight into the situation in urban South Africa from the Carletonville study. This important long-term study is based in the mining community of Carletonville, about 100 kilometres from Johannesburg and 50 kilometres from Soweto. It began in 1997, and aims to understand social and economic factors contributing to the rapid spread of HIV and AIDS in urban South Africa.

The rate of infection among adolescent girls in the study area is nearly 60% (Gilgen et al., 2000, p. 8). A large number of men in this community live in mine hostels. There are adjacent 'hot-spots' in which more than 50% of the women say they are commercial sex workers. The study shows that a range of factors raise individual susceptibility to infection: active or poorly treated STIs, the use of alcohol, and high numbers of lifetime sexual partners. Among men, protective factors were membership of a sports club and circumcision (about half the men were circumcised), while among the protective factors for women was membership of a burial society or church. For all, living in a squatter area raised the chance of exposure to infection (Gilgen et al., 2000, chapter 4). All the risk factors are associated with low levels of social cohesion, poor women and relatively better-off men.

These preliminary data from a long-term study are entirely predictable. They confirm that if you put people in circumstances where they cannot maintain stable relationships, where they are mobile, where life is risky and pleasures are few and necessarily cheap, then sexually transmitted diseases will be rampant. If, further, there are inadequate medical services and little is available in the way of immediate, accessible and effective treatment for STIs, then HIV will move in very fast indeed. Some of the people in Carletonville – the miners, the sex workers and others – had relatively good incomes. But they had these in a poor country and in a poor community.

Conclusion

Africa's history is one of abnormal normality. It differs from all other regions of the world in the sustained nature of disruption, exploitation and bad government – and the fact that Africans, in contrast to the indigenous populations of other world regions, have survived these experiences. In the last 30 years the misfortunes of this history have been compounded by a long period of economic crisis. The oil price hike in 1974 was soon followed by economic collapse. During this time, many of the recently independent states' wrong-headed policies took their toll. These policies had been generated from within by inexperienced and sometimes corrupt governments or imposed from without by, among others, the World Bank (Barratt Brown, 1995, pp. 65–6). Sometimes both of these things happened at once as Cold War alliances were made and broken across Africa.

As countries sought refuge from these difficulties with lenders of last resort, such as the International Monetary Fund, they were subject to structural adjustment policies (originating with the so-called Berg Report (World Bank, 1981)) imposed by the international financial institutions. A result of these policies was a huge out-migration of skilled people. In Zaire (now Congo), 80,000 teachers and health care workers lost their jobs in these decades; in Ghana the number of doctors fell by half; in Senegal the number of nurses fell sixfold. According to one estimate, 13,000 doctors and nurses left Zimbabwe for South Africa and Europe after structural adjustment was introduced in the early 1990s. The collapse of health services and introduction of user fees meant that sexually transmitted diseases were more likely to go untreated (Epstein, 2001, pp. 33–8).

Geographic disadvantage, disorder, relative deprivation, inequality and poverty: we have seen these in different ways in the case studies in this chapter. They are all characteristics of a risk environment where susceptibility is high. They are the horsemen of the twenty-first century apocalypse in Africa.

In the next part we turn to the social and economic impact of the epidemic, which is for the moment starkest in Africa.

Part III
Vulnerability and Impact

6
Introduction to Impact

Epidemic impacts are history-changing events. They terminate some lives, incapacitate others and stunt the capabilities of those who have to divert energy and time into care. In the end, sufficient numbers of deaths and illnesses make a society take a path other than that which it would previously have followed. This is impact. North America would have a different population composition, culture, economy and political system had 95% of the indigenous population not been wiped out by microbes originating in Europe (Diamond, 1999, p. 211).

The concept of differential susceptibility helps us understand the course of epidemics. In parts of the world, most notably Africa, prevention efforts have failed. Large numbers of people are infected, will fall ill and die. They will need health care and support, and leave behind families and orphans, many of whom will be impoverished. In the worst-affected countries economic growth may falter, provision of social services may become difficult and the epidemic may ultimately threaten political stability as the fabric of government is frayed.

In this chapter we outline concepts for understanding impact. We note that vulnerability to impact is differential; not all societies and nations will be equally affected. The most clearly discernible impact is demographic which is dealt with first. In the following chapters we look at impact as it affects different levels and aspects of society at large.

Impact, history and pragmatism

It is ironic that at a time when the importance of past epidemics is increasingly recognised and discussed by historians, there is very little appreciation of how AIDS impact is already affecting many societies now and into the future. After the optimism of the twentieth century, people are waking up to the fact that infectious diseases have not been beaten into submission. They are regrouping and searching out weaknesses in our defences. There is much talk of 'emerging' and 're-emerging' diseases. We confront new epidemics. Perhaps the reason humankind currently pays so little attention to disease is that the last global epidemic, the flu epidemic of 1918, occurred so long ago that it is now beyond collective memory. Whatever the reason, the false sense of security is exactly that – false – and HIV/AIDS is a harbinger of the global public health crisis.

Epidemics and their impact do not take place in isolation. They need to be related to other events – changes in political regime, new ideas, global warming, the global distribution of power. We cannot deal with these events in isolation from each other. We live in a world where perception of interrelated multiple long-wave events must be on the agenda of every politician and policy maker. We can no longer deal with issues piecemeal and sincerely claim that we have given them our full attention.

The impact of the AIDS epidemic can be studied for many reasons: because it is an interesting phenomenon; because of a pressing desire to help those in distress now and in the future; because it makes a mockery of international development goals and prospects for progress in some countries; because resulting poverty may be a threat to the national security of the US; or yet again because of a fear that 'AIDS refugees' may flood the countries of the north in a search for treatment. There is a premium on pragmatism as opposed to compassion. Pragmatism tends to capture resources.

What do we mean by impact?

This epidemic increases morbidity (sickness) and mortality (death) in populations at precisely those ages where normal levels of morbidity and mortality are low. This is shown in Figure 6.1

It is from these unusual events that other impacts flow. These impacts may be felt as an immediate and severe shock or they may be more complex, gradual and long-term changes. In some situations AIDS illness and death may threaten to overwhelm communities and perhaps whole societies; in others the shock is absorbed. Impact will occur at different levels: the household, community or nation. Table 6.1 provides a conceptual matrix for thinking about this. We note though that vulnerability to impact is only partly determined by the numbers of people infected and where they are located in society; difference in

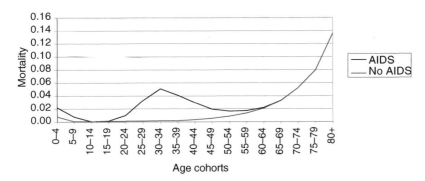

Figure 6.1 Age-specific mortality at 20% HIV seroprevalence in a population

degree will reflect differential resource endowments. Well-resourced communities and households will be better able to cope than poor ones, and the same is true for countries.

Sharp shock or slow erosion?

It is useful to begin thinking about impact as a continuum between a sharp shock and slow and profound changes.

An example of a sharp shock is the death of the main breadwinner or the main carer in a household or family. This results in immediate and marked decline in living standards and welfare. Similarly, the death of a strategically important and hard to replace individual in an organisation, for example an especially skilled worker whose skills are in short supply, will have a shock impact upon the operation of that organisation.

A slow but complex *series of changes* – some of them very subtle – results from gradual accumulation of impacts. This is illustrated by an example from the health system.

- TB is a frequent opportunistic infection associate with AIDS. It spreads to the wider population
- AIDS first affects the availability of treatment for non-AIDS illnesses in the health system
- There are additional pressures on health staff who suffer burn-out and emotional exhaustion
- Resources are constrained and the health of those who can't gain access to care for non-AIDS illnesses suffers. TB infection rates increase in the general population
- The result is an overall reduction of people's health status

Table 6.1   Understanding impact, by level, time and degree

Level of impact	Time of impact	Degree of impact	Does evidence exist that this happens?
Individual	Early	Always severe and variation by gender and age	Yes – death and illness
Household	Early	Severe emotional, variable financial depending on socio-economic status, gender, ethnicity and other social variables	Yes – household studies summarised in Chapter 7 Orphans and the elderly particularly affected
Community	Early, middle and late	Variable: dependent on scale, and resource base of community but likely to be long term and profound but not necessarily easy to see	Yes – evidence considered in Chapter 7 Orphans, the elderly and local service provision affected
Production unit/institution	Middle and late	Variable: dependent on the nature of an organisation or institution's activities or type of production and labour mix	Yes – evidence discussed in Chapter 10.
Sector	Late	Variable: dependent on location, production and use of labour	Yes – some evidence but limited, discussed in Chapters 9 and 11
Nation	Late	Economic probably slight, other may be greater. At present we have no evidence for these	No – only economic models and anecdotal evidence about effects on government infrastructure, see Chapter 12

- Society bears wider costs. These are either direct costs of care or indirect costs associated with decreasing health status and consequent knock-on effects to educational attainment, social functioning, and trauma associated with the premature deaths of relatives from TB.

This example of gradual change shows how:

- cumulative and linked effects may be severe but difficult to measure over the long term and that the chain of events does not stop there
- the combination of sharp shocks and slow changes affects all areas of social reproduction, production, livelihoods and governance.

Seeing impact

The curve of HIV infection is followed by the curve of AIDS illness and death which in turn determines the third curve, impact. For example, orphaned female children have a higher likelihood of infection, or if they are withdrawn from school we know their children will have higher mortality rates as female education is correlated with infant and child mortality rates. Thus AIDS impacts over three generations.

So, in considering impact, we are describing some events that we can see now, mainly the shocks, and discussing other medium- and long-term events, some of which we can only speculate about. However we believe that there is sufficient evidence to suggest that our speculations are justified and a cause for concern.

This epidemic is only 20 years old. In poorer countries the number of people infected continues to increase, the HIV epidemic curve has not peaked. The exceptions are probably Thailand and Uganda. However even here the 'impact curve' is rising as the cumulative infections of past years evolve into illness and deaths. (This is illustrated by Figure 2.5 in Chapter 2.)

Perception and estimation of impact will depend on:

- the perspective of those who are looking and the disciplinary, moral and political lenses they employ
- the degree to which those who are affected *count* in society. The impacts on marginal population are least likely to be counted and power holders are more likely to be able to say that these people do not count.

We have a fairly clear idea of the current scale of the HIV epidemic. From this we can make reasonable assessments of potential morbidity and mortality using modelling techniques. Demographic impacts can be estimated but others are speculative. One method of controlled speculation is to build scenarios. This approach has much to offer and has not been employed in relation to AIDS impact.

Looking into the future: building scenarios

Scenario building is widely used in business. In the 1980s, the large multinational Anglo-American projected possible futures for South Africa. The outcomes were presented to many thousands of people and played an important part in setting the scene for the negotiations that brought an end to the apartheid regime (Sunter, 1987).

Scenario planning works, as illustrated in Figure 6.2. This shows a 'Cone of Uncertainty' opening up into the future. For example, if we asked what the oil price would be in a week's time, we would get answers covering a range of a few cents. If we asked what it would be in ten years the range might be in the tens of dollars. This is true of any parameter: the further you look into the future, the less certainty there is.

The scenario planner aims to reduce the number of reasonable possibilities; hence the inner cone becomes what is most likely to happen.

With regard to AIDS impact, we start by looking at what we know now. For example, we can predict the numbers who will fall ill and die with some certainty over the next ten years. The next step is to look at 'key uncertainties' within the reduced cone. These are factors that are important for the future but whose movement cannot possibly be predicted, for example a very cheap and effective treatment becoming available.

Finally the scenario planner examines the interplay between 'key uncertainties' and writes the plausible scenarios. These are simple and

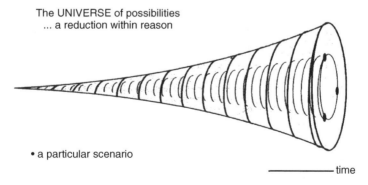

Figure 6.2   The universe of possibilities
Source: Sunter (1987).

consistent stories about the future which illustrate possible outcomes and challenges. Such hypothecations are more effective than single-line forecasts which offer no understanding of the interplay of forces within systems. Of particular importance is that they are able to take into account the complex interactions of multiple long-wave events. This is something which should be applied to AIDS impact, but which has not been done.

Three other points made by the Anglo team are important.

- Scenario plans seldom come true. For example, in the 1950s no one would have predicted that the Asian economies would take off and Africa's would stagnate.
- It is difficult to communicate bad news in a forecast. Indeed one rarely sees business predicting declining profits. People do not like being told that something bad is going to happen. It is preferable to put forward the *possibility* of bad news and offer a way out.
- Forecasts may be received as though they imply that the future is decided irrespective of any effort on the listeners' or readers' part. But as Anglo noted, there are two kinds of future: the 'active future' which you make happen, and the 'passive futures' which you let happen to you. With regard to AIDS impact, few if any governments have begun to consider their 'active futures'.

What do we know about impact?

There are a few literature reviews; some region-specific (Loewenson and Whiteside, 1997), some global (Chong, 1999; Barnett and Whiteside, 2000). What is particularly significant, and evident from these reviews, is how little original research there has been. The reviews tend to refer to the same studies again and again. Indeed, there is a general problem that reports of 'impact' are sometimes no more than recycled anecdotes, a game of 'Chinese whispers'.

As might be expected (and this is no criticism of researchers who are operating with limited funds and time), impact studies usually focus on one geographical area, one company or one community. The problem is that these results are then applied without discrimination to whole populations or nations. An example is the study done for the Zimbabwe Farmers' Union in one communal and small farm area. This found that any adult death had an adverse effect on output, but that in the case of AIDS this effect was worse. An adult death resulted in a 45% decline in marketed output of maize, but where the cause of death was identified as AIDS there was a 61% loss (Kwaramba, 1998). The study is good, 56 key informants and a survey of 544 households, well-analysed and clearly written up. The problem is that others then applied the finding simplistically to the whole country. On the basis of this one study in one area, another 'study' reported that there would be a decline in agricultural output not just in Zimbabwe as a whole, but more generally across Africa, and that this could be ascribed to AIDS. To save embarrassment we will not reference that study!

The few studies of impact that exist tend not to appreciate its full complexity. This should not surprise us. Many have been produced for policy purposes and national and international civil servants are often under pressure to work from minimum rather than maximum information. This means we understand impact very poorly. In particular, much impact is unmeasured: perhaps because it has not been appreciated yet; perhaps because it can't be 'measured' in ways which are recognised by policy makers, politicians and academics as legitimate, and are thus dismissed as 'anecdotal evidence'.

This section of the book looks at measured impact but we must remember that unmeasured impacts are of equal and possibly greater significance. Other points to consider are that:

- in some cases impact will not be apparent as individuals, households, firms and other socio-economic units disappear and their disappearance goes unremarked and uncounted
- evolving coping mechanisms are bound to confound predictions of the size, intensity and nature of impact. It is hardly surprising that households, firms and production units develop coping mechanisms; not to do so would be to cease to exist.

Differential vulnerability

In exactly the same way as not all people or communities are susceptible to infection (as discussed in Chapter 4) so not all will be affected in the same way or to the same degree. There is differential vulnerability to the impact of the disease.

The concept of vulnerability is most important in relation to a central concern of this book, the social and economic impact of the epidemic. *Vulnerability* describes those features of a society, social or economic institution or process that makes it more or less likely that excess morbidity and mortality associated with disease will have negative impacts. Like susceptibility, the concept of vulnerability applies at a number of levels. For example, a household with only one wage earner who is aged 25 is more vulnerable than one in which there are two or more wage earners, one of whom is more than 50 years old. A farming system in a dry region, with rainfall limited to six weeks of the year, is one in which any shortage of labour for key cultivation activities will result in restrictions of production for the entire season, and even starvation. An industrial process plant that depends upon one or two key pieces of equipment with very specialised operators who are in short supply is more vulnerable than one where large numbers of unskilled workers are involved in the same or similar processes.

It used to be that vulnerability of individuals, once infected, was not very variable. People could expect to experience episodes of ill health that would increase in frequency, severity and duration until they died. At best the wealthy could buy better diets and palliative care. With the advent of new anti-retroviral therapy this has changed. Those who have sufficient financial resources can literally buy extra days of life.

Thus relative wealth reduces vulnerability at all levels from the individual to the nation. The resources are not purely financial; they may include skilled labour, or access to care; or even a strong, cohesive and compassionate civil society.

The demographic impact of AIDS

Unusual levels of death alter population dynamics. Demography looks at populations and their dynamics. It is concerned with the numbers, growth rates and structure of populations. It measures and predicts size and growth rates, structure by gender and age, and key indicators like birth, death and fertility rates, life expectancy and infant and child mortality.

Demographers derive raw data from two main sources:[1] the census and vital registration statistics. Most countries conduct censuses every ten years. The purpose of a census is 'the total process of collecting, compiling, evaluating and publishing or otherwise disseminating demographic, economic and social data pertaining at a specific time to all persons in a country or a well delimitated part of a country' (Petersen and Petersen, 1985). The United Nations sets out what should be collected – and this includes data on age, sex, place of birth, citizenship, household and family structure, marital status, number of children and child deaths, literacy and educational qualifications, urban and rural domicile and economic status. Censuses have political implications. In Nigeria, Fiji and Malaysia, for example, the ethnic and religious make-up of the populations have implications for electoral roles and representation. South Africa based estimates of informal sector and rural populations prior to the 1996 census on aerial photographs of dwellings.

Vital registration is information about births, deaths and marriages. In many countries it is compulsory to register these events, but in poorer countries these data are rarely collected, there is little incentive for citizens to register births and deaths. An exception is South Africa, and we will draw on these data later.

There are three main problems in looking at demographic impacts. The first concerns the difference between an event and a process. The impact of AIDS is felt as a process: a person begins to feel unwell and so, perhaps, does not grow as much food, thus the family has less to sell and can't afford to send children to school. When the person dies household composition changes. The demographer records the death and its effect on household composition and dependency ratios. But the impact of the events leading up to the death and flowing from it are unrecorded. Demography is one of the most 'counting' of the social sciences (Greenhalgh, 1996); because of this it may insulate its exponents and readers of its reports from the underlying human processes.

Second, demographic indicators look at nations, provinces or areas. The impact of the disease may be very concentrated – cases will tend to cluster in households and among specific groups. A large-scale perspective, which concerns itself with averages, will not pick up small-scale impacts. This will only happen if the data are re-analysed in ways specific to the exploration of impact issues (see Figure 1.4, Chapter 1).

The third problem concerns the frequency with which demographic changes are measured. A census is carried out every ten years and analysis and reporting of the results may take several years. In the absence of vital registration, trends and changes have to be calculated on the basis of the census data alone. International compilations of data rely on national statistical agencies, central banks, and so on. The impact of a new and evolving disease will not be picked up and reflected in most national official data and has even less chance of appearing in international data sets.

Mortality

The most direct demographic consequence of AIDS is an increase in mortality.[2] In the absence of effective treatment the period from infection to illness is between seven and ten years (Stover and Way, 1998a). UNAIDS states that 'someone who has just been infected with HIV can expect to live nine years on average before falling seriously ill and to survive up to a year beyond that, even in the absence of anti-retroviral therapy' (UNAIDS, 2000f, p. 78).

Anti-retroviral therapies are unlikely to make a difference to life expectancy in the poor world. Even with recent price decreases and the withdrawal from recent litigation in South Africa by the multinational pharmaceutical corporations, these drugs are too expensive and need a fairly sophisticated delivery infrastructure. None of these conditions currently applies. This is not to say that access is impossible. Elites in many countries are accessing some form of treatment. For others there is a lottery of buying drugs when they can afford them and stopping when they can't. It may be that as prices fall – and they certainly will fall – the number of people accessing treatment will increase. However even at $350 per year for the drugs – the price offered by the Indian company CIPLA to NGOs in Africa in early 2001 – the cost of ART remains beyond the reach of most.

The bleak conclusion is that demographic impacts are largely unstoppable.

In countries where HIV is primarily spread through sexual transmission, the peak age of infection is 20–40 years and the peak ages of AIDS death are five to ten years later. Thus, AIDS increases mortality in adult age groups that would otherwise typically have the *lowest* mortality rates. Mother-to-child transmission, which is estimated to occur in about 30% of births to infected mothers (in the absence of interventions), accounts for increased infant and child mortality. (The effects of this were shown earlier in Figure 6.1.)

What evidence is there that the AIDS epidemic is causing increased mortality? To know the answer we need to measure mortality accurately. A meta-analysis found mortality rates in African adults and children has risen in the mid-1990s (Timaeus, 1998). However the data were limited, reporting slow and therefore mortality reflected the state of the HIV epidemic a decade previously. For most poor countries we are never going to have really up to date information about the demographics of HIV/AIDS. We will always be working with history. This should be a lesson to countries and societies not yet dramatically affected by the epidemic: get your vital registration machinery well-oiled so that you can know what is happening as soon as it begins! Train more demographers, do more surveys! Hardly a rousing cry to action for politicians but in this case very important indeed if politicians are to have the information they need in order to act. Alternatively, be prepared to accept and work with projections.

Data are however available for some specific sites and cohorts. AIDS has been identified as the major cause of deaths of adults aged 15–44 in Abidjan, Cote d'Ivoire, and of adults aged 15–59 in Tanzania (Adetunji, 1997; Boerma et al., 1997). More recent information on excess mortality for sub-national locations comes from Uganda. In Rakai, a team of researchers followed a cohort of 19,983 adults aged 15–59 at ten monthly intervals over four surveys. HIV prevalence in this cohort was 16.1%. Mortality in HIV positive people was 132.6 per 1,000 person years while in HIV negative people it was only 6.7 (Sewankambo et al, 2000). In other words HIV positive people were 19 times more likely to die than their peers who were not infected. South Africa's system of vital registration is good enough to estimate mortality and trends, as shown in Figure 6.3.

Box 6.1   South African mortality data: new evidence

Until recently mortality data were collected but not processed or released. One of the few good things to come out of the messy debate over the causes (and even existence of AIDS) that dominated South Africa in 2000 was release of these data.

A major contention was that there was no evidence of increased mortality in South Africa. In order to address this the Medical Research Council and Actuarial Society of South Africa collected and analysed mortality data from the Department of Home Affairs' Population register. The (reworked) data for male and female deaths in 1990 and 1999/2000 are shown in Figure 6.3. The message given at the panel meeting was there was evidence that there was something new, and it was killing people who should not have been dying.

Given the problems with official data, an obvious question is 'Are there alternative data sources?' A recent study in Swaziland used death notices from the local paper (Whiteside et al., 2000). Swaziland has high HIV prevalence. By 2000 this was 34.2% in ANC attenders (Swaziland Ministry of Health and Social Welfare, 2000).

Many people place bereavement notices in the local press. Increasingly, these notices include a photograph and some biographical details. The study reviewed death notices in the *Swazi Times* from 1 July 1994 to 30 June 1999. The total number of deaths rose substan-

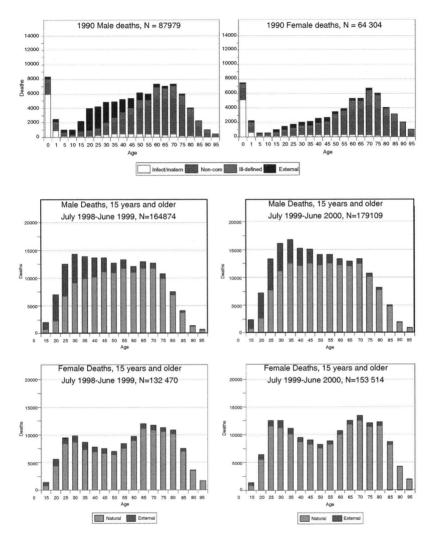

Figure 6.3   Male and female deaths, 1990, 1998, 2000: South Africa
Source: Dorrington et al. (2001), pp. 11, 15, & 16.

tially during the period and track the trajectory of deaths predicted from models.[3] This is shown in Figures 6.4 and 6.5. It is apparent that the majority of those dying are aged between 26 and 40.

Asian epidemics, with the exception of Thailand, are in the early stages so increased death rates are unlikely to be apparent. However in

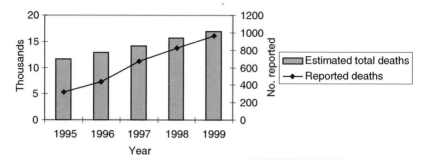

Figure 6.4   Modelled and reported deaths: Swaziland
Source: Whiteside et al. (2000).

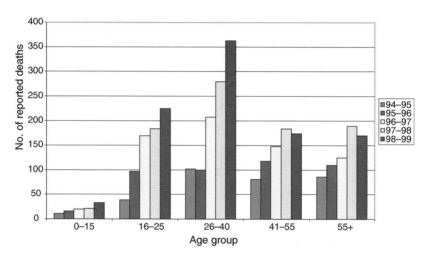

Figure 6.5   Reported deaths by age: Swaziland
Source: Whiteside et al. (2000).

India where mortality data were collected from the Mumbai Municipal
Corporation for selected years between 1986 and 1994, results showed
that there had been a small but significant increase in deaths among
prime-age adults. This might be attributed to HIV (Eliot in Godwin,
1998).

There is good evidence of increased adult mortality from Thailand.
Here there has been a marked increase in age-specific death rates of
men aged 15–50. This is shown in Figure 6.6 (World Bank, Social

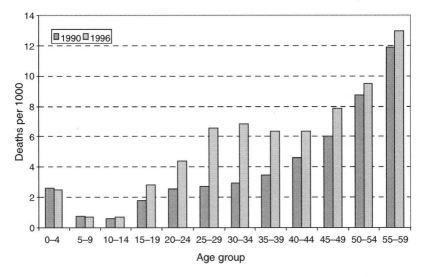

Figure 6.6 Thailand: age-specific death rates for men, 1990, 1996
Source: Van Griensven et al. (1998).

Monitor Thailand, 2000). In the north of the country the rate has quadrupled and 80% of the deaths in the 25–29 age group can be attributed to AIDS. The death rates for other groups are explored by Im-em (1999).

HIV/AIDS will affect not only adult mortality; mother-to-child transmission means increased infant and more particularly child mortality.[4] Between 13% and 45% of children born to infected mothers are infected, depending on the country and stage of the epidemic (Bryson, 1996). Many may survive beyond their first birthdays, but sadly most do not reach their fifth birthdays. Thus the greatest impact is on child rather than infant mortality.

Few data sets show these processes on a national level. Sewankambo's study in Rakai, Uganda, showed that infant mortality was 225 per 1,000 for children born to HIV positive mothers and 97.7 for children born to HIV negative mothers (Sewankambo et al., 2000). The real impact could be larger; children who are orphaned when their mothers die of AIDS often receive worse care than those whose mothers are alive. They will be less well-nourished, less well cared for and are less likely to attend school (see Chapter 8).

Life expectancy and infant and child mortality data

Human progress and development can be measured by a number of indicators. The most basic, and popular, are measures of life expectancy and infant and child mortality. In Japan the life expectancy of a citizen born in 1998 was 80 years. By contrast a Sierra Leonean born in the same year had a life expectancy of just 37.2 years. For every 1,000 Japanese babies born in that year four would die before their first birthday; in Sierra Leone 182 babies would not survive to age one (UNDP, *Human Development Report* 2000). Without any other information it is clear where most people would prefer to live. AIDS has a direct and immediate impact on life expectancy.

Box 6.2   Life expectancy

'Life expectancy' is a single index describing the level of mortality in a given population at a particular time as measured in years of life. Like infant mortality, it reflects something of the average 'standard of living' of a society. It is a health indicator that reveals more about deprivation than do indicators which measure average income.

It could better be called 'death expectancy' as it is based on death and is the age at which a person can expect to die. This more direct meaning would make the index self-explanatory.

Mortality rates crucially affect life expectancy indices. Life expectancy is dependent on specific mortality data, which include both childhood and adult mortality rates at a given point in time. The lower the death rates, the more people will survive through an entire age cohort, and thus the number of years lived will be greater. The higher the death rates, the fewer people will survive through an entire age cohort, and thus the number of years that a newborn infant can expect to live will be lower.

The ability to have children and see them grow up is for most people a basic expectation and a component of their identity. AIDS stymies these expectations. The relevant indicators are infant and child mortality rates, given as rates per 1,000 live births. Both are important because children in their first five years are particularly susceptible to a range of infectious diseases. Mother-to-child transmission of HIV, increased orphaning and economic and social stresses – all mean that AIDS has an adverse effect on these indicators.

What information do we have about the impact of AIDS on life expectancy and infant and child mortality? There are three readily available sources: UNDP's *Human Development Report*; the World Bank's *World Development Report and Development Indicators*; and the US Bureau of Census. The first two produce data purporting to show what has happened up to the present; the last uses models and projections to give current estimates and look into the future.

Each report starts from the same epidemic data but their results and interpretation are different. In some cases the difference is significant. For example UNDP puts Botswana's 1998 child mortality at 48 per 1,000; the Bank at 105. It is not clear whether and/or how AIDS impact is considered in these official figures. UNDP did not put AIDS into its population calculations before its 1997 report; even today it does not do so for all countries. The effect AIDS is having on the recorded indicators can be seen in the appendix to this chapter which show how life expectancy is falling with consequent effect on development as measured by the Human Development Index (HDI). (The importance of these data is explored further in Chapter 11.)

We should remember that according to models produced by the US Bureau of the Census the situation will get very much worse over the next ten years. This is illustrated in Figures 6.7, 6.8 and 6.9 for selected countries. The impact is devastating.

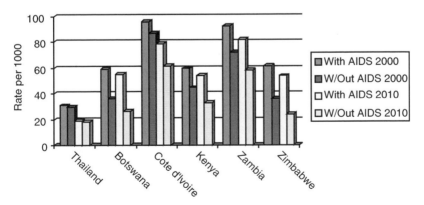

Figure 6.7 Infant mortality in selected countries, 2000, 2010
Source: US Bureau of the Census (forthcoming).

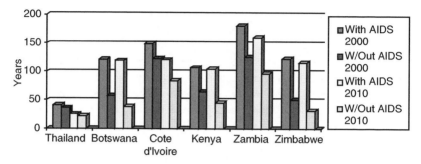

Figure 6.8 Child mortality in selected countries, 2000, 2010
Source: US Bureau of the Census (forthcoming).

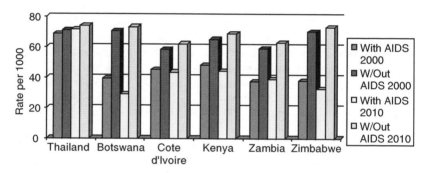

Figure 6.9 Life expectancy in selected countries, 2000, 2010
Source: US Bureau of the Census (forthcoming).

This bleak picture of decreased life expectancy and increased infant and child mortality is significant, especially in development terms. We shall return to this in Chapter 11.

Population growth and structure

Populations will grow more slowly and their overall structures will change. There will be fewer births. The number of births is affected as women die before reaching the end of their childbearing years. However, most births occur to women at young ages. The average age of a woman's death from AIDS is usually around 30. In Africa, only about one-third of lifetime births occur to women over that age. Births will also decrease because HIV infection substantially reduces fertility. In Uganda HIV infected women had lower fertility rates than HIV negative women. One study in rural Rakai District found that age-specific fertility rates for HIV infected women were 50% less than those for women who were not infected (Gray et al., 1997).

Another study in a rural population in Masaka (Carpenter et al., 1997) found that fertility rates were 20–30% less among HIV infected women. Since most women do not know their sero-status, the reduced fertility rates must be due to biological rather than to behavioural factors.

There has been much speculation about the impact of AIDS on population size and growth rates. Early in the epidemic some commentators argued that populations would be smaller than in the absence of AIDS, and it was possible that in some cases populations in badly affected countries would go into decline (Garnett and Anderson, 1992; Anderson et al, 1991; Rowley et al, 1990). At the time this view was contentious and was not generally accepted by UN agencies. Recent modelling, done for governments and by the US Bureau of Census, confirms that pessimistic view. Indeed, Bureau of Census figures suggest that population growth will indeed turn negative in some countries. By the year 2003, Botswana, South Africa and Zimbabwe will have seen growth rates of 1.1% per year to 2.3% per year in the absence of AIDS reduced to negative population growth rates of between –0.1% per year and –0.3% per year (Monitoring the AIDS Pandemic, 2000).

The dependency ratio is the number of dependants (usually children under the age of 15 and adults over the age of 64) per 100 adults of productive age 15–64 years. Dependency ratios should become worse due to AIDS because of the increased number of deaths among young adults. However, AIDS increases child deaths. These two tendencies roughly balance each other and the dependency ratio does not change dramatically in the presence of an AIDS epidemic (Stover and Way, 1998a). The dependency situation is adversely affected in other ways. AIDS will produce population structures never seen before, as shown in Figure 6.10 (US Bureau of Census)

AIDS increases the number of widows and widowers (Ntozi, 1997). When parents die children are often left in the care of grandparents and/or other members of the extended family or community. One of the worst consequences of the AIDS epidemic is the creation of orphans. UNAIDS estimates that about 2% of all children in developing countries were orphans before AIDS. By 1997 the proportion with one or both parents dead had risen to 7% in many African countries, reaching as much as 11% in some (UNAIDS, 2000f, p. 28) (see Chapter 8).

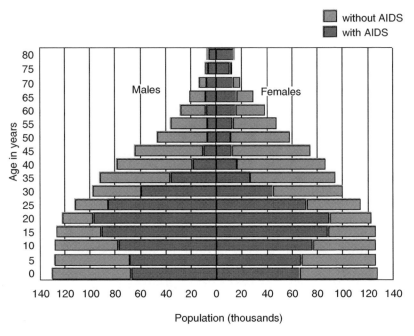

Figure 6.10   Projected population structure with and without the AIDS epidemic, Botswana, 2020
Source: UNAIDS 2000F

The demographic effects that we have outlined are the origins of the social, economic and political consequences of the epidemic that we explore next.

Appendix

Table 6A.1   Life expectancy and place in the HDI (selected countries)[5]

	1996 Report (1993 data)		1997 Report (1994 data)		1998 Report (1995 data)		1999 Report (1997 data)		2000 Report (1998 data)	
	Life Expect.	HDI (Rank)	Life Expect.	HDI (Rank)	Life Expect.	HDI (Rank)	Life Expect.	HDI (Rank)	Life Expect.	HDI (Rank)
Asia										
Cambodia	51.9	0.325 (156)	52.4	0.348 (153)	52.9	0.422 (140)	53.4	0.514 (137)	53.5	0.512 (136)
Myanmar	57.9	0.451 (133)	58.4	0.475 (131)	58.9	0.481 (131)	60.1	0.580 (128)	60.6	0.585 (125)
Thailand	69.2	0.832 (52)	69.5	0.833 (59)	69.5	0.838 (59)	68.8	0.753 (67)	68.9	0.745 (76)
India	60.7	0.436 (135)	61.3	0.446 (138)	61.6	0.451 (139)	62.6	0.545 (132)	62.9	0.563 (128)
Africa										
Botswana	65.0	0.741 (71)	52.3	0.673 (97)	51.7	0.678 (97)	47.4	0.609 (122)	46.2	0.593 (122)
Ethiopia	47.8	0.237 (168)	48.2	0.244 (170)	48.7	0.252 (169)	43.3	0.298 (172)	43.4	0.309 (171)
Cote d'Ivoire	50.9	0.357 (147)	52.1	0.368 (145)	51.8	0.368 (148)	46.7	0.422 (154)	46.9	0.420 (154)

Table 6A.1 Life expectancy and place in the HDI (selected countries)[5] cont.

	1996 Report (1993 data)		1997 Report (1994 data)		1998 Report (1995 data)		1999 Report (1997 data)		2000 Report (1998 data)	
	Life Expect.	HDI (Rank)	Life Expect.	HDI (Rank)	Life Expect.	HDI (Rank)	Life Expect.	HDI (Rank)	Life Expect.	HDI (Rank)
Kenya	55.5	0.473 (128)	53.6	0.463 (134)	53.8	0.463 (137)	52.0	0.519 (136)	51.3	0.508 (138)
Malawi	45.5	0.321 (157)	41.1	0.320 (161)	41.0	0.334 (161)	39.3	0.399 (159)	39.5	0.385 (163)
Namibia	59.1	0.573 (116)	55.9	0.570 (118)	55.8	0.644 (107)	52.4	0.639 (115)	50.1	0.632 (115)
Nigeria	50.6	0.400 (137)	51.0	0.393 (141)	51.4	0.391 (142)	50.1	0.456 (146)	50.1	0.439 (151)
South Africa	63.2	0.649 (100)	63.7	0.716 (90)	64.1	0.717 (89)	54.7	0.695 (101)	53.2	0.697 (103)
Swaziland	57.8	0.586 (110)	58.3	0.582 (114)	58.8	0.597 (115)	60.2	0.644 (113)	60.7	0.655 (112)
Zimbabwe	53.4	0.534 (124)	49.0	0.513 (129)	48.9	0.507 (130)	44.1	0.560 (130)	43.5	0.555 (130)

Table 6A.1 Life expectancy and place in the HDI (selected countries)[5]   *cont.*

	1996 Report (1993 data)		1997 Report (1994 data)		1998 Report (1995 data)		1999 Report (1997 data)		2000 Report (1998 data)	
	Life Expect.	*HDI (Rank)*	*Life Expect.*	*HDI (Rank)*	*Life Expect.*	*HDI (Rank)*	*Life Expect.*	*HDI (Rank)*	*Life Expect.*	*HDI (Rank)*
Zambia	48.6	0.411 (136)	42.6	0.369 (143)	42.7	0.378 (146)	40.1	0.431 (151)	40.5	0.420 (153)
Other countries										
Bahamas	73.2	0.895 (26)	72.9	0.894 (28)	73.2	0.893 (32)	73.8	0.851 (31)	74.0	0.844 (33)
Brazil	66.5	0.796 (58)	66.4	0.783 (68)	66.6	0.809 (62)	66.8	0.739 (79)	67.0	0.747 (74)
Guyana	65.4	0.633 (103)	63.2	0.649 (104)	63.5	0.670 (100)	64.4	0.701 (99)	64.8	0.709 (96)
Haiti	56.8	0.359 (145)	54.4	0.338 (156)	54.6	0.340 (159)	53.7	0.430 (152)	54.0	0.440 (150)

7
Individuals, Households and Communities

Changes in mortality and life expectancy result from the many hundreds and thousands of individual deaths. The impact of individual ill health and death depends on who the individuals are, their place in society and the resources they, their households, communities and societies have available.

There are dilemmas: in how we perceive health and its costs, a tension between the pressing and urgent demands of our own or our family's ill health and the more measured approach we adopt when confronted with the opportunity costs of aggregate health expenditure. We value others' health differently; or perhaps more rationally. We accept that some interventions are costly and cannot be available for all. Politics decides public health expenditure in the face of competing demands. A key question is the degree to which politicians and us consider that 'health' is a public good rather than a purely individual responsibility. This is an important issue because it raises two questions:

- Do we perceive individual health and welfare as just that, *individual*, or take account of the wider contributions – often non-economic – which individuals make to their societies?
- Do we limit ourselves to individual health or attend to issues of *public* health?

This chapter examines the impact of AIDS at the individual, household and community levels. This is where the impact is felt first and worst. But it is also here, beyond the obvious clinical and medical consequences, that it is hardest to measure.

182

Individual impact

In the absence of treatment, infected individuals can expect to experience periods of illness that increase in frequency, severity and duration. A few individuals may, through a combination of appropriate lifestyle, good nutrition and good luck, not fall ill. However for most, as CD4 cell counts decline, so does their state of health.

Thus individuals who are infected always confront an impact on their health. In most cases they also face an impact on the resources they have at their disposal. Your individual resources may not be affected if you are fortunate enough to live in a society where care is provided free by the state (and this is currently not the case in all poor and many rich countries) or if you have insured medical benefits.

Variation in individual impact was starkly illustrated by Judge Edwin Cameron in a speech to the XIII International Conference on HIV/AIDS. Cameron described how, although he fell severely ill, his access to good health care and drugs enabled him to pursue a vigorous, healthy and productive life.

I can take these tablets, because on the salary I earn as a judge, I am able to afford their cost … In this I exist as a living embodiment of the iniquity of drug availability and access in Africa … My presence here embodies the injustices of AIDS in Africa because, on a continent in which 290 million Africans survive on less than one US dollar a day, I can afford monthly medication costs of about US $400 per month. Amidst the poverty of Africa, I stand before you because I am able to purchase health and vigour. I am here because I can afford to pay for life itself. (Cameron, 2000b)

The reality for individuals is that, as with their chance of being infected, the impact of the disease will depend on their circumstances and the resources they can command.

But individuals exist in networks of relationships. How does the loss of an individual affect the broader society and community in which he or she lives and functions? The complexity is hinted at in Figure 7.1. Impact will depend on who that individual is, where he or she fits in the community and society and how replaceable he or she is. A key idea is 'social reproduction': the uncosted and literally invaluable labour and effort that goes into reproducing the life ways of our households, communities, institutions and even nations. And the same applies to all the other symbolic and practical activities that

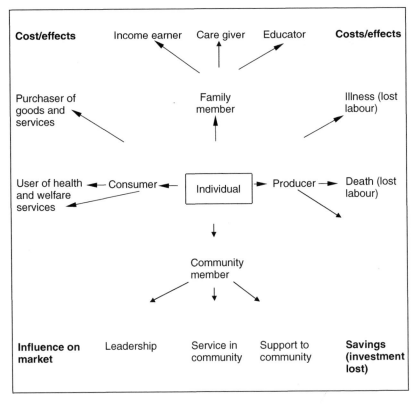

Figure 7.1   The individual as an economic and social actor

reproduce society and culture from day to day, year to year and across time.

Household impact

Because HIV is sexually transmitted, it clusters in households. This has given rise to some misconceptions about impact. Average households in communities will not be affected. This can be illustrated with a simple example. In a village of 100 households with an average of three adults per household, in a region with 10% HIV prevalence and a mature epidemic, we would expect to see three to five adult deaths per annum. It is likely that only one or two households will experience illness or death in any one year. It is possible that these households will dissolve and so not be counted.

Box 7.1   Households that disappear

Fieldwork in Uganda in 1989 found the following tragic case, a 'remnant household' which was on the verge of disappearance.

The man lived alone in a bare hut, sleeping on the floor. He possessed little beyond a blanket and the pot in which he was cooking a meagre meal. He was said to be 45 years old but looked considerably older. He was quite clearly demented and could not be interviewed. Information was obtained from others.

A few years ago, this had been a substantial household with a reasonable farm. His wife and eight of his teenage and adult children had died of AIDS within the last few years. He had no relatives living in the village, and supported himself by cultivating and selling some of his bananas. Onlookers said euphemistically of him, 'He is not expected to marry again.'

This case illustrates how, in extremes, the cost of nursing AIDS patients combined with disappearance of the family led to a state of utter poverty where life was barely sustained. Communal support systems could not cope, this man was destitute and isolated. (Barnett and Blaikie, 1992, p. 99)

Often the first sign is when the youngest child (infected in the womb) fails to thrive, dying after protracted illness. An infected mother is likely to have been infected by her partner. It is estimated that 60–80% of African women with HIV have had only one partner but were infected because they were not in a position to negotiate safe sex or prevent their partners from having additional sexual contacts (Colvin, 2000). The same is true in Asia. Marina Mahathir, daughter of Malaysian premier Mahathir Mohamad and head of the Malaysian Council of NGOs on AIDS, is quoted as saying: 'It is a fact not repeated enough that 90% of women who have been infected with HIV have only ever slept with one man in their lives, their husbands.'[1]

The effects of illness and death in households depend on:

- the number of cases the household experiences – this is where clustering becomes important

- the characteristics of the deceased individuals: age, gender, income and cause of death
- the household's composition and asset array
- the community's attitudes towards helping needy households and the general availability of resources – the level of life – in that community
- the broader resources available for assistance to households – from the state or from community-based organisations (CBOs) and non-governmental organisations (NGOs).

There is a limited number of studies of the effects of AIDS on households and most focus on economic impacts alone. They paint a bleak picture. The classic survey-based study was in the Kagera region of Tanzania in the late 1980s and early 1990s, conducted by the World Bank with Tanzanian co-investigators,[2] and its design and findings highlight important problems.

The measurement of impact on households during illness is difficult. Illness ranges from not feeling very well to complete inability to function. It is difficult to unravel these subtleties with survey methods because:

- even in the worst affected areas adult illness and death is comparatively rare
- the unit of measurement, the household, means that those that dissolve or disappear are lost to the research
- surveys of 'households' will not collect data on complex relations between clusters of households
- the epidemic and its impact are still evolving. The HIV epidemic has apparently run its course in Uganda and Thailand. In all other countries HIV prevalence continues to rise and the number of AIDS illnesses and deaths will follow suit some years hence. Thus surveys are trying to measure and quantify something that is still to happen.

What is a household?

A typical view of a household is that it will go through the following stages: formation when people come together to reproduce; maturity as they have children and bring them up; and dissolution as children leave home, the parents grow too old to work and finally die. There are many cultural variations, for example, adult children may remain in a household and be joined by their spouses, three generations may live in one household, or siblings may form joint households with their spouses and children.

It has been argued by some that an entity called 'the extended family' will absorb the orphans and destitute created through AIDS-related mortality. This view has been heard from people ranging from senior policy makers in international agencies to politicians in Africa and Asia and people in local communities. It is now heard less as the full effects of the epidemic become apparent.

The extended family:

- is a variable, it is dynamic and can become more or less extended depending on resource availability
- is ideological, it is something people want to believe because it validates their traditions
- is ideological because belief in it relieves politicians of responsibility for thinking through the implications of the epidemic
- reaches a point where it can no longer cope.

Household reproduction, size and structure

What effect does the epidemic have on household reproduction, the household's ability to sustain itself from day to day and to reproduce itself over time? The demographic impacts on households affect their ability to reproduce themselves at all. Households with adult female infections experience lower birth rates and higher infant and child mortality rates. In households where a parent or both parents have AIDS, the likelihood is that fewer children will be born and that a significant proportion of those who are born will die in infancy or early childhood. Inevitably this means that the personnel of the household are not replaced and that the life ways and traditions of that household are not carried forward.

It is axiomatic that death changes the nature of households. The loss of one unit – the deceased – reduces its size. However evidence from a number of studies suggests that in practice the change is hard to predict. In Kagera most households experiencing a death *added* at least one member when a previously absent member or non-member joined. The average size of these households declined by less than one – from 6.0 to 5.7 (World Bank, 1997a, p. 215). In Rakai, Uganda, by contrast, mean household size fell from 6.4 to 4.7 (Menon et al., 1998). People left the household, perhaps children were sent to stay with relatives or adults moved in search of employment. In Thailand the decline was from 4.1 people per household to 3.1, the decrease being equivalent to the death of the one person (Janjaroen, 1998). The significance of this has not been evaluated but it should draw to our attention the regional and national effects of large numbers of deaths in a community. These effects include the phenomenon of urban–rural migration which has been observed in western Uganda and the sending of children to rural relatives in Swaziland.

Deaths in individual households have implications for other households because of their interdependence. Rugalema (1999) shows how coping mechanisms become increasingly weakened as more households in a community are affected and communal support networks are less and less able to cope.

Affected households will try to adapt. One way in which they do this is by changing their composition. Three key points must be made:

- Societies where extended households are the rule or where clusters of households operate together to pursue a common livelihood strategy may be more robust in the face of adult death.
- Sending children to stay with relatives means the effect of the adult death will be felt beyond the sending family. Whoever takes care of the children can expect to expend resources.
- Orphans need care, either in other families or through some form of public support. Increasingly they do not receive this support.

Adaptations such as these depend on people's receptiveness to the idea that the traditional extended family system is still appropriate and care of orphans their responsibility. However, as early as 1992, a study in urban South Africa showed that 62% of Sowetans felt that AIDS orphans should be the responsibility of the state (Steinberg et al., 2000).

Mutangadura's (2000) study of 215 households in Manicaland, Zimbabwe, examined how adult deaths may cause the dissolution of households. She found that about 40% of the sample households had taken in orphans who had lost both parents. Mutangadura states that: 'Sixty five percent of households where the deceased adult female used to live before her death were reported to be no longer in existence in both the urban and rural sites' (p. 11). This lends weight to the supposition that often the worst impact is invisible because it is among those who are not counted.

New forms of household are developing as a response to the impact of HIV/AIDS, and include:

- elderly household heads with young children, grandparent-headed households
- large households with unrelated fostered or orphaned children attached

- child-headed households
- single-parent, mother- or father-headed households
- cluster foster care – where a group of children is cared for formally or informally by neighbouring adult households
- children in subservient, exploited or abusive fostering relationships
- itinerant, displaced or homeless children
- neglected, displaced children in groups or gangs (Hunter, 2000, p. 195).

Shell (2000) indicates that these types of new households (in which single parenthood and full orphanhood become common) are not as efficient as the more traditional family structure for passing on social values, producing a second 'lost' generation[3] within South Africa.

When household structures change, so does their internal organisation. Dependency ratios increase where households comprise children and the elderly (Menon et al., 1998). If dependants are reclassified to include adult people living with HIV/AIDS (PLWAs) then the dependency ratio will rise dramatically (Shell, 2000). This is demonstrated in Rakai where the number of households with no adult increased twelvefold in households experiencing the death of an HIV positive adult between 1989 and 1992 (Menon et al., 1998).

Income, consumption and expenditure patterns[4]

What effect does AIDS have on household expenditure and consumption patterns? An adult illness or death reduces household income. Less labour is available, not only because the affected individual can't work but also because time is diverted to care of the sick. Illness increases expenditure on medical care, food, washing materials, and so on.

Little quantitative work exists on the impact of illness at this level. There is rather more on the impact of adult death. The Kagera study (World Bank, 1997a) found that households experiencing an adult death spent less during the person's illness, but that a greater percentage of their expenditure was on medical care. They spent 33% less on non-food items such as clothing, soap and batteries and their food purchases decreased. Income was diverted but may also have been reduced as the number of hours worked was cut (World Bank, 1997a, p. 213).

Evidence from both Kagera (World Bank, 1997a) and Cote d'Ivoire (Ainsworth et al., 1998) indicates that households are resilient and there is a partial recovery in levels of consumption as time passes after the death. In other words households 'cope'. However our experience and that of others has been that anecdotal evidence often shows they do not cope, or that 'coping' may turn out to be another way of saying 'desperate poverty, social exclusion and marginalisation'. There is an unresolved problem: existing early quantitative studies indicate effective coping, while anecdote makes us believe otherwise – and recent work from Zambia supports this. A five-year retrospective study of 232 urban and 101 rural AIDS-affected families in Zambia found that 'One of the striking features of the economic impact of AIDS in affected families in Zambia is the rapid transition from relative wealth to relative poverty' (Namposya-Serpell, 2000, p. 1).[5] This was particularly marked where a father died (70% of the recorded urban deaths). Monthly disposable income of more than two-thirds of the families in this study fell by more than 80%.

Household surveys underestimate the degree of household dissolution and failure. This is because a particular survey design may not capture such information and also because the survey method itself may be incapable of capturing these kinds of data. By the time the survey team arrives for the first round of interviews some households have already disappeared. They are not there to be counted. Given the typical shape of the epidemic curve, the timing of a survey in relation to the phase of the epidemic may mean that the most acute phase has passed and the dissolved households have disappeared.

Death is expensive. In Kagera households, medical expenditures were higher when AIDS was the cause of death. But 'strikingly for all groups except men with AIDS, medical expenses were overshadowed by funeral expenses. On average, households spent nearly 50% more on funerals than they did for medical care ... In Thailand ... just as in Tanzania, the households spent much more on funerals than on medical care' (World Bank, 1997a, p. 211). It should also be remembered that while the state or employer may make some contribution to health care and medical expenses, the burdens of home care and funeral costs normally fall entirely on households.

Some households cope by the sale of assets. Table 7.1 summarises data from Kagera, Tanzania and Rakai, Uganda, on how adult death is linked to households' disposal of assets.

Around the city of Chiang Mai in northern Thailand, 41% of households where there had been an adult death subsequently sold land. Other forms of what economists euphemistically describe as 'dissavings' were reported by 5%, while 24% borrowed money (World Bank, 1997a, p. 218). In Zimbabwe, 24% of households said they had sold assets to cope with the death of an adult woman, with 'the main assets ... sold being cattle, goats, furniture, clothes, televisions, poultry and wardrobes' (Mutangadura, 2000, p. 15).

Table 7.1 Asset ownership in households with and without an adult death (% of total households)

Asset	Rakai District, Uganda		Kagera District, Tanzania	
	Households w/o adult death	Households with adult death	Households w/o adult death	Households with adult death
Bicycle				
First visit	34	39	27	26
Last visit	41	35	29	28
Radio				
First visit	30	40	31	36
Last visit	37	36	35	35

Source: World Bank (1997a), p. 217.

For the survival of rural and poor urban households, it is crucial that they retain the productive assets necessary for them to recover and rebuild. A household can sell a radio and survive; the sale of cattle indicates a phase change in their lives and in their ability to maintain and reproduce themselves. Indeed, it may be taken as a clear indication of failure to cope. Table 7.1 shows that percentage declines in asset ownership among those households selling assets is almost matched by percentage increases among households gaining assets. This may indicate that in impoverished settings death simply redistributes limited assets among the local population.

Two points should be noted. First, people who are driven to sell the clothes of the dead or their own clothes can hardly be said to be coping: these are the actions of the desperately impoverished. Second, following from this, we have to be aware that the very notion of 'coping' is deeply ideological and may smack of the rich telling the poor how to manage their poverty (Rugalema, 2000).

The limits of household studies

Existing household studies have their own limitations. The main ones are:

- most deal with Africa
- they concentrate on rural households. Why is unclear. It may arise from a basic paradox: foreign researchers want to work in rural areas, which, they believe, represent the 'real' Africa, and prefer to avoid places which are squalid or dangerous like poor parts of large cities. This rural bias among expatriate researchers combines with

local researchers' need to receive often generous overnight allowances while away from their urban base, and ensures the continued underrepresentation of the impact of HIV/AIDS on urban households. But in Africa and South Asia nearly one-third of the population lives in urban areas (UNDP, *Human Development Report*, 2000, p. 226)[6]

- as their titles indicate, these are mainly *economic* studies
- the problem is usually researched as a *household* study. This excludes information about relations between households
- survey methods fail to capture the most seriously affected households, those that have disappeared before the survey commences
- policy makers, politicians and agencies demand quantitative survey-based studies because they have the ring of a form of evidential 'truth' which coincides with the demands of funders' referees who are often academics. Such forms of 'truth,' although valid, are partial and do not tell of the underlying misery
- single or even multivisit surveys unsupported by ethnographic methods tend to underestimate impact
- commonly used survey methods fail to capture the dynamics of household and intra-household allocation and relations which underlie household decision making (Chong, 1999; Rugalema, 1999)
- AIDS may be seen as the major problem by the researcher – who has written and submitted a research proposal or is responding to a terms of reference or scope of work document. Communities and households may not have the same perception of its importance. This is illustrated by a Zambian study which looked at how children were valued in a situation of environmental and social change. The social change identified by the researchers in an area with 14.8% HIV prevalence among ANC attenders was increased morbidity and mortality due to the epidemic. They concluded that 'research methods used in the study villages found that there was almost no link made in people's minds between HIV/AIDS and either the value of children or fertility. At present AIDS is not seen as a major problem by the majority of people, despite its recognition as a worrying disease' (Barrett and Browne, 2000, p. 22).

Unmeasured impact

The study of households and their interaction has long been an area of research for sociologists and anthropologists. There is information on how households cope with shocks and respond to disease. However

AIDS is new and different. AIDS-affected households face the likeli-hood that they will have to cope with more than one death, because the disease clusters. They also have to deal with a long and debilitating illness that is costly in its use of resources – in terms of both finance and time, and which ends in death. In addition, the epidemic has a wider effect that weakens the ability of the community to lend support.

An in-depth study of the impact of the disease in Bukoba District of Tanzania (Rugalema, 1999) illustrates the stark impact on households. In the study community 32% of households were AIDS-afflicted – they had experienced direct illness or the death of one or more of their family members in the last ten years. A further 29% were affected 'in the sense that although they have not experienced direct death or illness of a household member from AIDS, they have experienced *ripple effects* ... include[ing] fostering orphans, providing labour or cash to help care for the sick person, and providing for survivors in an afflicted household' (Rugalema, 1999, p. 73). The disease has particular con-sequences for the old and the young, and this will be discussed in the next chapter.

The worst impacts will be felt in households and clusters of house-holds. It is here that costs of the disease have to be borne. It is here that mitigation interventions have to be located if they are to be cost effective and sustainable. It is here that social reproduction occurs at its deepest level: in the stories told by parents and grandparents to their children, in the giving and receiving of affection, in the taking and relinquishing of responsibility. It is also here that the state and large multilateral agencies have most difficulty responding. The scale is too small and the variability in circumstance too great to be covered by large programmes. The great danger is that it is here – where it is most needed and where the very long-term costs are stacking up – that response to impact will be impossible because there is no way of dealing with small-scale and large variability. This is a major policy challenge.

Community-level impact

In the same way that individuals make up households, households make up communities and communities make up nations. The impact of the HIV/AIDS epidemic on communities is neglected, yet increas-ingly agencies and governments see them as having 'the solution' to both prevention and impact issues.

Communities are seen as vital for successful prevention because:

- prevention efforts have by and large focused on biomedical and scientific interventions, and it has been apparent that these do not work if the socio-economic and community environment is not supportive.
- in settings where prevention has worked, for example in Uganda, community responses have been exceptional. These include openness and willingness to talk about the disease and to give support for those infected, as documented in the recent publication, *Open Secret: People Facing up to HIV and AIDS in Uganda* (Kaleeba et al., 2000)
- there is an ideologically driven trend to perceive the community as a nexus for implementation of currently popular beliefs in 'empowerment', 'stakeholding' and 'civil society' which all too often are the human faces of technical fixes for many of today's problems of poverty and exclusion.

The burden of coping with impact is shifting on to communities. Again the reasons are varied:

- the scale of the problem is such that governments recognise they have neither the financial nor human resources to deal with the impact
- communities will 'cope' (whatever this means), and so to argue that they are being given the task of doing so is to legitimise what is happening anyway.

There are no quantified studies of the impact of AIDS on communities. There are indeed no definitions of what 'community' is. We do know that not all communities are alike. Their definition will vary over time, space and according to who is looking at them. Those looking to communities as a resource in either prevention or impact mitigation see them as cohesive, interactive and mutually supportive entities. The utopian view is that people live in harmony with each other and adversity leads to increased cohesiveness and mutual aid and support. The reality is that a range of interrelated factors determines how individuals interact and if they collectively constitute a community, which include their history, cultural framework, the extent to which people as individuals and in kin groups know and routinely interact with one another, and levels of civil and social organisation.

Communities may develop or divide around specific issues. A central thesis of this book is that the level of social cohesion in a society determines susceptibility to HIV. We know that in some circumstances (and Uganda is an example) cohesion can be built around responding to HIV and mitigating AIDS impact. But where HIV/AIDS is concerned a further critical factor is whether the community sees this as something they can unite around or as something that divides them. Does it allow collective rather than individual or household action? Ugandan communities have often united in the face of HIV/AIDS. In South Africa's KwaZulu-Natal province, neighbours murdered Gugu Dlamini in 1999 for revealing her HIV positive status. They argued that she had brought shame on the community.

While communities inevitably have some role to play, they cannot be seen as 'the answer'. Rich communities may cope; poor ones may not be communities at all, lacking the resources to organise effectively. Collins and Rau note that

> caution is in order when talking about household and community coping mechanisms. Inventiveness in the face of adversity is now widely recognized and cited by many agencies. However, in too many instances, the rhetoric about coping mechanisms has become an excuse for doing little or nothing to reduce the pressures on communities. (2000, p. 40)

Furthermore, women may not have the same role and rights in the 'community' and may suffer active discrimination. 'Community', like 'civil society', can be a focus for conservatism, prejudice and active exclusion.

Where people lack material resources and do not have access to institutions and organisations beyond their limited and poor locality, they cannot be expected to take on extra costs and responsibilities in the absence of outside support. The great challenge for those who would assist communities, households, clusters and ultimately individuals to deal with the awful consequences of the AIDS epidemic is to face realities – to develop interventions and methods of support which recognise these realities, which can be effective at the local level and can take full account of the forces of globalisation which will otherwise only exacerbate the already established processes of poverty and exclusion. 'Community' is no easy technical fix to these complex problems. It is a word of great comfort, but only for those who would seek easy solutions. There is no easy answer.

8
Dependants: Orphans and the Elderly

The HIV/AIDS epidemic has altered and will progressively alter the demographic structure of many societies (Low-Beer et al., 1997; Stover and Way, 1998b). In Chapter 6 we showed how it is cutting away the middle generation of society. Population pyramids are becoming indented.

This chapter focuses on two of the most affected groups. The first has been widely identified and much has been written about their plight. They are the orphans and other vulnerable children created by the epidemic. The second group, the elderly, is largely ignored, yet this group often bears the burden of care.

Under normal circumstances the young are cared for by their parents, and later provide support for those parents. Some social scientists describe this as the 'intergenerational bargain' (Carmichael and Charles, 1999; Collard, 1999). In Greek tradition this has been likened to a vine, where the young adults stand straight and firm as the new shoots climb up and the old ones make their way down to the earth. If you take out the middle support the children can't climb and the old collapse.

This is one of the core and most important bargains made and maintained between people. It is a basis on which social order is constructed. In most societies there is no social pension or welfare provision, and while people may accumulate assets during their productive years these are often on their own insufficient to provide for old age.

Care of the aged is a global issue. In all societies people are living longer, or at least they were before the advent of AIDS. In wealthy societies there is increasing concern about how to respond to ageing populations. Here, the problem is the potential burden of care and support which the young face in caring for the increasing number of elderly. In the poorer AIDS-affected countries, life expectancy may be falling but this overall figure disguises the fact that people who reach their fifties

Table 8.1   Increased life expectancy (selected countries)

| Country | Disability-adjusted life expectancy (years) | | | |
| | Males | | Females | |
	At birth	At 60	At birth	At 60
Botswana	32.3	6.1	32.2	9.7
Uganda	32.9	6.2	32.5	7.4
Tanzania	35.9	7.8	36.1	9.2
Senegal	43.5	8.8	45.6	11.3

Source: WHO statistical annex 5, pp. 176–83.

and sixties have a much better chance of living into their seventies and eighties. The World Health Organisation has emulated other international agencies by including increasing quantities of data in annual reports. While most of the data in the 2000 report can charitably be described as impenetrable, there is some information on disability-adjusted life expectancies which is reproduced in Table 8.1.

AIDS impact is therefore being felt in a setting where ageing and care for the elderly were already issues of concern. It makes a bad situation worse.

Orphans and the elderly are not only AIDS affected, some will also be infected. (See the distribution of AIDS cases, Figure 2.8, Chapter 2). While it is true that individuals from either extreme of the lifecycle are less likely to become infected, cases do occur. In addition to those children infected through mother-to-child transmission the epidemic has brought into view early onset of sexual activity in many societies and underlined that older people have sex. It has also shown that some children are infected through instances of child abuse: this has been hard for many to accept.

Orphans

Orphans are part of all communities. There will always be children who have had the misfortune to lose parents. In many poorer countries families routinely took in children from the wider family. In rich countries institutions were available to care for these children. The scale of AIDS orphaning is such that these coping mechanisms are collapsing in the poor world. This stress is evidenced by the growing number of street children around the developing world.

Box 8.1   The vulnerability of young street children to sexual exploitation

Mpulungu, on the shores of Lake Tanganyika, is Zambia's principal inland port. An important trading and border post, it has high HIV prevalence (13.2% for the district in 1999). Poverty rates are high and school enrolments low. Living on the street, through economic necessity or because of AIDS, is a fact of life from an early age for a large number of children. Boys who live on the street – *mishanga* boys – are more obvious than girls. When they are very hungry or cold, young *mishanga* boys, aged eight to ten, go to their 'sugar mummies', giving sex in return for some material assistance and shelter. In the process, many contract HIV.

Local mores show little concern about sexual play among children of this age. One strongly held misconception is that a boy who is too young to impregnate a girl cannot transmit the AIDS virus. People believe that it is transmitted through sperm but not through other sexual fluids.

In these uninhibited but lethally misinformed circumstances, the infected *mishanga* boy spreads the infection received from his 'sugar mummy', infecting girls who are his own age or slightly younger.

How relevant is it to talk about safe sex for such children? Where will they get condoms? How can they use them? Will they fit? How can an educational programme protect such children? How can the erroneous views on HIV transmission be corrected when taboos prohibit factual discussion? (Kelly, 2000, p. 19)

How many 'orphans' are there?

So far, the AIDS epidemic has left behind 13.2 million orphans – children who, before the age of 15, lost either their mother or both parents to AIDS. Many of these children have died, but many more survive, not only in Africa (where 95% currently live) but also in countries throughout Asia and the Americas. By 1997, the proportion of children with one or both parents dead in some parts of Africa had increased to 7% and in some cases reached an astounding 11%. In African countries that have had long, severe epidemics,

AIDS is generating orphans so quickly that family structures can no longer cope. Traditional safety nets are unravelling as more young adults die of this disease. Families and communities can barely fend for themselves, let alone take care of orphans. Typically, half of all people with HIV become infected before they turn 25, acquiring AIDS and dying by the time they turn 35, leaving behind a generation of children to be raised by their grandparents or left on their own in child-headed households. (UNAIDS, 2000f, pp. 27–8)[1]

The bare statistics are troubling. They tell of a generation of children deprived of their childhood. Some of the earliest AIDS orphans are now in their mid-twenties and are themselves parents. Many of those orphaned by AIDS have lost their lives to it and never lived beyond early adulthood (see Figure 1.4).

There are two problems in estimating orphan numbers. First, estimates of numbers of orphans depends on estimates of numbers of AIDS deaths; second, estimates depend on how an orphan is defined. An example from Malawi will illustrate the first point. A study in 1997 found that government figures were based on old data and the number of AIDS deaths could have been underestimated by a factor of five (Hunter and Fall, 1998, p. 11). The question of definition is important for action and for policy. In making its estimates, the Government of Malawi defined orphans as 'children with mother or both parents missing'. A change of definition to include 'any child under 15 missing either one or both parents' increased the number of orphans and at the same time identified a wider range of children in need. This is not a semantics argument. It has important policy implications. Orphans who are not defined are not counted and provision cannot be made for them even if resources are available. Table 8.2 shows the difference between the old and the new estimates in Malawi.

Table 8.2   Estimates of orphan numbers in Malawi

	New Estimate	Prior Estimates	
		Total	of which AIDS
1995	980708	310000	140000
2000	1123947	660000	300000
2005	1429952	–	–
2010	1565818	–	–

Source: Hunter and Fall, 1998, p. 15.

A similar situation exists in Uganda:

> UNAIDS defines an orphan as a child under 15, who has lost either
> both parents (double orphan), or the mother (maternal orphan),
> and it is from this definition that the UNAIDS global estimation is
> made. Paternal orphans are disregarded in this definition, yet this ...
> is a great oversight, bearing in mind the large amount of absentee
> mothers for paternal orphans. If paternal orphans are included the
> figure will rise dramatically, for example in the research population
> 62.74% of orphans were paternal orphans. While the UNAIDS esti-
> mate of 11 million AIDS orphans world-wide, which is projected to
> rise to a staggering 40 million by 2020, is shocking to say the least,
> evidence from Uganda shows that this definition is wholly inade-
> quate and, therefore, the total number of AIDS orphans has been
> greatly underestimated. (Monk, 2000, p. 14)

Box 8.2   The significance of paternal orphaning

- In patrilineal groups when a child's father dies, the child is effectively a double orphan because the mother is sent away or leaves
  to remarry elsewhere
- Often both parents are infected, which means that the child will
  eventually become a double orphan
- Children over the age of five need the cash support for education
  and health care most often provided by the father. (Hunter and
  Fall, 1998, p. 15)

The point is that definitions are important and there is no final way
of deciding who is or is not an orphan, it is a social role and varies
from place to place and culture to culture. Whatever the numbers, it is
obvious that orphans run greater risks of many kinds: of social exclusion, of abuse and exploitation, than do children who have parents.

Social exclusion

Resources available in AIDS-affected households decrease because of
the deaths of productive members and the increased demand for
household expenditure – medicines, food, and so on. There are fewer
resources in two key areas:

- productive and financial resources
- time for caring, parenting and reflecting.

Children born to infected women may have only a 30% chance of being infected but they have close to a 100% chance of being orphaned. The consequences of an adult death will be apparent in the changed life chances of the child itself.

In Blantyre, Malawi, a study found that, controlling for household socio-economic characteristics, gender, birth weight, and the age and HIV status of the mother, young children whose mothers had died were 3.3 times more likely to die compared to children of mothers who did not die (Ainsworth and Semali, 2000). Maternal death, from whatever cause, results in higher mortality among children. Thus:

> The health and life situation of any woman is crucial to the health and life chances of her children, not only during pregnancy but throughout the entire childhood. A mother's capacity for child care – the time and energy she can devote to her children, the conditions in the home, her material resources, her skills and knowledge – continue to govern a child's passage from childhood to maturity, socially, physically and emotionally. (Mutangadura, 2000, p. 3)

AIDS-affected households tend to be poorer, consuming less food and with smaller disposable incomes; it is hardly surprising that children in these households are usually less well-nourished and have a greater chance of being stunted or wasted.

The World Bank's study in Kagera, Tanzania, in the early 1990s showed that even in 'richer' households (and we must not forget that these are all very poor communities) 29% of non-orphaned children were stunted (had a very low height for their age) while 50% of orphaned children were wasted (had a very low weight for their height). In poorer households 39% of non-orphaned children were stunted while 51% of orphaned children were wasted (World Bank, 1997a, p. 224). These figures point to the effects on all children of growing up in a poor society.

Stunting results from poor nutrition over an extended period. There are a number of pathways to stunting and orphanhood exacerbates these. Orphans may have been deprived of proper nutrition during the period that their parents were sick and dying. It is possible that a proportion of them are HIV positive and their poor physical condition reflects illness. They may have come from poor households and their stunting is an effect of their life with their previous household. They may be neglected in the household of their adoption.

Stunting has long-term effects. Foundations for future life are poorly built with poor physical condition, compromised immune systems and mental functioning. This will affect the ability of children to benefit from education and to function socially and economically later in their lives. It can affect a society for a generation or more.

Schooling

Orphans are less likely to have proper schooling. The death of a prime-age adult in a household will reduce a child's attendance at school (World Bank, 1997a, p. 225). The household may be less able to pay for schooling.[2] An orphaned child may have to take on household or income-earning work. Sick adults may have reduced expectations of the returns of investing in children's education as they do not expect to live long enough to recoup the investment. When a child goes to another household after his or her parents' deaths, the obstacles become greater as the child is not their own.

The standard of education that a child receives may be low. This is in part because of the under-resourcing of public education; it is also a result of the AIDS epidemic. AIDS increases teacher deaths and they may be difficult to replace, particularly in deprived, rural or otherwise remote communities. Teachers' illness is of particular importance. Classes remain untaught for extended periods and replacement is difficult while staff members are on sick leave.

In Zambia there is evidence of a fall in numbers of children attending primary school. This is at a time when the numbers of school-age children is increasing and numbers out of school are already large. The decline in school participation rates was thought to result from poverty, people's inability to pay the rising costs of schooling, and increasing parental disillusion with the low quality of education. It is likely that some of the fall in school participation is due to HIV/AIDS, its effects on poverty, levels of employment, and the quality of school provision (Kelly, 2000, p. 12).

In Zambia's Copperbelt – an area badly affected by HIV/AIDS – it was found that '44% of the children of school-going age were not attending school, but with proportionately more orphans (53.6%) than non-orphans (42.4%) not attending' (Rossi and Reijer, 1995, quoted in Kelly 2000, p. 12). A similar pattern was apparent in a rural area in the eastern part of the country where only 38% of the orphaned school-age children were attending school, compared with the provincial average of 51%. More recent data show that 32% of urban and 68% of rural orphans were not enrolled in school. These percentages are considerably higher than those for non-orphans who were not enrolled – 25% of urban non-orphans and 48% of rural non-orphans (Kelly, 2000, p. 12).

In Kagera, children from poor households had the lowest school enrolment rates whether they were orphaned or not. But orphaned children inevitably had lower rates than non-orphaned children. Differentials are striking. The enrolment rate for non-orphaned children between the ages of seven and ten from better-off households was 44%. But for orphaned children in the same age group and from poorer households, the rate dropped to 28% (World Bank, 1997a, p. 228). Figure 8.1 shows the differences in enrolment rate across a number of countries between children with and children without parents.

Enrolment rates varied with household assets, but they also varied with the gender of the deceased parent. In Zimbabwe, 99% of children attended school prior to the death of the mother. After her death, enrolment rates fell to 87% (80% in urban areas and 93% in rural) (Mutangadura, 2000, p. 17). When a mother died, children were expected to take on more domestic work to replace her labour contribution. Even those children who did not drop out of school attended less frequently because of the amount of domestic and farm work they

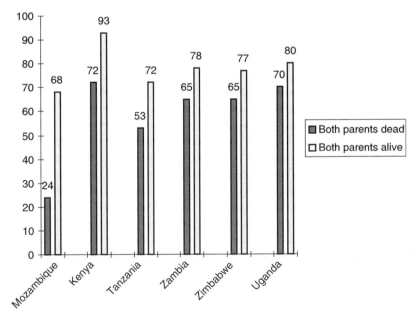

Figure 8.1   Percentage of orphaned and non-orphaned children (aged 10–14) in school
Source: UNICEF (2000), p. 30.

had to do. Girls carry a larger burden of domestic responsibility than boys and are more likely to be kept out of school.

It does not take any great leap of imagination to realise that even if they do manage to go to school these children's attendance will be less consistent, their progression rates will be more erratic and their academic attainment and results will be poorer. This is true whether they are living in an affected household, are orphaned and taken in by others, or orphaned and living on their own. A study in Botswana found that the present impact is limited:

> Teacher interviewees at the nine primary schools that were surveyed also indicated that, on average, only around one-third to one-half of the orphans they could identify in their class were having difficulties with their education and were in need of either material and/or emotional support. In their opinion, the remaining orphans were adequately looked after and were coping at school. The following written comment of a Headteacher neatly summarises the orphan situation at most of the survey primary schools: 'Generally performance goes down immediately after the death of a parent. Some remain depressed, but others are fine. It largely depends on the carer' ... Generally speaking, it is orphans from the poorest socio-economic backgrounds who appear to have most problems at school. Thus, while there are problems that relate specifically to orphanhood, it is the existence of endemic poverty, particularly in the rural areas, that is largely responsible for many of the difficulties faced by orphans as well as other 'needy children'. (Government of Botswana, 2000, pp. 49–50)

As with much else about HIV/AIDS, impacts are interrelated: poor nutrition, poor care, and poor or little schooling affects orphans. Other children in the community are affected by general household impoverishment.

The effects of orphans on non-orphans

Caring for children has costs. Taking in orphans increases demands on household resources. In societies affected by HIV/AIDS, many children live in households in which their own parents have fostered or are fostering orphans. In a study in Buganda, southern Uganda, in 2000 (Monk, 2000), 152 households were interviewed. A total of 342 non-orphaned children resided in these units. In addition there were 383 orphans. In the majority of cases there was no distinction between levels of care given to orphans or to the guardian's own biological children. Therefore, all children in the household suffer the same economic and other deprivations resulting from spreading resources more thinly as a 'coping' response to the epidemic. Boxes 8.3 and 8.4 show a little of the complexity of orphaning and orphan care in Uganda in 2000.

Box 8.3   Buganda, Nabutaka village

In this household a husband and wife, aged 30 and 27 respectively, are caring for eight children; their own 5-year-old girl and 1-year-old boy plus six orphans:

16-year-old boy, a nephew, paternal orphan; the wife's brothers aged 12 and 6 (double orphans); a 6-year-old boy, nephew, double orphan; a 5-year-old girl niece, paternal orphan; and a 5-year-old boy, nephew, paternal orphan.

The dependency ratio of this household has increased dramatically as a result of fostering of children from five different deceased relatives. The 16-year-old boy is in secondary school, but the foster parents are struggling to find the school fees. The guardian is trying to persuade him to change to a technical school, as he thinks that this will be better for the household in the long run. (Monk, 2000)

Box 8.4 Buganda, Kabanyi village

There are 11 people in this household. In addition to the husband, 65 years, and wife, 40 years, there are nine children, six of whom are orphans: a 14-year-old boy; a 12-year-old girl; a 10-year-old boy; a 6-year-old girl; and a 5-year-old girl. These are all paternal orphans, grandchildren of the household head and children of his deceased son. They have lived in this household for four years, since their mother remarried. In addition there is a 6-year-old boy, a grandchild who has lost both parents to AIDS.

Fostering has caused enormous financial strain on this household. The children show signs of malnutrition, not surprising when the dependency ratio has increased three times. (Monk, 2000)

Taking adult roles

AIDS disrupts social roles, rights and obligations. For the orphaned child there is often a premature entrance to burdens of adulthood, all without the rights and privileges – or the strengths – associated with adult status.

Becoming an orphan of the epidemic is rarely a sudden switch in roles. It is slow and painful, and the slowness and pain have to do not only with loss of a parent but also with the long-term care which that parent's failing health may require. Children who care for adults may experience a world gone seriously awry. A young girl of eight or nine may be used to caring for younger siblings: she is unprepared to care for her mother, father, or both of them. As well as the physical difficulties there are inevitably difficulties of culture and sensibility. Coping with a parent who is weak and requires food to be cooked or water to be brought is one thing. Coping with a parent's severe diarrhoea, declining mental function and mood changes is quite another. Children also become uncommonly familiar with death. A man from Buganda remarked:

> When I was young there weren't many burials like today. When our parents had gone away to sleep at the house of someone who had died we children would be afraid that the person who had died would come out of the sitting room of his house, where he was lying, and eat us! But children of today know who is ill, who is dead and who is weak. They go to burials at a young age and are used to them. They may have seen the body of an aunt, and then the father dies and they see his corpse, then the mother and a stepmother, so they are used to it, and used to dead bodies. (Williams, 1998, p. 247)

It is not only in relation to their own parents that children take on new and premature roles. When they become orphans, they go to their grandparents or to another relative. An aunt or uncle may also die of HIV/AIDS, or a grandparent from old age. Successive orphaning is not unknown. It is all too common for quite young children or early adolescents to be caring for aged and infirm grandparents.

One respect in which orphaned children will most probably not accede to adult status is with regard to property and land. Early research on these issues (Barnett and Blaikie, 1990, 1992) indicated that on the death of a parent or parents, children were quite likely to be disinherited.

The challenge of care

'Our extended family system will cope with orphans', people used to say in Africa in the early 1990s. In Uganda it was realised and accepted by the mid-1990s that 'the extended family' system was (a) various and variable, and (b) often not coping. Institutional care is unacceptable to people in Uganda and in most other parts of Africa. It is necessary to find ways to care for orphans within family and household systems that have been increasingly stretched, using institutional care as a last resort. Institutional care has a bad name in some places where 'orphan farming' has developed as an income-generating activity (Barnett and Blaikie, 1992).

An assessment of the costs of orphan care in South Africa looked at six different approaches. The costs are summarised in Table 8.3.

Table 8.3   The cost of orphan care in South Africa ($1 = R11)

Care Model	Annual cost (minimum standard)	Increase	Reason for increase
Community-based support structures	276	–	–
Home-based care and support	306	+30	Process for identification Process for placement and grant access
Informal fostering/ non-statutory foster care	325	+19	Higher degree of supervision Smaller scale
Statutory adoption and foster care	410	+85	Security of accommodation Quality of accommodation More administration
Unregistered residential care	956	+546	High staff to child ratio Provision of emergency care Care of sick children
Statutory residential care (caring mainly for HIV positive children)	2590	+1634	Very high staff to child ratio Care only for sick children Meet statutory requirements for a children's home High overheads On-site medical care On-site preschool education

Source: Gow and Desmond (forthcoming).

There is a wide range of care options, from the less costly informal care to the more costly formal care models. Although community-based care and home-based care and support appear to be the most cost efficient ways of caring for orphans, these models are not always appropriate or feasible. Appropriate resource allocation – a political and practical issue – is a major limitation to be addressed if the basic needs of the children are to be effectively met by informal family-orientated care models. In addition, the appropriateness of less formalised care options in caring for children who may be sick or who have suffered abuse needs to be considered.

It is difficult to know how to support households with AIDS orphans. Targeting them is neither practical nor desirable and is potentially stigmatising. It could also mean that other orphans and their carers – with the same needs – would be excluded from benefits. The majority of orphans are in poor countries where even the better-off households are poor by the standards of rich countries. The problem is how to support all orphans and other vulnerable children more effectively in such contexts.

Botswana provides a revealing case study.[3] Once again we begin with the question of how many orphans there are. The Ministry of Finance and Development Planning predicted that there would be 85,000 orphans in Botswana in the year 2000 (Government of Botswana, 1997). The 1995 Sentinel Survey on HIV infection rates in Botswana projected 65,000 AIDS orphans by this date (Government of Botswana, 1995). Yet a recent publication puts the number at only 46,032 (Hunter and Williamson, 2000). The situation is made more complex by the difficulty in defining an orphan for practical as opposed to statistical purposes. In 1991, 47.1% of the country's households were said to be 'female headed'. What that means in practice is that if a mother dies the father is no longer on the scene and these children are effectively orphans, even if their father is still alive. Whether the number of AIDS orphans is 46,000 or 85,000, this is a considerable challenge to existing support systems.

The majority of orphans in Botswana are children whose parents have died from AIDS-related infections. A rapid assessment of orphans in 1998 estimated that the cause of parental death was HIV/AIDS in 51% of cases, but in addition, 13% of parents were recorded as having died from TB, 7% from other illnesses and 12% from unknown causes. It is likely that many of these were in fact AIDS deaths (Rajaraman, 2001).

In this situation, some dispute over whether state intervention or institutional care is appropriate remains. As in Uganda ten years ago, so in Botswana today, they say that fostering and institutional care are not part of the tradition; that the extended family will cope (Jacques, 1998, quoted in Rajaraman, 2001). But

> [t]he Rapid Assessment on the Situation of Orphans in Botswana tells a different story ... of orphan suicides, destitute children eking their living out of garbage dumpsites, and a growing number of child-headed households. In a context of intense social and economic pressures, orphans are increasingly reported to be mistreated and abused by caregivers; deprived of their inheritances by opportunist relatives and neighbours; forced to drop out of school to perform domestic labour or bring home wages; pressured into entering commercial sex work and vulnerable to sexual abuse. (Rajaraman, 2001, p. 9)

Although the government offers some additional support for orphans, carers are sometimes reluctant to accept this assistance, particularly if acceptance may identify the dead parent as having died of AIDS; or it may suggest that the family cannot cope – another stigma. Given the possibilities of abuse, neglect and poverty, Rajaraman (2001, p. 9) suggests that 'the Government has an obligation to intervene, in order to protect the human rights of the children involved.[4] This does not imply overriding traditional systems of caring for orphans; it will, however, mean developing institutions to monitor, support and supplement them.' But despite considerable rhetoric and funding, the Government of Botswana has not mobilised sufficiently to develop a structure of care for orphans. NGOs and particularly the churches are bearing the heaviest load. The government has not yet introduced an effective system either for registering orphans or for ensuring that different ministries' activities are co-ordinated to provide effective support. This is the situation in one of Africa's wealthiest countries; it is far worse in the poorer countries.

As the epidemic's range increases, these problems will appear elsewhere. In Calcutta, India, there have been reports of numerous AIDS orphans for some years[5], while in the Ukraine, the predicted number of AIDS orphans in the next five years may well overwhelm existing institutional provision (Barnett et al., 2000b, p. 1,399). The Ukrainian case is of particular concern as the situation there is replicated in all of the former Soviet Union – implying a vast orphan population from the Polish border to Vladivostok.[6]

Orphans, states and war

The unmeasured consequences for the orphan generation are of great concern. We are talking about unsocialised, uneducated and in many instances unloved children struggling to adulthood. The cost to them as individuals remains unmeasured. The costs to the wider society are potentially enormous and are already being seen and felt.

It has been speculated that the huge amount of orphaning will lead to an increase in crime. This has been spelt out as follows for South Africa:

> AIDS and age will be significant contributors to an increase in the rate of crime over the next ten to twenty years. There will be a boom in South Africa's orphan population during the next decade ... Growing up without parents, and badly supervised by relatives and welfare organisations, this growing pool of orphans will be at greater than average risk to engage in criminal activity. (Schönteich, 1999, p. 1)

At worst there may be increased political instability with orphans swelling the ranks of the child soldiers (Zack-Williams, 1999). In a society which is already stressed and where government may offer very little, large numbers of 'youth' who have been orphaned from an early age can easily become armed youths, easy recruits for millenarian cults or prey to unscrupulous politicians.

Most orphans do not become child soldiers. Not all child soldiers are orphans – some of them are abducted from their parents. But in some parts of Africa, south-east Asia and the borderlands of the world, there are substantial numbers of orphans among the child soldiers. Some of them, particularly in Africa, are AIDS orphans. Of the 30 or more current or recent armed conflicts involving child combatants, 13 were or are in African countries. These include Liberia, Sierra Leone, Uganda, Ethiopia, Angola, Rwanda, Algeria, Eritrea, Democratic Republic of Congo, Congo Brazzaville, Burundi, Somalia and Mozambique (Brett and McCallan, 1998).

It has been estimated that in Sierra Leone the government utilised between 1,000 and 2,000 child combatants among its fighting forces, whilst the rebel Revolutionary United Front had between 3,000 and 4,000 (Brett and McCallan, 1998, p. 222). These are most probably underestimates as anti-government forces abducted several thousand children after the report was compiled (Zack-Williams, 1999, p. 2). Perhaps half of all the combatants in Sierra Leone are in the age range 8–14 years (Peters and Richards, 1998, p. 186). There are no data concerning numbers of child soldiers fighting in the Great African War in the Democratic Republic of Congo. But there is little reason to think that the situation there should be any different. Formally recruited, or forced, these children are exposed to terrible conditions. Infection with HIV is but one of the risks that they run.

The epidemic has vastly increased the numbers of orphans in Africa. Caring for them within the 'extended family' is desperately hard. Levels of care are variable, and some end up on the streets of the cities, while others are drawn into soldiering. In either case these lives are hardly a preparation for the future as a member of a household or a community, least of all as a citizen. As these orphans grow into youth and adulthood, there are serious implications for the societies in which they will live their lives.

Children's rights

Orphanhood threatens many aspects of children's lives. The International Convention on the Rights of the Child in principle provides a protective framework for children.[7] It accords them the following rights which are to be protected by signatory governments:

- To be cared for by his or her parents (Article 7)
- To preserve identity, nationality, name and family relations (Article 8)
- To maintain regular contact with parents if separated (Article 9)
- To freedom of expression (Article 13)
- To freedom of association (Article 15)
- To be brought up by parent or guardians whose basic concern is his or her best interests (Article 18)
- To protection from physical or mental ill-treatment, neglect or exploitation (Article 19)
- To conditions of living necessary for his or her development (Article 27)
- To education (Article 28)
- To rest, leisure, play and recreation (Article 31)
- To protection from economic exploitation and performing any work that interferes with his or her education or is harmful to his or her mental, spiritual or social development (Article 32)
- To be protected from all forms of sexual exploitation and sexual abuse (Article 34)
- To be protected from abduction, sale or trafficking (Article 35)
- To be protected from torture or other cruel, inhuman or degrading treatment or punishment (Article 37).

In normal circumstances many of these rights are violated; HIV/AIDS increases the numbers of children at risk. Beyond governments' failures to protect childrens' rights, the ways in which these rights will be violated are determined by:

- Age and sex of child – boys and girls are treated differently; older boys are more able to stand up for themselves; older girls may be subjected to sexual abuse
- Age of guardian – the stage of the guardian's lifecycle will influence whether or not there is competition between the orphan(s) and her/his own children, whether or not the guardian is sufficiently active or has sufficient resources to engage with the needs of the child
- Relationship of guardian to child – the degree of closeness and the particular relationship will influence the outcome of the adoption/fostering
- Number of parents dead – if both parents are dead then the child is more dependent
- Kinship – this will affect the degree to which the orphaned child is accepted as part of the guardian's group
- Proportion of children orphaned in the community – orphan overload in a poor community may result in people being unable to take on more responsibility.

In extreme cases, which are all too numerous, orphans turn to the street, where their physical needs and financial desperation make them vulnerable to crime, substance abuse and sexual exploitation. This places a significant number at risk of contracting HIV through virtually inescapable income-generating prostitution. AIDS orphans are at greater risk of malnutrition, illness, abuse and sexual exploitation than children orphaned by other causes. They must grapple with the stigma and discrimination so often associated with AIDS, which often deprives them of basic social services and education (Kelly, 2000). A recent study of the situation of orphans in Tanzania sums up their circumstances (Conroy et al., 2001). This survey looked at the lives of AIDS orphans, 'ordinary' orphans and excluded 'paternal' orphans, and found that:

- child-headed households are more frequently found among AIDS orphans than among others
- AIDS orphans attended school less frequently than did other orphans
- AIDS orphans are more likely to drop out of school than others

- numbers of orphans are swamping household and community ability to cope
- girls are more vulnerable than are boys to abuse and ill treatment
- in a sample of 2,786 AIDS orphans, there were 128 incidents of attempted suicide; in a sample of 2,420 other orphans, there were none.

Older people

Population ageing is now a global phenomenon and is set to accelerate over the coming decades (Kinsella and Tauber, 1992–93). The population is ageing for two reasons. First, the proportion of older people to younger people is changing. In the past, high mortality and fertility meant the proportion of the population reaching old age was relatively small (Velkoff and Lawson, 1998). Second, people are living longer. In poor countries, improvements in average life expectancy are achieved primarily because infants survive the initial high-risk years of life, whereas in rich countries this is achieved primarily through declines in mortality in the older age groups (Kinsella and Ferreira, 1997).

Even though, proportionally, the numbers of people reaching older age may not appear dramatic, the absolute numbers are. A 7% increase (from 12% to 19%) of the population reaching age 60 and over between 1950 and 1998 within rich countries,[8] resulted in absolute numbers growing from just over 100 million to 355 million (Velkoff and Lawson, 1998).

Since 1980 the majority of older people have been living in poor regions. In Thailand, Brazil and South Africa, the rates of increase are among the highest in the world (see Table 8.4). Velkoff and Lawson (1998) suggest that by 2025 there will be 500 million more older people living in developing countries than the developed countries.

Not only are more people living into old age, but the older population is itself ageing. The 'oldest-old'[9] is the fastest-growing segment of the older population, growing faster in poor than in rich countries (see Table 8.5) (Velkoff and Lawson, 1998).

The standard definitions, population aged 65 years or over, do not reflect the nature of old age in most of sub-Saharan Africa (Apt, 1996, 1997) and other poor regions of the world and in poor communities. Limited life expectancy, poverty, hard work, frequent illness and, in the case of women, childbearing, all result in relatively early onset of 'old age'.

In contrast to children who are orphaned or otherwise at risk, older people are less appealing to donors. There is prejudice against older

Table 8.4 Population indicators by age and sex

| Country | Population aged 80 and over (000s) | | | | % change aged 80 and over, 1998–2025 | | Aged 80 and over as % of 60 and over | | | |
| | 1998 | | 2025 | | | | 1998 | | 2025 | |
	Male	Female	Male	Female	Male	Female	Male	Female	Male	Female
Afghanistan	35	27	100	94	183.5	250.4	6.0	5.1	7.0	7.0
Algeria	75	86	178	257	138.0	199.0	9.0	9.2	7.7	10.3
Argentina	278	492	555	1044	99.6	112.5	12.9	17.1	15.4	22.2
Australia	188	348	482	727	155.9	109.0	13.8	20.9	17.7	22.8
Bangladesh	220	127	457	431	107.6	240.6	6.2	4.2	5.3	5.0
Brazil	429	854	1531	2982	257.1	249.4	7.9	11.4	11.0	15.8
Canada	311	596	746	1187	139.9	99.1	14.0	21.1	15.4	20.9
China	3866	6595	10152	15805	162.6	139.6	6.5	10.4	7.7	10.8
Colombia	85	119	300	576	252.2	381.8	7.2	8.4	8.5	12.6
Egypt	99	142	253	500	156.5	251.3	5.6	6.7	5.9	9.2
Ethiopia	69	94	129	224	85.8	137.2	5.8	6.8	8.2	10.1
France	679	1519	1330	2352	95.9	54.9	13.3	21.8	17.1	23.8
Germany	789	2206	2195	3785	178.1	71.6	10.7	20.4	18.4	26.6
India	2956	2790	8309	9674	181.1	246.7	8.5	8.4	10.2	11.0
Indonesia	313	473	1351	2314	330.9	389.2	4.9	6.1	7.9	11.2
Italy	746	1498	1466	2622	96.6	75.0	13.2	19.6	19.1	27.0
Japan	1439	2899	3936	6734	173.5	132.3	11.9	18.4	22.5	30.5
Kenya	43	57	99	184	132.1	224.0	8.2	8.7	11.8	14.8
Malaysia	44	69	146	271	233.6	294.8	7.4	9.5	8.3	11.9
Mexico	245	371	830	1428	238.9	285.0	8.7	11.1	11.1	14.3
Morocco	82	97	201	325	145.2	235.2	9.1	9.2	9.0	12.2
Nepal	36	39	126	172	248.3	338.0	5.6	6.1	8.8	10.8

Table 8.4 Population indicators by age and sex *cont.*

Country	Population aged 80 and over (000s)				% change aged 80 and over, 1998–2025		Aged 80 and over as % of 60 and over			
	1998		2025				1998		2025	
	Male	Female	Male	Female	Male	Female	Male	Female	Male	Female
Pakistan	342	353	670	933	96.0	164.2	8.2	8.5	8.1	9.9
Peru	71	102	265	377	274.2	268.6	8.5	10.8	11.7	14.8
Philippines	166	210	419	644	152.8	206.1	8.5	9.0	8.2	9.8
Poland	223	532	519	1103	132.6	107.2	8.9	14.1	11.8	18.7
Romania	147	262	347	661	136.1	151.8	8.2	11.1	15.6	21.9
Russia	593	2427	1213	3561	104.5	46.7	6.7	14.1	9.5	16.6
South Africa	110	227	226	469	104.6	106.9	9.0	13.3	10.4	14.4
South Korea	105	289	642	1189	512.7	311.0	5.4	10.5	11.1	17.1
Spain	461	928	884	1593	91.7	71.6	12.8	19.3	17.8	25.0
Sri Lanka	89	94	210	340	135.4	261.8	10.7	10.6	11.6	14.1
Sudan	48	36	129	154	169.3	327.9	6.8	6.2	8.0	7.8
Taiwan	126	140	416	625	229.6	346.9	9.4	11.6	13.9	18.2
Tanzania	48	60	88	165	81.8	172.7	7.5	8.0	8.8	10.7
Thailand	188	319	646	1220	243.9	282.4	7.5	10.5	10.6	15.1
Turkey	218	352	810	1256	272.0	256.7	8.4	12.0	12.3	17.1
Ukraine	261	894	461	1290	76.6	44.3	7.4	13.9	11.0	18.6
United Kingdom	730	1627	1278	2208	75.1	35.7	14.1	23.6	16.6	23.7
United States	2881	5835	5631	8766	95.5	50.2	15.2	22.8	14.8	19.7
Uzbekistan	55	126	118	223	116.0	77.0	8.0	13.2	7.7	10.9
Venezuela	84	116	231	345	175.7	197.9	11.9	14.4	11.0	13.7

Source: Velkoff and Lawson (1998).

Table 8.5   Percentage of population in older age groups, 1997–2025

Region/country	Year	Age group		
		50+	60+	70+
Southern Africa	1997	12.0	6.2	2.5
	2010	14.1	7.5	3.2
	2025	15.5	9.1	4.2
Botswana	1997	9.7	5.4	2.4
	2010	9.8	5.3	2.5
	2025	9.1	5.6	2.8
Lesotho	1997	11.7	6.7	2.8
	2010	12.1	6.5	3.0
	2025	14.1	7.7	3.3
South Africa	1997	13.3	6.8	2.8
	2010	16.2	8.6	3.6
	2025	18.0	10.8	5.1
Zimbabwe	1997	8.5	4.3	1.7
	2010	8.6	4.7	2.2
	2025	8.4	4.9	2.4

Source: Kinsella and Ferreira (1997)

people and rapid social change and 'development' often places them in positions of severe disadvantage. For example, the migration of young adults from rural to urban areas means that old people's adult children will not be around to look after them. The changed status from respected elder to burdensome old person is particularly likely when the children's generation ceases to take traditional responsibilities seriously as they pursue new individualistic lifestyles. The HIV/AIDS epidemic magnifies all of these problems, and older women face more difficulties than older men. Rural old women are among the populations most adversely affected. A measure of the degree to which the impact of HIV/AIDS on older people has been neglected is that we are aware of only one scientific study and indeed few other publications on this express theme.[10]

The main problem confronting the elderly in a society affected by HIV/AIDS is poverty. An inevitable second problem is grief: 'I am not OK because of thinking about the death of my son. At times I don't eat well, not because I am ill, but because of sadness about the loss of my son' ('Grace Nanteza', quoted in Williams, 1998, p. 245). Grief and poverty go together for the old because the epidemic affects them through the death of one or more of their adult children. Older people are likely to be among the poorest in poor societies. Their failing powers makes it more difficult for them to work on a farm or earn a living in some other way. They become increasingly dependent physically and financially in all societies, and once again 'the extended family' and its strengths can turn out to be more myth than reality (Laslett, 1965; Gubrium, 1973; Foner, 1984).

Poverty and frailty are made worse by the loss of adult children in two respects: the loss of financial and other support that older people could have expected and might have received, and the unexpected burden of orphaned grandchildren who come to live with them.

Rich older persons can buy their way out of the worst material effects of the death of an adult child or children. Fieldwork in rural Uganda in 1989 identified an apparently prosperous elderly couple. In-depth interviews elicited the following story. The couple had worked hard and saved by investing in their children's education. For many years they had enjoyed the fruits of their investment in remittances from their son the headmaster, their daughter the nursing sister and their other sons, both government officials. Then one by one and in quick succession their children all died. The couple found themselves hosting 15 grandchildren from under two years of age to mid-teens. Their solution was for the old man, now in his eighties, to take a young woman of 26 as his second wife. This is one way of coping, but it is restricted to the relatively rich. The reality for the majority of the elderly is quite different.

Old age: poverty exacerbated

A detailed study of older people in Buganda (Williams, 1998) graphically illustrates the conditions which the elderly endure in a rural society in Africa. They have poor housing and are often unable to build anew or to repair what they have. Poor housing means poor security and loss of food and other valuable items to insects, animals and theft. Preparing and cooking food can present challenges. Within their homes, poor old people may not have sufficient bedding to stay warm at night. One of Williams's respondents told him: 'I sleep on a bark cloth on the ground and I cover myself with my dress. I'd sleep better if I had a blanket' (Williams, 1998, p. 140). Another said:

> The problem is that I don't have the strength to carry pots from outside and I am afraid I will fall over. I used to have it (the kitchen) outside, but it was hard to get in and out of the door at

night, and once I fell over. So now I have it in here, but I still fall down sometimes. When I cook near my bed I can cook lying down and that is easier. (Williams, 1998, p. 138)

Old people living alone face considerable difficulties obtaining water for washing, cooking and drinking. These are all the greater if people do not have a watertight container to take to the well or pool and thus spill some on every arduous journey they make. If you are no longer strong enough to go to the well yourself, water supply requires people, and people are not dependable. To ensure an adequate supply of water a person must either pay somebody to do the work or maintain an active network of social investment. Failing adequate water supply, the results for the elderly may include: thirst, hunger because there is no water with which to cook, dirty clothes, lack of personal hygiene, and intestinal worms associated with poor sanitary conditions (Williams, 1998, p. 143).

Another constraint is fuel wood. This is a very labour intensive and demanding task and old people often find it hard to obtain enough. The result of this combined with falling ability to produce food from the farm or purchase it is inadequate diet:

> Sometimes I don't eat any supper. Last night my granddaughter who lives with me went to her mother to get food because we did not have any. She came back with some cassava, but we couldn't cook it because we hadn't got any firewood. ('Edith Manube', quoted in Williams, 1998, p. 152)

The elderly are dependent; dependence requires support; support is found in social life; social life requires energy and inputs if it is to be maintained and reproduced – the elderly lack the energy to make these investments, that is why children are important and why, when they die and their work, remittances and other support cease, the circumstances of an old person can decline dramatically. What then happens when the grandchildren come to live with them?

Old age and orphans

Williams suggests that 'Old people are affected by the epidemic more through the fulfilment of their parental obligations than the loss of their children's support' (Williams, 1998, p. 230). First of all they care for their children who are sick, then they bury them; finally, they care for their grandchildren.

In Uganda as long ago as the late 1980s, aged grandparents had increasingly assumed responsibilities for rearing orphans.[11] Lack of energy to work in the fields meant that the range of food available to them and their dependants became smaller and their nutritional status became worse. The implications were summed up by a teacher, who said: 'We have over 80 orphans in this school and you can tell those from grandparent homes. Their noses are always running and their uniforms are often not clean, ironed or repaired.' Many grandparents with orphans said they had problems with discipline. Young people were to be found playing truant in the nearby town and were identified by members of the community as orphans coming from grandparent homes.

Attendance at Parent Teacher Associations by grandparents is important because households without orphans need to be informed of the reduced economic status of orphan families in order to enable the headmasters to commute the PTA fee. In 1989, many orphans in the research area had dropped out of school because their grandparents could not afford these fees. A teacher and a grandparent independently pointed out that 'grandparents are often ignorant of how, or lack the energy, to go and defend their wards, or at least enable them to get a fair hearing and treatment in cases involving insubordination to school authorities'.

On the other hand, older grandchildren may provide practical and emotional care for a grandparent. So the effects of orphan care on the elderly and the ability of the orphans to contribute to the household is sensitive to personalities and to specific age distributions in a household. A young child or children require constant physical care and attention but may soon begin to help with domestic chores. An older orphan may turn out to be a help for the grandparent but he or she may also be trouble. Adolescence or its approach may signal a time of extreme tension between the generations, sometimes ending in the departure of the orphan. But sometimes it is the sheer numbers of orphans who come to rest in the grandparent(s) household which overwhelm their capacity to offer material and emotional care.

Burial and memory

Talking in the early 1990s about the death of an adult child or children, elderly people in Uganda and Kenya often returned to the theme of 'proper burial'. The concern among the old is that their funerary rites should be correctly carried out. If you lose your adult children then it is difficult to believe that your burial will be performed according to

custom and that you will be treated with the respect that you deserve.
An old man said:

> We produce our children to ensure that our clan continues. They
> would have been caring for us in our old age, but now we die like
> someone who has produced no children. For example, that land
> there was owned by a man who had some children, but two went
> away and the rest died. Then he and his wife died and the house
> collapsed. Now the land is fallow as if he hadn't produced children.
> Look at George Kabongo! He produced two children, one of them,
> Ndawula, is still here, and owns most of the land now. When
> Kabongo dies people who go by will know that this land belongs to
> his son. They will know he died leaving someone on the earth. It's
> important that people remember you, and it means the clan will
> continue. ('Noah Serawadda', quoted in Williams, 1998, p. 246)

Conclusion: young trees make a strong forest (Kiganda proverb)[12]

It is estimated that by 2005 just over 30% of Malawi's children will be
orphans because of AIDS and other reasons: by 2010 that figure will
have risen to 35% (Hunter and Fall, 1998, p. 7). The situation in Malawi
is no worse than in any other country of east, south and central Africa;
indeed it may be better. There will be fewer young trees in the forest
because they will themselves be cut down by the epidemic. Those who
survive will not necessarily have been adequately nurtured.

The breakdown of intergenerational dependency and support is not
unique to an HIV/AIDS epidemic. It has been commented on in many
countries of Europe (Carmichael and Charles, 1999). Provision can be
made through the market or the state in rich countries. Poor countries
have not and cannot provide safety nets for their people. There is little
in the way of public provision. People cope by caring for themselves in
households and in communities as well as they can.

The HIV/AIDS epidemic confronts us with a new situation. Societies
remain poor and will be further impoverished by the epidemic itself.
The growth of dependent populations and the disappearance of mature
adults erode the possibilities of 'coping' at the local level and nationally. This is apparent all over Africa but also elsewhere, for example in
the Ukraine. Ukrainians have the oldest average age in Europe, and per
capita one of the largest numbers of pensioners. Under the Soviet
system a pension was provided by the state. Money did not come from

investments but from current revenue. The dramatic decline in government revenues since 1991 has been reflected in a decline in the real value of pensions as well as delays in paying them. Not only are the old poor and without any substantial social safety nets, but because of the unfavourable dependency ratio they are unlikely to have either family or state provision in their final years. Our calculations suggest that as a result of the HIV/AIDS epidemic, there will be an additional 30,000 totally unsupported old people in the Ukraine within ten years (Barnett and Whiteside, 1997).

The evidence from Africa and from the Ukraine – which is representative of much of the former Soviet Union – shows that a serious situation exists in both places. Throughout Africa the intergenerational bargain is becoming progressively harder to maintain. The outcome is awful for the people themselves; its long-term effects have to be imagined as one and possibly two generations of children grow up with inadequate care.

9
Subsistence Agriculture and Rural Livelihoods

> Even if [rural] families are selling cows to pay hospital bills, [one] will hardly see tens of thousands of cows being auctioned at the market ... Unlike in famine situations, buying and selling of assets in the case of AIDS is very subtle, done within villages or even among relatives, and the volume is small.
>
> (Rugalema, quoted in Topouzis, 2000, p. 26)

Agriculture, farming and rural livelihoods

Agriculture is the cornerstone of human life. Farming feeds agricultural workers, other rural dwellers and those living and working in urban areas. Agriculture accounts for only 4% of value added to global domestic product, in contrast to industry's 32% and the 62% contributed by services (World Bank, 2000b, p. 189). However these bald statistics do not reflect the real importance of the agricultural sector. Without this sector there would be no industry, no services and no urban areas. We all have to eat. Seed production, plant breeding, food production, processing and marketing have been interlinked worldwide activities for thousands of years.

In the last 100 years, and particularly in the last 50, all of these activities have become parts of globalised flows of information, finance and marketing. Plant genetic materials are now patented, owned by multinationals and manipulated to suit cultivation regimes, marketing goals and consumer preferences. Consumers living in rich countries can buy almost all products throughout the year, while often their local varieties disappear in the global competition. South African grapes replace Italian in the northern hemisphere's winter, Mexican squashes jostle for shelf space with Kenyan beans and pineapples. At the end of this value chain[1] are people who till the soil, tend and harvest the crops. An example is a farm household producing green beans in Machakos, Kenya in 1991.[2] These people cultivated about 3 hectares of maize and vegetables, mainly for themselves but also for sale. They grew about half a hectare of beans for the agent of a supermarket in Europe. The price paid to the farmer was less than one-eighth the price European consumers paid. The woman of the household said that her husband had to work as a migrant labourer for part of the year to make ends meet. There are millions of such farmers. They survive from year to year solely on their own efforts and the produce of a few hectares of land. They are dependent on their own labour, are price-takers and are most immediately threatened by the epidemic.

Difficulties with food production lead to poor nutrition: both protein-energy malnutrition and deficiencies in micronutrients such as iron, zinc and vitamins. Poor nutrition leads to compromised immune systems, making individuals more susceptible to infection in general (Morris and Potter, 1997; Chandra, 1997; Beisel, 1996; Scrimshaw and SanGiovanni, 1997). These links are a facet of a risk environment with links back to the global economy. HIV infected individuals have higher nutritional requirements than normal, particularly with regard to protein (up to 50% increased), and energy (up to 15%). Illness may precipitate appetite loss, even anorexia, thus reducing dietary intake at a time when requirements are higher. Such interactions are thrown into stark contrast for the poor, and particularly the rural poor, who are more likely to be malnourished prior to becoming infected. Onset of disease and death might be delayed in well-nourished HIV positive individuals. Diets rich in protein, energy and micronutrients help in resisting opportunistic infections (Haddad and Gillespie, 2001). Thus for rural populations, the impact of HIV/AIDS on farming, farming systems, rural livelihoods and nutrition is potentially serious. It has been largely overlooked in the focus on prevention.

Despite its apparent low share in global output, agriculture is probably the main livelihood of more people than any other economic activity. If we consider urban and rural residence as a partial indicator of involvement in agriculture, then the picture is clear. Globally, 54% of the population lives outside urban areas. In low-income countries 70% of people live in rural areas; in South Asia and sub-Saharan Africa the percentages are 72% and 67%, respectively. FAOSTAT estimated that globally 2,575,456,000 people lived and worked in agriculture in 1999 (the last year for which information was available). The agricultural population of Africa in 1999 was estimated at 430,962,000, that of

India 553,227,000. These figures may underestimate the numbers of people for whom subsistence agriculture is the main prop of their livelihood strategy and also those for whom it is a minor but important part. Figure 9.1 shows that Africa is the continent in which people are most food-insecure.

In late 2000, of the 32 countries in the world recorded as facing exceptional food emergencies, 16 were in Africa. Table 9.1 shows for each country the reason for the food emergency and the most recently recorded HIV/AIDS data (where these were available). It is important to note that these latter data are likely to be less accurate and to underestimate the scale of the epidemic where civil strife is a factor in food insecurity. There is a predictable association between HIV/AIDS, poor data, civil unrest and food insecurity.

Diversity in livelihoods

For most rural producers, farming is rarely a sufficient means of survival. Practically all rural households have to juggle a diverse portfolio of activities and income sources. To a degree this is so for highly capitalised farmers in the EU or North America. It is vitally so for smallholders in Africa, India and Latin America. To do this they must

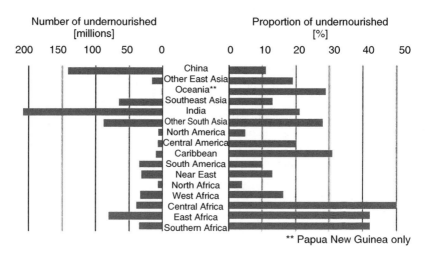

Figure 9.1   Number and proportion of undernourished, by region and sub-region, 1996–98
Source: FAO (2000).

Table 9.1 Food emergencies, causal factors and HIV/AIDS in Africa[3]

Country	Reasons for food emergency	Most recent HIV data	
		UNAIDS 2000 – national adult seroprevalence	*United State Bureau of the Census year and population group as indicated – Rural population groups = 'normally healthy people' and pregnant women*
Angola	Civil strife, population displacement	UNAIDS Adult rate 2.78%	no rural data
Burundi	Civil strife	UNAIDS Adult rate 11.32%	1994 Rural rates 7.3–12.4%
Congo, Democratic Republic	Civil strife, internally displaced people, refugees	UNAIDS Adult rate 5.07%	1997–98 Rural rates 2.5–5.3%
Congo, Republic	Past civil strife	UNAIDS Adult rate 6.43%	no rural data
Eritrea	Internally displaced people, returnees and drought	UNAIDS Adult rate 2.87%	no rural data
Ethiopia	Drought and internally displaced people	UNAIDS Adult rate 10.63%	1995 rural rate 0.4–3.0%
Kenya	Drought	UNAIDS Adult rate 13.95%	1995-98 rural rate 4.0–27%
Liberia	Past civil strife, shortage of inputs	UNAIDS Adult rate 2.98%	no rural data
Madagascar	Drought and cyclones	UNAIDS Adult rate 0.15%	1995 rural rate 0.0%

Table 9.1 Food emergencies, causal factors and HIV/AIDS in Africa[3]   *cont.*

Country	Reasons for food emergency	Most recent HIV data	
		UNAIDS 2000 – national adult seroprevalence	*United State Bureau of the Census year and population group as indicated – Rural population groups = 'normally healthy people' and pregnant women*
Rwanda	Drought in parts	UNAIDS Adult rate 11.21%	1996–97 Rural rate 5.0–12.0%
Sierra Leone	Civil strife, population displacement	UNAIDS Adult rate 2.00%	no rural data
Somalia	Drought and civil strife	UNAIDS Adult rate not available	no rural data
Sudan	Civil strife in south	UNAIDS Adult rate 0.99%	no rural data
Tanzania	Food deficits in several regions	UNAIDS Adult rate 8.09%	1995–98 rural rate 1.5–44.4%
Uganda	Civil strife in parts, drought	UNAIDS Adult rate 8.3%	1995–98 rural rate 1.9–28.3%

nurture 'the social networks of kin and community that enable such diversity to be secured and sustained. Thus livelihood diversity has both economic and social dimensions ...' (Ellis, 2000, p. 3).

In many poor communities (and as we have seen in the case of Rajasthan), farm work is interwoven with occasional short-distance or regular long-distance migration. It may be linked with petty trade in handicrafts and farm produce; it can combine work on the smallholding and wage labour on an adjoining commercial estate. Rural livelihoods can involve non-farm and non-rural activities – including work in factories, coal mines and ports. In a village near Giridih in Bihar, India, most lower-caste men worked away for several months of the year. They went to Calcutta as labourers, and to the small coal-mining towns situated along the railway from Bihar to Calcutta.[4] They could not survive from rural activities alone; annual migration was essential to household survival. In the context of an HIV epidemic, such livelihoods become risky.

When illness strikes it is the domestic–farm–livelihood labour interface which experiences the stress of impact. Not only that, but these diverse activities have implications for susceptibility to infection and the growth of an epidemic.

Most of the examples in this chapter are from Africa, but the indications are clear for rural societies in other parts of the world. India has large numbers of HIV positive people. The picture in China is unclear; there is one report of 20% seroprevalence in a rural community. This is impossible to confirm and is almost certainly atypical.[5] Even such an isolated report is indicative of a growing epidemic.

The rural impact of AIDS

The rural impact of HIV/AIDS is insidious. For the most part it goes unnoticed by agencies and politicians. The seasons and other natural rhythms that frame rural existences mean the pace of this long-wave event's impact will be slow. Each turn of the cultivating seasons will see a small, significant and usually negative change in farming, household relationships and the social fabric of the community. At times there will be step changes when household or community life undergoes marked transition from one level to another: the remaining parent in a household, probably the mother, dies and the family unit is finally dissolved. Most change will be more gradual. Leaving an area uncultivated will be reversible in the short term. But after a point it will be extremely hard to reclaim from the bush – or from others who may have laid claim to it, particularly easy where weak forms of property are common. Property disputes may surface easily when there are opportunities to contest inheritance because landholding is complex and unregistered. Land or equipment sale may well be irreversible and herald a new way of life, for example, permanent migration to town.

For the last two decades HIV/AIDS has affected the ability of increasing numbers of households to access food in quantities and of a quality necessary for active and healthy lives. The impact on food supply and on subsistence agriculture continues and affects ever-wider swathes of Africa. It is neither emergent nor is it something of the past: it has happened to many communities and will happen to others. The process is beginning in Asia.

We have few studies of continents other than Africa; none will tell us very much about the impact of AIDS on agriculture and rural life. Often we have to infer what is happening to agriculture from what is happening to rural households. A recent study of AIDS impact on 600 households in northern Thailand (Kongsin and Watts, 2000; Kongsin, 2001) shows that households where somebody is sick with AIDS are under stress. What it does not show is the agricultural and livelihood implications of this impact. This was not the remit for this particular study. However, the research area, Phayo Province bordering Laos, is very rural. One must conclude that the results of the household study are but the tip of an iceberg which reaches into the rural livelihood systems of this region of Thailand (total population 60.8 million and agricultural population 30.25 million) and those of neighbouring countries. In Laos itself, 4.057 million of the total population of 5.297 million is agricultural (FAOSTAT) and the country has low levels of seroprevalence. This is not true of its immediate neighbours, Thailand and Vietnam, which have much more serious epidemics (UNAIDS, 2000c). It is to be expected, then, that rural areas in all these south-east Asian countries will be affected by the impact of HIV/AIDS.

In those parts of sub-Saharan Africa where the epidemic appears to have peaked, rural households are facing health care costs they cannot meet without selling assets or going into debt. They face labour shortages on their farms. And as the cost of death and illnesses rises, so they see reduction or liquidation of any savings they may have as well as a reduction in their asset base of equipment and animals. And when we speak of 'savings' and 'asset base' in this context we need to recall that in most cases we are speaking of a few dollars, a bicycle and one or two animals.

These material losses are a faint indication of deeper events. Rural households and communities are not only losing material things. People who are sick and troubled call in their social and familial obligations. The effect is breakdown of social solidarity and social bonds (Rugalema, 1999); a thinning of the social fabric. This does not happen equally because such events have gender and class dimensions. Men will have more access to assets than women. The wealthy have more resources to call on, and for longer, than the poor; and these resources are of a different order. The poor call on credit; the wealthy can call on more informal transfers with extended or even indefinite repayment periods because they are known to be people of substance (Lundberg and Over, 2000).

The systemic effects of death and illness

There are wider effects of death and illness. We are not only concerned with households and individuals. The epidemic also affects physical and environmental systems through its effects on the human population. A household has a farm. A farm has internal organisation of crops, labour, livestock, soils and flows of resources such as manure. In each particular climatic and ecological zone, a certain type of farming is possible given the technical capacity and numbers of the human population. This is a 'farming system'.

In subsistence agriculture all is dependent upon timely availability of competent labour. Illness and death bring downshifting in cropping systems and livestock management: a smaller range of crops is grown on a smaller area and husbandry is less punctilious. Livestock are less well-protected from hazards such as straying and theft or from insect pests and predators. A small, inexperienced boy or girl cannot know the best pasture land and does not have the energy to take the animals long distances. In time, the livestock diminish in quantity and quality.

Rural infrastructure is also affected. Labour and skill shortages or disruption of work periods to attend funerals, all have effects on activities that create and maintain the rural environment. Terraces, bunds, irrigation and drainage channels, soil maintenance, cleared areas, bridges, tree planting, erosion defence works, fencing, storage facilities – the list is very long, and all these and more are affected. Failure to maintain water sources and sanitation threatens health further. Studies show that the range, variety and yield of cultivated crops may decline due to labour constraints (Barnett and Blaikie, 1990, 1992; Barnett and Haslwimmer, 1993; Rugalema, 1999). The infrastructure effects may have knock-on consequences: the irrigation works, the drainage channels and terraces decay and so the farming system becomes unsustainable.

When this stage is reached, it is not the household or individual alone which has experienced impact: the agricultural system has undergone a change from which it may not recover. Different agricultural systems, mixes of rainfall, crops, livestock and climate will have different levels of vulnerability to the epidemic. It is likely that dryness, periodicity of rainfall, labour intensity and seasonal concentration of agricultural tasks are key markers of relative vulnerability.

In arid areas such as central Sudan, Mali, parts of northern Kenya and eastern Ethiopia, all planting and weeding has to be completed soon after the end of the rains which come once a year. In contrast, in parts of west and central Africa, there may be two generous rains per year plus high humidity for much of the remainder. The former farming systems are more vulnerable to shortage of labour supply because key cultivation activities are concentrated in the brief rainy season. In contrast, wetter areas can grow a wider range of crops over a longer period. These wetter farming systems are less vulnerable and more resilient. However, by 1989 and 1993, such farming systems in areas of high seroprevalence were already showing signs of stress (Barnett and Blaikie, 1990, 1992; Barnett and Haslwimmer, 1993).

Similar differences in vulnerability of farming systems may be seen in Nepal. Here, cold, high-altitude cropping systems that produce potatoes, barley and some vegetables are more vulnerable than those of the humid tropical *terrai* on the border with India. In the *terrai*, the range of crops is broad and moisture availability more dependable for longer periods. Nepal may be facing a considerable and generalised epidemic; high-altitude farming systems are more vulnerable to labour loss than those of the *terrai*.[6]

Rural livelihoods and local knowledge

There are issues of local knowledge and quality of labour. Labour-intensive irrigation systems may be vulnerable because they are knowledge, experience, administration and politics intensive. Box 9.1 explores such a farming system and how it might be affected by HIV/AIDS. HIV/AIDS will probably have similar effects on any rural system where the management of common property resources is important. This might include forest reserves and rural infrastructure such as terraces and fishponds.

Paul Richards (1985) has pointed out the importance of indigenous experimentation and knowledge for agricultural change and development. He notes much of what may be thought of as 'knowledge' in the

Box 9.1   **Indigenous irrigation systems in Sanpatong District, Thailand**

Indigenous irrigation systems, locally known as *muang fai* are characterised by a weir built across the river to raise water levels, thus allowing water to enter a main canal and pass to the fields. These systems are communally managed, providing water during the rainy season and making cultivation possible in the dry season.

Each *muang fai* has its own organisation. This is headed by a leader who is elected by all water users in the local association. He appoints one or more assistants who act as his *laam* – messengers. Farmers using the system contribute labour and materials to maintain it.

In 2000, a study of the impact of HIV/AIDS on one of these systems, Fai Tacumpa, showed the following changes to cropping:

- a shift away from labour-demanding crops such as rice and chilli to less labour-demanding soya and onions
- a reduction in the areas of wet rice and conversion of these to production of longan fruit – at the time of the study, the area under rice cultivation had decreased from 2,062 *rai* (1 *rai* = 0.6 hectares) in 1990 to 1,460 *rai* in 2000. Approximately 50% of this change was directly attributable to HIV/AIDS.

In addition there were impacts on irrigation organisation and infrastructure:

- in one irrigation association, 50% of water users died of AIDS
- as a result of these levels of mortality, the organisation had to alter its system from demanding labour from its members to demanding money for essential maintenance work
- canal maintenance previously carried out by water association members had now to be done by hiring a bulldozer
- frequency of some canal maintenance fell from twice a year to only once a year. (Thangpet, 2001)

sense of rules and techniques is not that at all. It is the ability to improvise and respond to events. People do not work from a rulebook, they 'manage', using a bit of 'commonsense' here, a little social influence there, a tad of technique, and finally they improvise (Richards, 1993). This knowledge is handed down through families. AIDS can mean that the basic community and family knowledge of how to do farming in these ways in a particular environment disappears. People become ill, others look after them. Soon individual energies are sapped. Knowledge of soils, climate and how to bring people together to co-operate disappears or becomes less widespread. So the rural system is confronted with stress and become increasingly vulnerable to further shocks. This will be so particularly when continuing shocks are combined with declining nutritional status.

There are effects on people's abilities to market surplus or cash crops. Going to market and knowing what to do there is often culturally differentiated between men and women. A widow may find it impossible for reasons of skills, social mores, child care obligations or lack of knowledge to travel from her village to the market centre. For example, in western Uganda in the late 1980s, women did not ride bicycles, it was considered culturally inappropriate. Whereas their husbands had been able to cycle off frequently along the narrow rutted track to the main road 10 kilometres away to sell a small amount of surplus produce, such an undertaking was not within women's socially and culturally defined capabilities.

Subsistence agriculture and AIDS impact: the problem of 'the household'

Commercial agriculture and the commercial sector in general are more able to economise on and minimise the quantity of labour employed (discussed in Chapter 10); small-scale agriculturalists cannot do this.

The domestic–farm interface of production, consumption and reproductive work is complex. Economists and other social scientists may isolate these into individual activities. But for subsistence farmers, farm work, family life and domestic work are not distinguished in practice. People may make sharp distinctions when they talk about their lives. They may say, 'Men never weed the crops – that is women's work; men do the heavy work, ploughing', or 'Men provide the protein, women the starch.' The impact of a death or an illness on such a household goes right to the core of its labour economy, as shown in Figure 9.2.

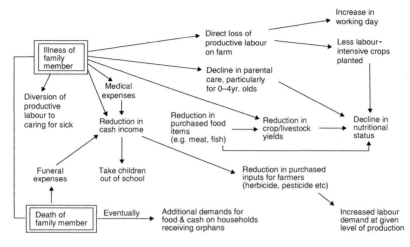

Figure 9.2   Household coping mechanisms in the face of AIDS: impact on the domestic labour economy
Source: Barnett and Blaikie (1992), p. 105.

In Chapter 7, we saw that households are often interdependent and should be considered as 'clusters'. This means that the complexities of AIDS impact are substantial. Rural households do not operate in isolation.

The land

Land is 'owned' in many different ways. There is a continuum from exclusive and enduring use to seasonal rights in communally 'owned' land. We can speak of 'strong' and 'weak' forms of property. Where land tenure is weak and inheritance rules unlegislated, customary and probably fluid, illness and death of a farmer can mean difficult times for household survivors. They face competition from other kin and interested parties. Women and orphans may find themselves thrown off the family's land and on occasions forced to migrate to town to seek a living. This is also an impact of HIV/AIDS and such events have been reported from many parts of east and central Africa.

For subsistence agriculturists there can be no livelihood without labour. But in some circumstances other factors intervene to make agriculture more or less possible. In dryland areas such as Rajasthan in India, where irrigation is practised side by side with dryland cultivation, availability of irrigated land may be the first constraint (Barnett,

1998). Scarcity of such land means that people without irrigation have already relegated agricultural production to a secondary place in their livelihood portfolio, depending primarily upon labour migration (Barnett, 1995). Here it was the poorer 'tribal' Bhil or Adivasi people who were least likely to have irrigated land and most likely to be labour migrants. In upland Nepal, environmental conditions are so unstable as a result of progressive soil erosion, and the climate so demanding, that even if people own land it is insufficiently productive. The result is that labour migration, particularly by young women, has become of the greatest importance in maintaining livelihoods. Both these examples show how availability and quality of land has implications for the relative susceptibility of such communities to HIV/AIDS infection (see Chapter 3) and vulnerability to its impact.

The environment

'Agriculture' does not take place in a predictable environment in either the physical or the policy sense of that word. It is subject to both abrupt and slower long-term changes. The impact of HIV/AIDS on agriculture is likely to be a medium-term but profound change. The main sources of change affecting the agricultural and rural environment are national politics, land tenure rules and laws, climate, disease – both human and animal – and terms of trade for produce.

These contextual considerations may mask the relationship between HIV/AIDS impact on agriculture and rural livelihoods and other events. We may be confronted with people's reports of major changes in their way of life which either they or an observer associates with the impact of HIV/AIDS but where definitive data are not available and where it is not even clear what might constitute 'definitive' information. In that situation it is hard to decide whether HIV/AIDS is a key factor in the reported change, but it is necessary at least to consider this possibility.

For example, in Rakai in 1989 and again in 1993 people complained that since the coming of AIDS they had been increasingly plagued by biting insects in their farms and their homes. They also reported more wild animal damage to crops than had hitherto been the case. We do not know for sure that these were objective events or that they were the result of AIDS. Local accounts of the connection seemed logical: more deaths, more illness, more funerals, less time to devote to cultivation, less land cleared, the bush encroaches on the village providing access for insects and animals. In the absence of contradictory data – for example, satellite images indicating the absence of substantial changes in land use and/or decline in cultivated area – we cannot dismiss these accounts. In any case it is difficult to disentangle these processes from others, particularly when we consider the numerous 'crises' which are said to afflict Africa.

African 'crises' and the difficulties of disentangling the agricultural/rural impact of HIV/AIDS

Chapter 5 outlined the nature of Africa's 'abnormal normality' from an historical perspective. Here we examine contemporary processes happening alongside the HIV/AIDS epidemic. All have major consequences for rural life and economy; many are very slow and difficult to plot and measure. They include:

* structural adjustment policies
* long-term food insecurity
* environmental and/or climatic change
* the absence of a 'green revolution'
* the crisis of state legitimacy.

'Structural adjustment policies' (SAPs) have been described in Chapter 3. The amplitude of their impact is between 10 and 50 years. There was more than one form of structural adjustment. The earliest, most extreme forms were replaced by structural adjustment 'with a human face' (Mehrotra and Jolly, 1997). These tried to target safety-net assistance to those most disastrously affected (Davies and Sanders, 1988). The effects of these policies have been widely discussed and debated (Cornia et al., 1988; Bassett and Mhloyi, 1991; Bijlmakers et al., 1998; Mehrotra and Jolly, 1997; Demery and Squire, 1996). The resulting and undoubted increases in both rural and urban poverty may actually have assisted the spread of HIV by increasing communal susceptibility to infection.

SAPs may have had some positive impacts at the national level and in urban areas. Most rural areas and communities were not able to respond to price signals because of institutional, infrastructural and political obstacles. In some cases, structural adjustment raised agricultural output prices, mainly by removing parastatal middlemen, but it also increased input prices. The net effect was that rural commercial producers were probably marginally worse off, having paid the price of increased uncertainty and adjustment as the policies came into force. But rural subsistence households and communities (who were not selling in the market) faced dramatically increased prices for all their purchases.

Table 9.2   Per capita agricultural production,[7] Africa, 1965–2000

Agriculture (PIN) Net Per-Cap PIN 89–91			Year on year change					
	1965	1970	1975	1980	1985	1990	1995	2000
Africa developed	105.3	104.6	110.1	113.3	99.4	98.0	77.4	89.1
Africa developing	111.7	114.1	107.8	98.2	96.4	98.0	99.4	100.5

Source: FAOSTAT Database, (various years).

Africa is the only continent in which overall per capita food supply has fallen over the past 30 years, Table 9.2 (FAOSTAT).

Few observers see any hope of medium-term improvement, even without the HIV/AIDS epidemic. The problem for many communities is not an overall food shortage, it is insecure and maldistributed food supply.

In Asia the 'green revolution' – a combination of improved seed varieties, fertiliser and irrigation – resulted in increased yields when it was introduced some 30 years ago. It enabled commercialisation of agriculture with consequent increases in productivity and yield. No similar package has been successfully developed for Africa, the institutional, political and economic structures to enable such change have not been present. In the absence of a green revolution, the following two points become more pressing as background to the impact of the HIV/AIDS epidemic on agriculture in Africa: first, the continuing evidence of climatic change; second, the issue of legitimate government.

In recent years, climate change[8] has manifested itself as decreased and less predictable rainfall in parts of Africa. Opinions differ as to whether this is a long-term or cyclical change. Whatever the case, the effects of global climate change are likely to hit Africa hard. African agriculture is 85–90% rain-fed, typically makes up 40% of GDP and is a major component of most countries' export earnings. The continent is vulnerable to short-term climatic variation. This seems to be increasing in southern Africa and has considerable costs for poor households. Southern Africa is likely to experience more extremes: droughts and floods. Other parts of the continent will also experience wider climatic fluctuation than has previously been the case. The major river basins, with the exception of the Congo, may become water-scarce. Increased evapo-transpiration in the arid north of the continent may lead to further and more rapid desertification. This will mean shorter growing seasons and thus increased vulnerability to loss of labour as the timing of agricultural operations becomes less flexible. In west Africa, more frequent and longer dry periods are expected. In east and central Africa agricultural capacity will decline and increased temperature and humidity is likely to create conditions for expanded ranges for malaria, sleeping sickness and other infectious diseases of plants, animals and humans. In Africa, climate change appears as an additional factor, another long-wave event, which will combine with HIV/AIDS impact to challenge the agricultural base of the continent.

The issue of political legitimacy and what governments can do for agriculture is fundamental. Agriculture policy change has to be 'induced' (Hayami and Ruttan, 1971). This requires two basic political conditions: that government *is* able to act and that it *be perceived* as legitimate so that it may act.

Political legitimacy is a long-term problem in most parts of Africa. States are not necessarily competent. The writ of government may not run far from the capital and its right to govern may be contested. At worst, as in the Democratic Republic of Congo, Liberia, Somalia, Sierra Leone, Angola and other countries, war or extreme civil unrest may have been a 'normal' condition for decades. This makes it difficult for societies to respond to any problems or crises; and the polity[9] itself may be and often is the source and focus of crisis. Political uncertainty makes it hard for small farmers to cultivate, improve land and animals and market produce.

What is to be done?

Given the difficulties of disentangling the effects of HIV/AIDS on rural communities in Africa or anywhere else from other environmental, political and economic events, pragmatic responses are needed. We cannot await conclusive scientific proof of how these processes interrelate. It is necessary for agencies, governments and communities to work practically and listen to those people who are living the experience of epidemic impact. Anecdotal evidence may be less conclusive but it is also sometimes a long way ahead of the 'scientific' evidence that moves politicians, donors and multilateral organisations. Experience with AIDS and agriculture lead us to think that the time lag between significant anecdote and quantitative 'evidence' may be as long as 20 years. For example, the first desk study of the impact of HIV/AIDS on agriculture was undertaken in 1988 (Gillespie, 1989); the first field studies were completed in 1990 (Barnett and Blaikie, 1990) and 1993 (Barnett and Haslwimmer, 1993); yet neither the United Nations Food and Agriculture Organisation (FAO) nor the United Kingdom Department for International Development (DfID) – the funders of these early field studies – takes proper account of the disease in its programming. USAID has only begun to incorporate HIV/AIDS into its agriculture sector programming in the last three years.

HIV/AIDS impact and food security

We can summarise the ways in which the HIV/AIDS epidemic appears to be affecting agriculture, household livelihood strategies and hence food availability and security.

To the extent that HIV/AIDS morbidity and mortality impoverishes households, it threatens food security, which consists of a number of components:[10]

- food should actually be available
- people should have access to sufficient food
- supplies should be stable
- food should be of good and dependable quality.

Households are 'food secure' when all four elements are in balance. Instability in one or more elements renders households vulnerable to food insecurity.

Food security is the outcome of food production using mainly family labour, land and other resources; food purchase using household income; and the availability of assets and social claims – being able to borrow an implement or a worker at short notice. Own production takes precedence and provides the bulk of the food consumed by most rural households. However, food purchase or acquisition of food from the market is an important source of food, especially for complementary and nutritious foodstuffs (which includes protein sources such as fish or meat; minerals, like salt; and vitamins, found in fruit and vegetables) which cannot be produced at farm level. Assets such as livestock can be turned into food or cash if need be, while social claims facilitate non-market interhousehold exchange of food and other goods and services.

Adult morbidity and mortality may affect one or all of the elements of food security. Even minor health problems such as sprains, cuts or scorpion stings may have significant knock-on effects if they incapacitate the household member long enough to disrupt the farming cycle.

Illness of productive adults is especially feared among farm house-holds; it reduces the labour supply suddenly and has short- and long-term consequences. This is particularly so when considering the crucial seasonality of agricultural work.

HIV/AIDS affects food security by reducing household ability to maintain a diverse portfolio of activities and to produce and buy food. It results in loss of assets and a severe decline in the insurance value of social networks. The sicker your family member becomes, the more money you may have to borrow from relatives and friends, the more you may seek their assistance. In the end, they say 'No more.'

A farming household's first response is to adopt 'downshifting' mea-sures, changes to the number and range of crops grown. Observed choices have been to sacrifice cash crops for food crops and leafy crops and fruits for starchy root crops. In Uganda in the late 1980s, people reduced their work on coffee that required pruning and marketing in favour of their staple, bananas. Then they cut down on the bananas and vegetables and concentrated on easily cultivated, easily stored and starchy cassava. This is a classic survival change in cropping systems where high value and nutritious crops are progressively substituted for poor-value root crops. Figure 9.3 summarises this transition as reported in rural communities in Buganda in the late 1980s. The figure does not show one actual case; rather, it illustrates a general process.

Most societies discriminate between men and women and older and younger in relation to food access. The effects of the downshift are borne unequally. Chronic food insecurity and high levels of malnutri-tion among children are the results of such change in cropping patterns.

Livestock

The HIV/AIDS epidemic compromises the accumulation, care and husbandry of livestock. They are disposed of to generate cash for care and treatment of the sick, slaughtered for consumption during funer-als, taken away from survivors by other family members, deliberately de-stocked because of shortage of labour, or they may die because of poor management. Loss of livestock implies loss of manure for the farm and loss of products such as milk, meat and eggs for the family. It also means liquidation of important savings for many households.

In many cattle-keeping communities, people share the care of their animals with friends and relatives over a wide geographical area. This reduces the risk of loss in the event of disease or theft. As with reduced

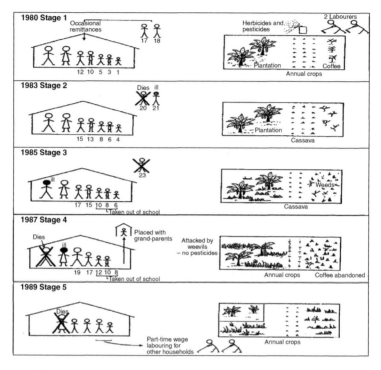

Figure 9.3   The impact of illness and death on cropping patterns in rural Uganda, 1989
Source: Barnett and Blaikie (1992), p. 89.

crop range on the arable side, so reduction of the range of domestic animals kept or withdrawal from such risk-pooling arrangements are all symptoms of the way that AIDS impact makes a household, cluster or community more vulnerable to the next traumatic event.

The interaction between human and plant disease[11]

HIV/AIDS may adversely affect the care of livestock and expose them to disease. The same may be true of crops, where poor human health means poor cultivation and ultimately poor disease and pest control.

Mycosphearella musicola causes a viral disease of bananas called Black Sigatoka. Savoury bananas are the staple for many people living in central and east Africa. This disease has been gaining ground in the region for about 20 years. There is a possible but unexamined relationship between human and plant disease with feedback to human nutrition. It is a relationship to be expected in areas where human populations are affected by major epidemics. The bananas grown in Uganda are tended by stripping off the leaf sheaths which surround the stem of the plant. Local people say that if this is not done the weevil population gets out of control and weakens the plant. When this happens its resistance to disease is reduced and the Sigatoka virus finds a ready host.

This hypothesis points to another channel through which HIV/AIDS may affect entire farming systems and human nutrition. Such changes may go unnoticed and unreported. Those whom these affect have little influence; and government and agencies lack the perspective to track events of this sort. It is of greatest importance that governments, multilateral and bilateral agencies take seriously the need to monitor farming system changes as a result of HIV/AIDS. This is necessary if one of the long-term effects of the epidemic is not to be a steady reduction of rural communities' ability to provision themselves.

As in so many other respects, Africa has suffered worst and earliest from the impact of HIV/AIDS on its agriculture and rural livelihoods. Particularly because of existing and long-term food insecurity it is necessary to confront that impact immediately. But we must be aware of the probability of rural and farm impact in other regions of the world with large rural populations. Here, although food security may not be so critical, rural impact could be serious.

In a 2001 publication entitled *Sustainable Agricultural/Rural Development and Vulnerability to the AIDS Epidemic*, FAO/UNAIDS called upon governments to pay more attention to the real burden of HIV/AIDS on local communities and to ensure that rural development also aims at combating the epidemic. The FAO has finally recognised that HIV/AIDS is not only a health but also a development problem. The report concludes that the rural epidemic has been underestimated.[12] As of December 2001, the FAO, in association with other donors, was beginning to put effort and funds into this problem. The difficulty is that HIV/AIDS shows up the inadequacy of much that this and many other development organisations have been doing for decades. It challenges us to find novel responses.

10
HIV/AIDS and 'For Profit' Enterprise

> The misery of being exploited by capitalists is nothing compared to the misery of not being exploited at all.
>
> (Robinson, 1964)

This chapter looks at how HIV/AIDS affects large organisations mainly using examples from commerce and industry. Many principles can be applied to any large organisation, from a government ministry or department through parastatals to NGOs. Organisations survive by providing services or producing other kinds of output. Business organisations aim to make a profit.

At its simplest, profit is made by selling goods and services for more than the cost of production. The cost of producing goods is a function of inputs including labour, materials and utilities. HIV/AIDS raises costs, reduces the productivity of individual workers and alters the firm's operating environment through:

- increased absenteeism, the result of employee ill health or because staff, particularly women, take time off to care for sick members of their families or because funeral ceremonies are frequent and time-consuming
- falling productivity: workers whose physical or emotional health is failing will be less productive and unable to carry out more demanding jobs
- employees who retire on medical grounds or who die have to be replaced and their replacements may be less skilled and experienced
- recruitment and training of replacement workers incurs costs for an organisation
- employers may increase the size of the workforce and hence payroll costs to cover for absenteeism

- as skilled workers become scarcer, wages rates may increase
- the business environment may change with investors reluctant to commit funds if they think AIDS and its impact will compromise their investments and returns.

Impact of illness and death

There is a normal level of illness and death in the workforce of any organisation. Mortality rates among workers unaffected by AIDS are around 0.4% or 4 per 1,000. This is explicitly and implicitly built into management assumptions about workforce fitness, human resource planning and provision of benefits.

Companies are ill equipped to measure increased levels of mortality and morbidity resulting from this epidemic. It is hard to identify which employees have died of AIDS. The stigma attached to the disease often means that cause of death will be deliberately hidden, sometimes by medical practitioners who defer to family feelings. Without these mortality data, the cost of the disease cannot be calculated.

Some studies have looked at trends in deaths in organisations, correlated these with HIV prevalence in the general population, and assumed increased mortality was due to AIDS. In Zambia (Baggely et al., 1993), the general mortality rate among formal sector employees rose from 0.24% in 1987 to 2.1% in 1993. In the absence of other marked mortality events, the most likely explanation of this increase was HIV/AIDS. By the mid-1990s, the Uganda Railway Corporation had an annual employee turnover rate of 15%. There were suggestions that more than 10% of its workforce had died from AIDS-related illnesses. In Kenya, 43 out of 50 (86%) employees of the Kenya Revenue Authority who died in 1998 died from AIDS. A 1996 study for the Makandi Tea Estate in Malawi showed a sixfold increase in mortality from 1991 to 1995 – from 4 per 1,000 workers to 23 per 1,000 (Jones, 1996).

There is consistent evidence of AIDS impacts in companies across Southern Africa. Table 10.1 shows death rates attributable to HIV/AIDS in Swaziland, Zimbabwe and Zambia are all similar. The slightly lower rates in Zambia and Zimbabwe are because these data are earlier than those for Swaziland (Coutinho, 2000).

A further problem is that people die after they have left the company. Sick employees leave, are medically retired or dismissed before they die. It is not in the interests of an employer to retain workers who are unable to perform and who are chronically sick. Legal

Table 10.1   Comparison of AIDS attributable death rates

Industry	Year	HIV/AIDS attributable death rate
Fridgemasters (manufacturing) Swaziland	1999	7.5/1000
Hippo Valley (sugar) Zimbabwe	1997	5.0/1000
Nakambala Sugar Estate Zambia	1992	6.75/1000
RSSC (sugar) Swaziland	1999	9.41/1000

Source: Coutinho (2000).

protections provide most employees with days of paid and unpaid sick leave. Once these are exhausted the person is dismissed. So, a person is ill for a period and then leaves the organisation. Later they die. How can the organisation know the costs it bore during the period of illness and as result of the death should be ascribed to AIDS?

The broader question is how can an organisation gain a picture of its potential liabilities and the long-term implications of the epidemic for its operations? There have been a number of studies of the cost of AIDS. At first these used accountancy methods and were restricted to costs, they did not engage with the long-term structural and human resource implications of the disease. This chapter begins by considering the accounting approach and its results.

Absenteeism

Work in the early 1990s suggests (Roberts et al., 1996) that the greatest problem confronting companies is absenteeism. A study of African enterprises found that HIV-related absenteeism accounted for 37% of increased labour costs, and AIDS absenteeism accounted for a further 15% (Figure 10.1).

Absenteeism is not only the result of employee illness. It occurs because employees are caring for sick family or friends or attending funerals. In Zambia between 1992 and 1995, absenteeism for funeral attendance increased by a factor of 15 at the country's largest cement company (Smith, 1995). In addition to condoned absences there are those taken without permission, where people simply do not come to work. A company may wish to track absence but will always find it difficult to establish why people are away. Finally there are people who

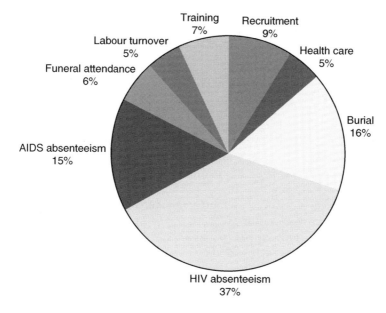

Figure 10.1 Distribution of increased labour costs due to HIV/AIDS by category
Source: Roberts et al. (1996).

are not absent but who are unproductive while they are at work. Employees may force themselves to come to work because if they don't they will lose their jobs. But they are not effective while they are there. In one company where workers operated as 'teams', we were told of people who, with the connivance of their co-workers, spent a shift in the toilets because they were too ill to work. All knew that these workers would be medically discharged if they took more sick leave.

Benefits

The cost of benefits depends on, among other things, conditions of employment, level of staff, local legislation, shopfloor agreements and worker representation. The more regulated an economy, the less likely it is businesses will be able to unload or 'outsource' risk. Where government regulation is weak, companies will offer little in the way of benefits, will rarely be called to account for violation of whatever legislation exists, and will be able to sack workers who are likely to be expensive or disruptive. Thus, in some countries, and in some sectors of most countries, companies are relatively invulnerable to HIV/AIDS impact risk – they can avoid it. Where regulation is more firmly implemented and labour organisations are stronger, company vulnerability increases. This has implications for the global distribution of exposure to vulnerability and ties together the large multinationals and the local household across the globe.

Depending on the environment, on their position in the value chain, on the political milieu, companies may have room to manoeuvre. Benefits are negotiable and it is not axiomatic that they will increase or necessarily cost the firm more. For example, in South Africa many companies offer group life insurance: if an employee dies in service for any reason, the estate receives a multiple of annual salary. This multiple is negotiated with the insurance company annually and can be altered to take account of changing actuarial calculations of risk. If claims go up in any year then premiums rise and employers and employees have the choice of paying more for the same cover or reducing benefits. Some companies in southern Africa have reduced group life payments in response to this. Medical aid and medical insurance provision have been affected. The simplest response is to exclude AIDS from the conditions that are covered under the scheme or to cap the cover provided.

Companies have three choices in the face of increasing costs of benefit schemes:

1. to bear the cost themselves – effectively an increase in the cost of labour
2. to negotiate that the costs are borne by their employees – effectively reducing take-home pay
3. to reduce benefits – paying the same for less.

It is certain that companies will have to adapt. The Chief Medical Officer of the Indian Tata Corporation, annual turnover mid-2000, $215 million,[1] told the authors with great pride how his company offered health care to all its workers, from the CEO to the most recently employed unskilled labourer, and in some cases even offered benefits to whole communities in which it had major activities. The company employed many hundreds of thousands of workers. Its potential risk exposure for HIV was great.

A major South African insurance company's estimate of potential benefit liabilities to the corporate sector is shown in Figure 10.2 (Kramer, 2001). This shows how three benefits – a lump-sum payment on death, a spouses pension and a disability pension – rise in the face of increased mortality and morbidity. In 1995 the cost of these benefits comprised about 7% of payroll costs. By 2010 the figure could rise to 18%.

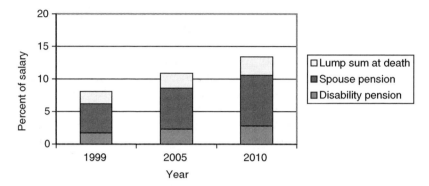

Figure 10.2 Illustrative impact of AIDS on employee benefits in South Africa
Source: Kramer (2001).

At present most companies are not really aware of the impact that AIDS is having on their operations and benefits. Few have management information systems capable of recording and reporting these changes permitting adequate corporate planning. Where life insurance or medical insurance are managed outside a company, then these service providers tend to have a better idea of trends and adjust their policies accordingly.

The impact on markets

Companies want to sell their goods or services. What is the effect of AIDS on the market? Little has been published on this issue and company studies are commercially sensitive and generally unavailable. Informed speculation is necessary.

In certain circumstances, HIV/AIDS could reduce the absolute number of potential customers by altering 'the demographics' of a society. If a market is already relatively saturated with a product and its sustainability depends on increasing population size and growth as well as increasing household and individual disposable income, this market is vulnerable to the epidemic. What should a CEO do when confronted with the following prediction?:

By the year 2003 ... Botswana, South Africa and Zimbabwe will be experiencing negative population growth: down to –0.1 to –0.3% from the 1.1 to 2.3% it would have been without AIDS. This is the first time ever that negative population growth has been projected for developing countries. (Stanecki, 2000)

The demographics of HIV/AIDS reduces numbers of consumers in the 25–49 year age groups. If demand for consumer goods remains strong – because people who are consumers but who die are replaced in employment by those who were previously unemployed – then this does not much matter to companies. If GDP and consumption expenditure are affected, demand falls. Chapter 7 showed that HIV/AIDS reduces household disposable income as treatment and burial costs and the loss of earners use up savings and reduce income. HIV/AIDS may decrease employment as companies choose to mitigate their dependence on labour by increasing capital intensity, using less-skilled labour which is cheaper to replace and has poorer benefits packages, or ultimately relocating to another country. Any of these responses could affect markets by reducing the *number* of consumers or their *capacity* to purchase products.

This has been observed in South Africa where clothing chains offer credit which is written off in the event of the customer's death. Store cardholders may also be offered funeral benefits in the event of their or their dependants' deaths. Such marketing inducements become less sustainable when claims rise. An insurance company in Durban, which underwrites claims on the death and funeral benefits of a major retail chain, reported a 50% increase in the number of claims in 1998. Premiums increase to reflect this (Michael, 2000).

A major South African furniture and household appliance retailer, the JD Group (JDG), looked at the potential impact of AIDS on its consumers. The company estimated that the overall HIV prevalence rate among their customers was 15% at the time of the study, rising to 27% by 2015. The implications of this were:

- the South African customer base would grow slowly until 2010; thereafter the demographic impact of AIDS would be felt, resulting in an 18% decline in customers by 2015 in all provinces bar the Western Cape
- other countries such as Swaziland, Lesotho and Botswana would experience a reduction in market size of about 14% by 2010
- the increase in illness and death meant that consumption patterns would change as consumers reallocated income.

The company concluded that strategic repositioning would be required before 2005. The Group has expanded into Eastern Europe, opening stores in Poland and the Czech Republic (Whiteside and Sunter, 2000, p. 107).

ING Barings and Deutsche Bank endorse this pessimistic view of the southern African market. In 2001, Deutsche Bank looked at soft drinks manufacturer Amalgamated Beverage Industries (ABI) and found that:

- the epidemic will adversely affect demand for the company's products
- ABI's principal products appeal to the young and the wealthy: both of these segments (but in particular the young) will be affected by HIV/AIDS, and it is estimated that a shrinking 'young' population will reduce sales growth by 12.5% over the next ten years
- because the wealthy market is more protected from the impact of HIV/AIDS than the less affluent, ABI has launched new products aimed at them
- increasing capital intensity of production means that the company depends heavily on skilled and educated employees: these are particularly vulnerable and expensive to replace (Deutsche Securities, 2000).

ING Barings forecast reductions in household and government demand in all sectors except health, the greatest effects being on semi-durables, durables and residential buildings (Quattek, 2000, p. 41).

Proactive responses cost money

Companies are not passive in the face of the epidemic. Growing evidence suggests that many are responding. At the least this involves some form of prevention programme, provision of education and condoms. The other extreme is the Debswana example (discussed later in this chapter) where decisions have been taken to provide ART at 90% subsidy for infected workers and their spouses, and to step up prevention programmes and insist that companies doing business with Debswana have anti-AIDS activities in place.

Responses and their associated costs may be accepted voluntarily by companies, or the companies may be forced to take them on by legislation. Voluntary expenditure would include company-supported prevention and control programmes as well as efforts to mitigate the impact. These activities may be motivated by a cost-benefit analysis – where the company takes a hard look at the impact of the disease and establishes that prevention or mitigation activities make economic sense, the returns outweigh the costs. This type of activity has a long history. In the early part of the last century the Rockefeller Sanitary Commission carried out an intensive campaign against hookworm in the southern states of the US. The US-owned United Fruit Company, with its vast, labour-intensive, central American estates, realised that 'it was, in effect, getting the labour from one-half to three-quarters of a peasant, with hookworm taking the profit from the other one-quarter to one-half. In the early 1920s the United Fruit Company began to emulate the Rockefeller antihookworm strategy' (Desowitz, 1997). A review of the programme in 1924 concluded that it had improved both the health of the workers and the profit of the company.

A second motive is social responsibility: the company and/or management feel they have a stake in the society and should respond to the threat of AIDS. At minimum this might include only prevention activities aimed at the workforce, but in some instances could extend to local communities.

Finally, companies may see publicity benefits in being associated with an issue, or conversely do not want bad publicity arising from their failure to act or from seeming to do the wrong thing. For example, Molsens, a Canadian-based brewer, played a key role in sponsoring the business sector satellite meeting at the international AIDS conference in Vancouver in 1996. A reason they gave for this involvement was that their market was young adults, who identified AIDS as one of their concerns. It was therefore important that the company engage with this issue.[2]

Company involvement may not be voluntary. All businesses operate in a legal environment. This regulation extends from shopfloor agreements through the regional and national legislation to international conventions. It may also include international standards or ISOs. ISO is the short name (not acronym) of the International Organisation for Standardisation's benchmarks or standards. ISO is derived from the Greek 'isos' or 'equal'. The international standards of particular interest are:

- ISO 9000 – provides businesses with a framework for quality management and quality assurance
- ISO 14000 – a similar series to the one above, providing a framework for environmental management. <www.iso.ch>

Legislation may require that companies respond to AIDS. One overt (and costly) example was in November 1999 when the Government of

Zimbabwe announced a 3% AIDS levy on individual and company taxes. This money was to be paid into a discrete fund, administered by the Ministry of Health and Child Welfare, and was to be used wholly and exclusively for AIDS activities.

All these responses cost companies money and have to be included in the expenses they incur as a result of the epidemic. But the responses will have benefits that should be offset against the costs.

The business environment

Two studies from South Africa suggests that bankers and brokers are beginning to consider the impact of AIDS for investment (there may have been other and earlier studies but the ones we cite are in the public domain). High HIV prevalence is a disincentive, lack of clear leadership in addressing it compounds this. This is important in the light of the globalisation of production. Only firms which are resource- or market-based have reason to remain in countries where costs to business are increasing.[3] The options of moving or not investing have to be assessed. If the decision is to invest then AIDS increases the risks and decreases the returns.

Methods for describing the impact of HIV/AIDS

Private sector activities are profit driven. Private enterprise does not provide welfare services, although most large companies recognise the relation between employee satisfaction and provision of benefits. Senior managers have to address the following:

- What is the effect of this disease?
- How do we measure it?
- What can we do about it?

This section looks at how, practically speaking, the impact of HIV/AIDS can be understood not only on business organisations but on organisations in general. This is the technique of the Institutional HIV/AIDS Audit.

Table 10.2 summarises the results of four studies which adopted an accountancy approach – using either the wage bill or the operating profit as the main indicator of impact. They looked at costs and tried to ascribe AIDS costs by department, activity or cost centre. These were then added together to provide an estimate of present costs and then projected forward to give an estimate of future costs.

Table 10.2   The impact of AIDS on private sector companies

Country	Company	Impact
Cote d'Ivoire	3 manufacturing companies	0.8–3.2% of the wage bill (Aventin and Huard, 1997)
Malawi	Makandi Tea Estate	6% of operating profit (Jones, 1996)
South Africa	Company 'A'	7.2% of total salary bill (Thea et al., 2000)
Swaziland	Royal Swaziland Sugar Corporation	1.1% of operating profits, 3.4% of pre-tax profits and 4.6% of after tax profits (Coutinho, 2000)

These types of study show that:

- HIV/AIDS has the potential to increase organisational costs over both the short and the long term. These may be significant if management does not act early
- actual costs to an organisation will depend on the stage of the epidemic, the employee profile, the structure of the work, and available benefits
- measuring costs in an individual company is a complex procedure, but it can be done
- the studies are not necessarily comparable because of differences between companies, countries and methodologies
- companies respond both to studies and to their own perception of the epidemic.

This last point is important. Companies are not passive. Because they are profit-focused and competing, and because they have resources, they are able and willing to commission impact studies. The findings of these studies – perhaps the outcome of a scenario planning exercise (see Chapter 6) – become the 'reality' within which the company makes strategic decisions.

The general approach takes the following three components:

1. 'direct costs' – impacts that involve increased financial outlays by the company

2. 'Indirect costs' – reduced workforce productivity less output for a given level of expenditure on labour, including reduced productivity by both the infected employee and by other employees who are diverted from their normal responsibilities
3. 'Systemic costs' – resulting from cumulative impact of multiple HIV/AIDS cases

The method for completing such a study is summarised in Figures 10.3 and 10.4. These are taken from a methodology developed by staff of the Harvard Institute of International Development (Simon et al., 2000). It shows how, through a number of discrete accounting steps, it is possible to arrive at an estimate of the workforce-related costs of the epidemic.

In one company where this approach was applied (Thea et al., 2000), the HIV/AIDS cost was the equivalent of 7.2% of the 1999 salary bill. That is the same as employing more people but without any output or profit benefit. On the contrary, this is a drain on resources and has been described as 'an AIDS tax'.

This is a robust, valuable and coherent method for looking at the problem, but has the following disadvantages:

• it is enormously time-consuming, requiring either that there is an excellent management information system or that resources are committed to going through records and systems and extracting the information
• it does not go far enough: it does not look at the structure of production or administration characteristics of any particular organisation, but restricts analysis to costs associated with the workforce.

Institutional audit

Such questions and many others can be considered through the *institutional audit* methodology. This approach begins from the notions of susceptibility and vulnerability developed in Chapters 4 and 6. It uses these concepts to assess the susceptibility of an organisation's workforce to infection and then employs conceptual and analytical techniques to evaluate organisational vulnerability. (The approach is discussed in detail in Barnett and Whiteside, 2000.) It has been developed with a number of organisations over the past ten years and emphasises a 'troubleshooting' perspective, in contrast to the long-term cost-benefit analysis favoured by others.

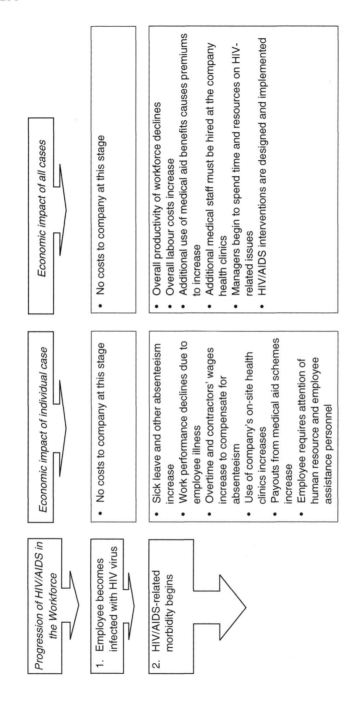

Progression of HIV/AIDS in the Workforce

1. Employee becomes infected with HIV virus

2. HIV/AIDS-related morbidity begins

Economic impact of individual case

- No costs to company at this stage

- Sick leave and other absenteeism increase
- Work performance declines due to employee illness
- Overtime and contractors' wages increase to compensate for absenteeism
- Use of company's on-site health clinics increases
- Payouts from medical aid schemes increase
- Employee requires attention of human resource and employee assistance personnel

Economic impact of all cases

- No costs to company at this stage

- Overall productivity of workforce declines
- Overall labour costs increase
- Additional use of medical aid benefits causes premiums to increase
- Additional medical staff must be hired at the company health clinics
- Managers begin to spend time and resources on HIV-related issues
- HIV/AIDS interventions are designed and implemented

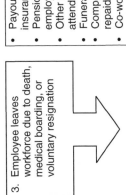
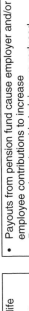

3. Employee leaves workforce due to death, medical boarding, or voluntary resignation

- Payout from death benefit or life insurance scheme is claimed
- Pension benefits are claimed by employee or dependants
- Other employees are absent to attend funeral
- Funeral expenses are incurred
- Company loans to employee are not repaid
- Co-workers are demoralised by loss of colleague

- Payouts from pension fund cause employer and/or employee contributions to increase
- Returns on investment in training are reduced
- Morale, discipline, and concentration of other employees are disrupted by frequent deaths of colleagues

4. Company recruits a replacement employee

- Company incurs costs of recruitment
- Position is vacant until new employee is hired
- Cost of overtime wages increases to compensate for vacant positions

- Additional recruiting staff and resources must be brought in
- Wages for skilled (and possibly unskilled) employees increase as labour markets respond to the loss of workers

5. Company trains the new employee

- Company incurs costs of pre-employment training (tuition, etc.)
- Company incurs costs of in-service training to bring new employee up to level of old one
- Salary is paid to employee during training

- Additional training staff and resources must be brought in

6. New employee joins the workforce

- Performance is low while new employee comes up to speed
- Other employees spend time providing on-the-job training

- There is an overall reduction in the experience, skill, institutional memory, and performance of the workforce
- Work unit productivity is disrupted as labour turnover rates increase

Figure 10.3 Progression of cases and costs of workforce HIV/AIDS

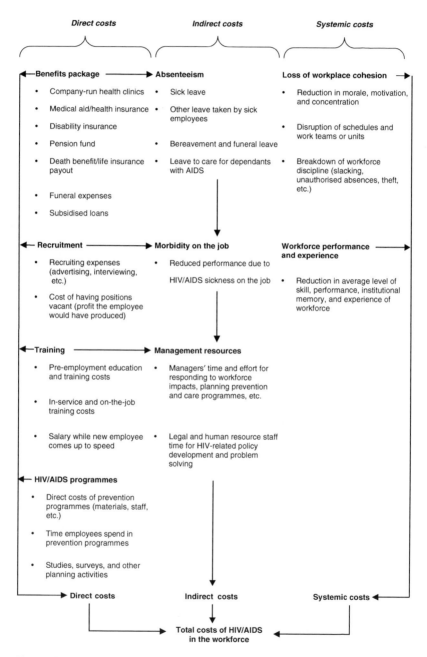

Figure 10.4   Economic impact on the workforce of HIV/AIDS

An institutional audit consists of the following components:

- personnel profiling
- critical post analysis:
- assessment of organisational characteristics
- estimate of organisational liabilities
- productivity
- organisational context

Below we discuss each of these components in turn.

Step 1: Personnel profiling

What kinds of people are employed?

Susceptible groups. Are there particular groups among employees who may be particularly exposed to infection? Why are they exposed? Can/should the organisation do anything to reduce this exposure? Will undertaking such programmes benefit the organisation? Should all employees be included or only those who are most difficult to replace?

Skill levels. What skill levels are there in the organisation? How many at each level? What are the costs of training/replacing these people? Given the known and predicted rates of seroprevalence, how many people might be expected to become ill or die in each year over the next *x* years in each category of employment?

Ease of training and replacement. How easy will it be to train or recruit personnel at each skill level, considering costs and time for training and also the state of the national and regional labour market?

Step 2: Critical post analysis

Are there key personnel whom it will be particularly difficult to replace, on whom a production or administrative process depends (for example the 'institutional memory' or the person who knows how to use the computer)?

Step 3: Organisational characteristics

Size of organisation and 'depth'. How easy will it be to replace or retrain within the organisation? Are there sufficient people to allow for internal training? Should the organisation introduce 'shadowing'? How big is the organisation? Does it have sufficient internal resources to be able to undertake replacement and/or training or replacement of personnel? Is it big enough to move people around to take over other people's jobs? What is the lead-time for training or recruiting a replacement for different skill levels?

Step 4: Liabilities

The potential or actual liability of the specific organisation will be determined by some or all of the following factors.

Level and type of employee benefits. This relates to contracts of employment and considers the benefit packages.

Level of labour value added. For a production organisation or a commercial organisation, this measures the part of gross profit attributable to the work done by labour.

Variables are: the quantity of labour/quality of labour (seen in levels of pay), and labour as a proportion of all inputs to product. In a software design enterprise, the labour value added will be large; in a bottling plant labour value added will be small.

Step 5: Productivity

Reduction in the quality and quantity of labour supplied will be the result if employees fall sick or have to care for sick dependants. Absenteeism may result in slow and hardly detectable decline in output in any organisation. How is this going to be detected and coped with?

Labour/capital substitution. Can capital be used to replace people who are sick or those who die, so as to avoid that risk in the future? Could larger numbers of unskilled workers replace the lost skilled workers?

Out-sourcing and multiskilling. Can non-core functions (for example security and cleaning) be out-sourced? This is a possible solution for the enterprise but it must be noted that while such tactics will shift the problem from the company, it will not solve the problem at a national level. Can staff be trained to have multiple skills enabling them to do their own and others' jobs should the situation demand it?

Step 6: Organisational context

What is the legislative and industrial relations framework? What must an organisation do for its workers in the way of invalidity benefit, keeping them at work while they are HIV positive but are not ill, or when they have AIDS but are not so sick as to be unable to work?

The steps and activities of an institutional audit are summarised in Table 10.3.

Experience with institutional audits: case studies

A number of case studies of institutional audits are discussed below and some key features of the process and outcomes noted.

Critical post constraints: Zambia – Chilanga Cement Company and Nakambala Sugar Estate

These two cases show how critical posts affect a large integrated production unit. Chilanga operates two kilns for manufacturing cement. These are huge, inclined pipes through which a water and limestone slurry is poured and heated, and from which it emerges as pellets that are powdered to make cement. These kilns take several days to heat up and cool down, and, once operating, run continuously 24 hours a day. Each kiln needs one full-time operator. This means that an eight-hour shift requires three operators per kiln, a total of six operators to operate both kilns 24 hours a day. The people are not highly qualified employees. But, according to the company, the more experience they have the better. At the time of the study the company had eight kiln operators to allow for unforeseen exigencies. Even so, if two operators were injured in an accident and one became sick, the equipment could not be operated at full capacity, and in a closely linked continuous chain production process such interruption could adversely affect the entire operation.

At Nakambala (Haslwimmer, 1994), a sugar estate with satellite smallholder outgrowers, a number of major problems were identified. First, this estate produced over 100% of Zambia's sugar requirements. It not only saved the country foreign exchange, but also earned a small amount from exports. Second, the central cane processing plant served the entire complex and needed to operate around the clock during the harvest season. Its routine and emergency maintenance was of the highest importance. This meant that maintenance engineers were key to sugar production in Zambia. Replacement of these key individuals was made more difficult by increased demand and higher wages offered in the South African labour market.

These examples show the importance of critical posts in any institutional audit – quite junior posts may be crucial to the operation of an enterprise. Impact on a small but vital national economic enterprise can have serious knock-on effects to the wider economy. In poor countries where there is limited diversification, HIV/AIDS can have major effects on national economic vulnerability.

Table 10.3 Steps and processes of an institutional audit[4]

Activity	Justification	Outcome	Resources	Challenges and assumptions
1 Internal (and if necessary external) performance/impact appraisal of the organisation	Increase productivity Establish base profitability Establish base sustainability	Identify the necessity and nature of institutional audit In particular: –whether and how many of the next steps are necessary –whether and how many of the steps set out in the text are necessary	Annual financial statements, sectoral legislation, mission statements, strategic plan and previous budget	Systematic organisational management/monitoring tools are used and reports are available
2 Establish the current profile of the organisation – e.g. use SWOT analysis (identify Strengths, Weaknesses, Opportunities and Threats)	Identify new opportunities and possible threats, minimise impact of weaknesses, maximise potential of strengths	Potential susceptibility/vulnerability are agreed and prioritised in the order of their potential impact on institutional productivity and/or sustainability	Consolidated management information system [MIS][5] reports and performance appraisals Independent facilitators and arbiters	MIS and/or performance and/or appraisal systems exist and can be used

Table 10.3 Steps and processes of an institutional audit   *cont.*

Activity	Justification	Outcome	Resources	Challenges and assumptions
3 Detailed Diagnostic Assessment	To define and cost the impact of vulnerabilities which have been identified	Establish baseline for measuring future productivity/ sustainability and/ or organisational growth potential	Outcomes of steps 1 and 2 above	The organisation has come this far in its analysis and still believes that it has a role, a potential market, and an effective workforce
4 Environmental Survey	To quantify the potential market(s), agree strategies for and risks involved in continuing in same market, expanding into another market or ceasing to operate in this market	Agreed strategic objectives, targets and performance standards	Paper/Time consultants and other specialists	That the previous steps have been completed

Kenya: the estate sector

Rugalema's study in Kenya makes important observations about the nature of critical posts in the high-value export-orientated estate sector.

> Examples of units and operations sensitive to loss of labour abound in agro-industry. In *horticulture*, agronomic operations are sensitive to loss of labour and nursery management; weeding and pest controls are very sensitive operations that may result in a total loss of the product. In sugar processing, *pan boiling* and *centrifuging* are crucial and more sensitive to loss of labour than any other operation in a sugar factory. Qualified personnel who work in shifts constantly man the two processes. In case of the absence of qualified personnel, the rest of the sugar processing operations are compromised. In the processing of sisal fiber, *brushing* is very sensitive to loss of labour. Only experienced personnel can do this, the beaters being the most important. Without qualified/experienced fibre beaters, production targets cannot be reached. (Rugalema, 1999, p. 30; original emphasis)

This illustrates the relation between critical posts, enterprise vulnerability, investment climate and national vulnerability. The estate/agro-industry sector is export oriented. Enterprises are either managed or owned by large multinationals or their subsidiaries, and their main markets lie with major foreign companies. Given the substitutability and price volatility of such primary products, the inevitable question is: 'At what stage does HIV/AIDS make production too costly for the enterprises to remain viable?'

Market perception: an NGO[6]

This case highlights issues of market perception and investment climate in a non-production context. It concerns a major NGO working with vulnerable children and orphans through child sponsorship. The organisation has a strong religious core and its supporters in the US and Western Europe are perceived as conservative.

The audit demonstrated that in many ways the organisation was robust. In part it was thought that because of the strong religious orientation of many of its staff, they were less susceptible to infection than the general population. The organisational managers were not unduly worried about potential benefit liabilities and there were no indications of critical posts that might impact negatively upon organisational operations.

As the audit proceeded, it became apparent that the organisation was vulnerable in a curious way that could not have been predicted. Its income stream depended upon retaining long-term donor sympathy. HIV/AIDS had implications for this income stream. Children were being orphaned in increasing numbers; some were infected and were dying in infancy or childhood; older orphans were being infected in their early to mid-teens. These were not messages and images the conservative donor community wanted to see or hear and senior management felt that this presented a marketing problem.

Debswana: process and drug therapy[7]

Ownership of the Debswana Diamond Company is split equally between the Government of Botswana and De Beers. The company is crucial to the country, contributing 33% of GDP, 65% of government revenue and over 70% of foreign exchange earnings. It is one of the major employers and provides a substantial portion of technical training.

The operation includes diamond mines, Jwaneng, Orapa and Letlhakane (these two managed together as the Orapa mine); the Botswana Diamond Valuing Company (BDVC), which sorts and values the diamonds; the Teemane Manufacturing Company, which cuts and polishes diamonds, and Morupule Colliery. The company's head office is in the capital, Gaborone.

Between 1996 and 1999, HIV/AIDS-related morbidity and mortality increased. Ill-health retirements and AIDS-related deaths rose. In 1996 40% of retirements and 37.5% of deaths were due to HIV/AIDS. By 1999 the proportion had risen to 75% of retirements and 59.1% of deaths. The company hospitals recorded an increase in the number of patients with HIV-related conditions; while in the workplaces there was anecdotal evidence of workers going absent or underperforming because of HIV/AIDS.

It was at this stage that the company took a bold decision: to ascertain seroprevalence among the workforce by means of a survey. This was possible because at that time the first saliva-based HIV tests were becoming available. Protocols for the study were discussed extensively with employees and unions. The company made it clear that, as well as giving a picture of the HIV prevalence rate, the results would be used to help determine what form of treatment it could and should provide to infected employees and their dependants.

The results of the survey were shocking. HIV prevalence across all employees stood at 28.8%, highest at Jwaneng mine and lowest at head office. By job band, the prevalence was highest in A and B bands (the bands with the lowest skill requirements) and among the 30–34 year age groups. This is virtually the same prevalence found across the country, indicating that the company HIV/AIDS education campaigns had had neither more nor less impact than national ones.

The foci of the audit were:

- the skill levels in the organisation and their relative infection rates
- the ease of training and replacement of these skills as well as related costs of training and lead times for new recruits to come up to speed
- an analysis of the critical posts to see which groups of workers constituted the focus of vulnerability
- risk reduction strategies in relation to critical posts
- estimating liabilities and costs associated with sickness, death benefits and pensions – bearing in mind that some employees had benefits which would be paid earlier than expected. This has implications for insurance
- developing systems of productivity monitoring
- consideration of potential treatment options and costs.

The audit took place over 15 months and identified the following key issues.

- An overall HIV/AIDS strategy was urgently needed for the group
- Development of a group information system: identification and organisation of information to provide data on the impact of HIV/AIDS had been a major problem during the audit process. The management information system had to be restructured if it were to enable the company to extract accurate and reliable data in relation to HIV/AIDS prevention, treatment and impact mitigation
- Provision for future costs: the company had to be aware of evident and likely future costs
- Enhancement of manpower planning was important for the long-term welfare of the company
- Lifestyle training: as part of the prevention programme, training/educating employees had to be done in new ways. Lifestyle training would also reach out to communities and create a culture of communication about sexual relations

- Restructuring employee benefits: these needed to be flexibly structured. For example, there might be a choice between a gratuity and a pension depending on employee needs. The benefit system should provide incentives for people to stay HIV negative
- Medical issues: treatment, testing and counselling all depend on affordability at individual level, and sustainability at company level. People had to be encouraged to go for voluntary testing
- Legal issues: managers and employees had to be sensitised to legal issues relating to management of AIDS in the workplace
- Productivity issues: the company had to monitor productivity to identify AIDS-related declines
- Critical posts – two sets of workers were identified:
  - dump truck drivers in the mine. These huge trucks, each with a capacity of 170 tonnes, require skilled and experienced drivers. The trucks ideally operate 24 hours a day. In this mine there were 20 trucks and 80 drivers.
  - diamond valuers – who are in short supply and require long training and experience.

By the end of the audit, Debswana had a clear idea of its problems, potential liabilities to its employees, and its obligations and commitments. This enabled the company to take some strategic decisions. Among these was the decision (a path-breaking one) to cover 90% of the cost of ART for workers and their spouses.

Lessons from institutional audits

A wider frame of reference is required if companies and other organisations are to gain a useful understanding of the epidemic for their continuing operations. This is what the institutional audit approach offers. Here we draw out some of the main lessons to be derived from experience with this approach.

Application

Few organisations have management information systems which are adequate to the task of an accountancy approach or institutional HIV/AIDS audit. In one study which included a number of multinational companies, the MIS was so poor that there was no proper record of workers' daily attendance at the workplace (Clancy, 1998). Institutional audits show the benefit of such an MIS.

Implications

Many organisations, particularly businesses, are most interested in the implications of the epidemic for their 'bottom line'. They try to make a simple calculation, balancing the cost of undertaking prevention efforts within the organisation against the potential cost of not doing so. But as all the case studies show, the impact of HIV/AIDS on organisations is not at all limited to the bottom line. Impact may be far more complex than that and potential responses have to more varied and creative as the institutional audit allows.

Response and responsibility

The simplest response for business organisations to increased levels of infection in the population is to avoid the problem. This can be achieved by:

- Moving to an area where there is no AIDS
- Excluding people with HIV from the workforce by testing all applicants and employees and not employing or firing those who are infected. A more subtle response would be to employ people who are less likely to be infected, for example, women over 40 years of age
- Reduce the size of the workforce and/or move to more capital-intensive production methods
- Transfer the problem by out-sourcing all but core functions
- Stopping employees from becoming infected through prevention programmes.

Companies with data on the full economic impact might conclude that the HIV/AIDS prevention programmes can be justified on financial as well as moral, ethical and social grounds. Unfortunately, they may also find that this is not the case. It may be cheaper to replace less skilled employees than undertake prevention programmes or prolong life.

If companies accept that they have and will continue to have infected employees, then a second response is cost avoidance. This strategy has been neglected but it needs to be recognised that

> Transferring costs to government, to household, and to a lesser extent to other companies is a rational response by profit-maximizing businesses, and it should be expected. Of all those affected by the epidemic, private firms have the greatest flexibility in containing and avoiding its costs. Companies will avoid costs because they can; governments and households will bear those costs because, in most

cases, they cannot avoid them. (Simon et al., in Commonwealth Secretariat, 2000, p. 76)

But if this is to be an option, then governments have to take on additional responsibilities. The question is whether they have the ability to do so.

Cost avoidance may involve many of the strategies outlined for avoiding HIV infections – for example, out-sourcing means that all liabilities for worker benefits will be borne by the company that provides the labour. However, additional strategies can come into play, including:

- A change in the structure of benefits which will protect the company from increased costs by increasing employees' contributions or reducing benefit payments
- Ensuring that employees who are ill are medically discharged when they are no longer able to work
- Changes in government provision so that the burden on companies is reduced.

The small business sector

The small business sector is a crucial employer and component of national economies. It includes many 'informal' sector activities that mesh with the activities of larger enterprises. These are at the end of the value chain, the final subcontractor of a subcontractor to a multinational company.

Typically, these small-scale enterprises, which may be one-person or family businesses (and thus they overlap with the household issues discussed in Chapter 7), are engaged in a wide range of economic activities on the margins of the 'formal' or mainstream economy. Their operations are frequently unlicensed and unregulated.

High unemployment in poor countries and the absence of adequate social protection schemes force many (particularly women) to engage in informal sector activity as a survival strategy. In many countries, structural adjustment programmes and neo-liberal economic policies have caused significant socio-economic dislocation, resulting in an expansion of the sector. Trends towards the 'casualisation' of formal sector employment, or the 'informalisation' of production by subcontracting work to lower-cost informal enterprises, have also contributed.

People working in this sector may be more susceptible to infection. They tend to be relatively youthful and therefore sexually active (Soonthorndhada, 2000); they are poor; low education means they are less likely to know how to protect themselves. It is also possible that people entering the sector through choice rather than necessity are, by their very nature greater risk takers in all facets of life, including their sexual behaviours. Furthermore, women in informal enterprises are more likely than women in more affluent households to have to resort to risky survival strategies such as sex for cash in order to supplement household income.

Informal enterprises may individually be particularly vulnerable to the impact of AIDS. This is charted in Figure 10.5, which details the interaction of key elements at the levels of the operator's family, the enterprise and the wider community. The flowchart highlights the impact on the enterprise operator and his or her immediate family, but is also applicable to non-family employees of such an enterprise.

Conclusion

This chapter has shown that consideration of the impact of HIV/AIDS on business organisations and large organisations in general is complex. It is not a simple accounting exercise. The case studies show that impact can be unexpected and go far beyond the 'bottom line'. Indeed, one of the results of institutional audits is to show that the key vulnerability of the organisation lies less in the bottom line than in the production process itself or in the investment or market climate.

For the small business at the end of the value chain, vulnerability issues overlap with those of the household. The smaller the business, the deeper its location within the unregulated, 'informal' sector, the greater its vulnerability to illness and death of its proprietor, sole worker or employees.

Just how limited poor world responses have been is illustrated by the recent publication, *The Business Response to HIV/AIDS: Impact and Lessons Learned* (UNAIDS, 2000h). This gives 17 profiles of business activities in response to HIV/AIDS. There are only eight from the poor world: two each from Thailand, South Africa and India, and one each from Brazil and Nigeria. The rest are international organisations or from the rich world. Only two responses go beyond education and pre-vention. In Brazil, Volkswagen focused on prevention, control and treatment of people living with HIV/AIDS. The care programme resulted in a 90% decrease in hospitalisation and a 40% reduction in the costs of treatment and care. In Thailand, American International Assurance introduced an innovative evaluation and accreditation pro-gramme. Companies with programmes accredited by the Thailand

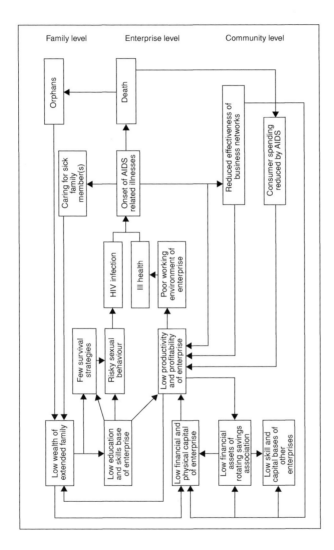

Figure 10.5 Vulnerability of the informal sector to HIV/AIDS

Business Coalition on AIDS are rewarded by credits on group life assurance premiums.

Global production processes mean that companies are more and more mobile and less and less liable to be called to account in any one country. HIV/AIDS shows how the costs of disease and its consequences can be shifted on to households and governments in poor countries.

11
AIDS, Development and Economic Growth

AIDS and development

Economic growth is the promise that governments offer to people. Continued delivery of growth affords legitimacy to government. Economic growth is the means; 'development', improved living standards, better quality of life – all these are the ends. But what is development?[1]

We don't know how to describe development, but we know it when we see it. And, perhaps more importantly, people who want it know when they don't have it! And exactly what development is will depend on peoples' perspective. For a poor villager in remote Rajasthan, development may mean clean water and a good education for his or her children plus not having to migrate in search of an income for half of each year; for a Malaysian it might mean his or her own vehicle and satellite television.

Development implies either tangible improvement in individual or national circumstances, or belief in change for the better. People need to be able to look to the future and have something to aim for – some goal, some promise. Individuals, communities, societies and nations set goals and have projects. Having a view of the future depends on individual health, well-being and capabilities.

Evidence suggests that in some societies the epidemic means that individuals are rethinking their personal goals (MacPherson et al., 2000). Poverty and absence of hope for the future have paradoxical and apparently contradictory effects on attitudes to risk. People may take short-term health risks to earn a living, for example, the rubbish pickers on the burgeoning garbage tips of many major cities.

Box 11.1   What is development?

Development cannot be defined in any simple way. It is a political and cultural term in everyday use. It is therefore heavily disputed. A product of 'Western' thought, culture and political interests, it has often been used as though it were technical, neutral and merely descriptive. In this sense it is used to describe the goals of higher levels of life, improved efficiency of production and distribution, increased social and economic scale and continuing growth, and in some respects of 'Westernisation', repetition of the supposed direction and narrative of Western history to become 'modern'. Recently, when used in this way, efforts have been made to put issues of distribution to the fore. This is seen in the use of the Human Development Index and of human rights as part of the approach advocated by the United Nations Development Programme. In contrast, many commentators from the both the 'north' and the 'south' and from within the environmental movement now question it as a goal. This is particularly true of those writing from a postmodern perspective. The result is a paradox. Many governments, intellectuals and ordinary people in the 'south' still aspire to these goals while some intellectuals in the 'north', and to some extent in the 'south' and from the environmental movements, would discard it as desirable or possible. Some would now reject development as a goal, placing the emphasis on 'sustainability' and environmental conservation. Others would continue to seek it for the future it promises.

While intellectuals, some ordinary people and some politicians reject the goal or even the possibility of development, other intellectuals, other politicians, swathes of the world's poor and many states continue to demand it in its simplest forms: clean water, enough food, civil order and a future for their children. The conflicts between economic growth, environmental sustainability, equity and distribution can only be resolved by political negotiation and compromise. This is the greatest challenge for relations between and within societies and most difficult to meet in a context of globalisation. (Barnett, 2001)

'The idea of development was once a towering monument inspiring international enthusiasm. Today, the structure is falling apart and in danger of total collapse.' (Wolfgang Sachs, quoted in Hoogvelt, 2001)

They are also quite risk averse; the poorer you are the less likely you are to take risks with the few resources you may have accumulated. The shorter the timeframe that people have, the more short-term risks they take with their health and the less willing they are to risk their limited assets which must be used for short-term survival. They are unwilling to invest for the future. A Zimbabwean who believes he or she will live only 40 years will not invest in education, housing and savings. What are the consequences for economic growth and development of such AIDS-induced stances towards risk?

The goals and projects of governments in the poor world are articulated in their national development plans. These set targets for areas such as education, health and transport and detail how the goals are to be achieved. HIV/AIDS means these development targets will not be achievable. Over the next few decades, gains will be slowed and some past achievements reversed.

International development targets

The international community has a set of development goals. Donor agencies and multilateral organisations subscribe to these general goals while differing as to the means to achieve them. There is no evidence at international levels that the impact of HIV/AIDS has been appreciated or that those development goals have been rethought or strategies reworked.

The Development Assistance Committee of the Organisation for Economic Co-operation and Development (OECD) articulated a set of global and international development goals in 1997. These are supposed to be 'ambitious but realisable'.[2] The specific goals are:

Economic well-being:
- a reduction by one-half in the proportion of people living in extreme poverty by 2015.

Social development:
- universal primary education in all countries by 2015;
- demonstrated progress towards gender equality and the empowerment of women by eliminating disparity in primary and secondary education by 2005;
- a reduction by two-thirds in the mortality rates for infants and children under age 5 and a reduction by three-fourths in maternal mortality, all by 2015;

- access through the primary health-care system to reproductive health services for all individuals of appropriate ages as soon as possible and no later than the year 2015.

Environmental sustainability and regeneration:
- implementation of national strategies for sustainable development in all countries by 2005, so as to ensure that the current trends in the loss of environmental resources are effectively reversed at both global and national levels by 2015. (OECD, 1997)

These targets have influenced the public stances of most of the major donor agencies.

Attacking poverty is the goal that resonates best with donors and in their policies. The World Bank articulated its 'poverty reduction policy' in 1998 (World Bank, 1998) and in 2000 began its Development Report with the statement:

Poverty amid plenty is the world's greatest challenge. We at the Bank have made it our mission to fight poverty with passion and professionalism, putting it at the centre of all the work we do. And we have recognised that successful development requires a comprehensive, multi-faceted, and properly integrated mandate. (World Bank, 2000/01, p. v).

The European Union's new co-operation agreement with the African Caribbean and Pacific states has, as its cornerstone, poverty alleviation. Britain's Department for International Development 1997 White Paper recognises that development is 'first, and most importantly, about the single greatest challenge which the world faces – eliminating poverty'.

The HIV/AIDS epidemic means development goals and the way development is carried out need to be rethought. The consequences of HIV/AIDS have not been properly considered by anyone. Development organisations, NGO, bilateral and multilateral, have come late to this problem and then only paid it lip service, often in the form of the twenty-first century's substitute for action – a website or a CD rom. Worse, existing development indicators do not reflect the impact of AIDS nor can they measure its complex adverse consequences. Table 11.1 summarises the OECD goals and how HIV/AIDS might impact on them.

Table 11.1 HIV/AIDS and international development targets

Development goal	Effect of HIV/AIDS	Global and national impact
Reduction by one-half of proportion of people living in extreme poverty by 2015	AIDS increases poverty especially at the household level, has serious impact on human capital	Will slow global progress, some national impact but population decline reduces this, main impact at community/household level. Goal hard to achieve
Universal primary education in all countries by 2015	Impact on supply of education through teacher deaths and resources, on demand side through uptake especially female students	Worst affected countries will see declining enrolment especially among most vulnerable groups. Goal harder to achieve in some countries
Demonstrated progress towards gender equality, women's empowerment by eliminating disparity in primary and secondary education by 2005	Girl children most likely to be kept out of school to provide care or when resources are limited	Disparity will not be reduced with out targeted intervention. Goal harder to achieve
Reduction by two-thirds in the mortality rates for infants and children under age 5 by 2015	Infant and child mortality will continue to increase for the next decade and possibly longer	The target will not be met and in some countries there will be deterioration over the period
Reduction by three-fourths in maternal mortality by 2015	Little impact recorded to date	No impact recorded
Access through the primary health-care system to reproductive health services for all individuals of appropriate ages and no later than 2015	Demand from HIV/AIDS patients will put pressure on the public health-care system, additional human and financial resources required	Will require more resources than previously envisaged. Goal may be more difficult to achieve
Implement national strategies for sustainable development in all countries by 2005, to reverse the loss of environmental resources by 2015	Little impact recorded to date, but may be some – and surprising, e.g. loss of skills, increased demand for wood for cremation or land for burial	Not yet known

AIDS and poverty

The overarching international goal is poverty reduction. The 2000/1 World Development Report 'seeks to expand the understanding of poverty and its causes and sets out actions to create a world free of poverty in all its dimensions' (World Bank, 2000/1, p. v).

Since 1996 there has been a slight decrease in the percentage of global population living in poverty, but the absolute number has risen (Table 11.2). There are wide disparities between regions and within countries.

Table 11.2   Global population living on less than US$1 per day

	1987	1990	1993	1996	1998
People (million)	1183.2	1276.4	1304.3	1190.6	1198.9
Share of population (%)	28.3	29	28.1	24.5	24

Source: World Bank, *World Development Report* 2000/01.

The relationship between poverty and HIV/AIDS was explored in Chapter 5, where we suggested why and how poor people are more likely to be infected. The converse relationship, how HIV/AIDS contributes to and exacerbates poverty, has been examined in the last four chapters. Vulnerability to impact will be determined by the relative wealth of people, households and societies. Poverty assists the spread of HIV and AIDS pushes people into poverty or makes it harder for them to escape from it.

Poverty is more than financial deprivation. This was recognised by the UNDP, which began publishing a *Human Development Report* in 1990. The first report opened with the statement: 'The real wealth of a nation is its people. And the purpose of development is to create an enabling environment for people to enjoy long, healthy and creative lives. This simple but powerful truth is too often forgotten in the pursuit of material and financial wealth' (quoted in UNDP, *Human Development Report*, 1999, p. 1). The Human Development Index (HDI) introduced in 1990 is designed to capture as many aspects of human development as possible in one simple composite index, producing a ranking of human development achievements. This is described in Box 11.2.

The UNDP recently introduced a new index, the Human Poverty Index (HPI), and this is intended to provide a measure of poverty. This combines the following components:

Box 11.2:   The Human Development Index and Life Expectancy

The goal of development is that people should be enabled to live long, informed and comfortable lives. The HDI determines how nations and regions of nations compare with each other and over time. It is constructed from three indices:

- life expectancy which is a proxy indicator for longevity
- educational attainment which is measured by literacy and enrolment rates
- standard of living which is measured by real GDP per capita

The 'Life Expectancy Index' was devised using the highest life expectancy value as 85 and the lowest as 25. It is calculated by taking:

Actual value – minimum value
Max. value – minimum value

In other words, the HDI life expectancy at birth has a maximum value of 85 years and a minimum value of 25 years. Thus, if life expectancy at birth is 65 years in a particular country, then the life expectancy index for that country would be calculated as follows:

$$\frac{65 - 25}{85 - 25} = \frac{40}{60} = 0.667$$

- percentage of people expected to die before 40 years of age
- illiteracy
- percentage of people without access to health services and safe water and percentage of children moderately or severely underweight for their age.[3]

How are these indices affected by the AIDS epidemic? Do the HDI and HPI provide insights into the current and potential impact of HIV/AIDS? The answer is a qualified no.

One of the most measurable impacts of AIDS is on mortality rates.[4] Adults and many infants and children are dying prematurely. This impact is measured in the HDI through the life expectancy component. Table 11.3 shows how AIDS mortality has affected both life expectancy and HDI scores and rankings for selected countries. Botswana is worst affected

Table 11.3   Life expectancy and place in the HDI (selected countries)

	1996 Report (1993 data)		1997 Report (1994 data)		2000 Report (1998 data)	
	Life expect.	*HDI (rank)*	*Life expect.*	*HDI (rank)*	*Life expect.*	*HDI (rank)*
Cambodia	51.9	0.325 (156)	52.4	0.348 (153)	53.5	0.512 (136)
Thailand	69.2	0.832 (52)	69.5	0.833 (59)	68.9	0.745 (76)
Botswana	65.0	0.741 (71)	52.3	0.673 (97)	46.2	0.593 (122)
Cote d'Ivoire	50.9	0.357 (147)	52.1	0.368 (145)	46.9	0.420 (154)
Kenya	55.5	0.473 (128)	53.6	0.463 (134)	51.3	0.508 (138)
Malawi	45.5	0.321 (157)	41.1	0.320 (161)	39.5	0.385 (163)
South Africa	63.2	0.649 (100)	63.7	0.716 (90)	53.2	0.697 (103)
Zimbabwe	53.4	0.534 (124)	49.0	0.513 (129)	43.5	0.555 (130)
Zambia	48.6	0.411 (136)	42.6	0.369 (143)	40.5	0.420 (153)
Haiti	56.8	0.359 (145)	54.4	0.338 (156)	54.0	0.440 (150)

Source: UNDP, *Human Development Report* (1996–2000).

and fell from 71st to 122nd. Even Thailand, where the epidemic is under control has been affected. Life expectancy has fallen slightly and this has contributed to the fall from 52nd to 76th place in the HDI rankings.

The UNDP data are a couple of years old and in a rapidly evolving epidemic they do not pick up its full impact. The alternative source of life expectancy data, the US Bureau of the Census, gives grim figures projected to 2010. It compares life expectancy 'with AIDS' and 'without AIDS'. Table 11.4 shows this for selected countries. The figures speak for themselves.

Table 11.4   Life expectancy, 2000, 2010 (selected countries)

	2000 life expectancy		2010 life expectancy	
	With AIDS	*Without AIDS*	*With AIDS*	*Without AIDS*
Cambodia	56.4	60.2	59.8	64
Thailand	68.6	71.2	71.7	73.8
Botswana	39.3	70.5	29	73.2
Cote d'Ivoire	45.2	58.1	43.4	62
Kenya	48	64.9	44.3	68.4
Malawi	37.6	53.3	35.8	57.3
South Africa	51.1	65.7	35.5	68.3
Zimbabwe	37.8	69.9	32.2	72.8
Zambia	37.2	58.9	38.9	62.8
Haiti	49.2	56.6	51.5	60.4

Source: US Bureau of the Census, (forthcoming).

Social development goals

International social development goals include universal primary education by 2015 and 'measured progress' towards gender equality and the empowerment of women by eliminating disparities in primary and secondary education by 2005. These goals will be hard to achieve in AIDS-affected countries. Children will miss education. Once children are orphaned their chance of education slips away. Female children are most likely to be taken out of school, widening gender disparities.

Worst affected will be the goal of a two-thirds reduction in mortality rates for infants and children under the age of five. In the absence of interventions an infected mother has about a 30% chance of transmitting HIV to her infant. Most infected children will not reach their fifth birthdays. In addition, some mothers of uninfected children will die of AIDS, and evidence shows that orphans have higher mortality rates. The economic and social stress associated with having AIDS in a household further reduces life chances of infants and young children.

Table 11.5 shows child mortality with and without AIDS. The effect of AIDS on this basic indicator is horrifyingly apparent. Effective and cheap interventions are available, a single dose of Nevirapine considerably reduces the chance of transmission. This is the only area where a quick, inexpensive and achievable intervention could significantly influence an international development target. However, this leaves unresolved the cost of additional orphans. While these children are

Table 11.5   Child mortality, 2000, 2010 (selected countries)

	2000 Child Mortality rate per 1000		2010 Child Mortality rate per 1000	
	With AIDS	*Without AIDS*	*With AIDS*	*Without AIDS*
Cambodia	107.7	98.5	83.5	73.2
Thailand	41.9	36.8	29.3	25.5
Botswana	136	38.9	169.5	27.1
Cote d'Ivoire	155.6	125.8	129.1	83.5
Kenya	110.1	70.1	107.4	50.9
Malawi	219.6	175.4	202.6	137.3
South Africa	119.6	65.6	146.6	47.6
Zimbabwe	132.8	41.3	153	28.8
Zambia	168.8	106.5	145.7	79.9
Haiti	155	137.8	124.7	106.3

Source: US Bureau of the Census, (forthcoming).

Table 11.6   Comparative infant and child mortality rates, 1998

Country	UNDP *Human Development Report 2000* (1998 data)		World Bank *World Development Indicators 2000* (1998 data)	
	Infant mortality	*Child mortality*	*Infant mortality*	*Child mortality*
Botswana	38	48	62	105
Kenya	75	117	76	124
Malawi	134	213	134	229
South Africa	60	83	51	83
Uganda	84	134	101	170
Zambia	112	202	114	192

saved from premature death due to HIV infection, they lose their mothers.

Data from the UNDP and the World Bank are equivocal. Table 11.6 shows that:

• there are unexplained data incompatibilities
• it is not clear whether either organisation takes the impact of AIDS into account, and if so, for which countries.

This is further discussed in Box 11.3.

Box 11.3   Data problems

The Bank and UN are producing different figures. It is not clear where the demographic impact of AIDS is being considered. It is factored into UN data for some countries. The UN included HIV/AIDS in its 1997 *Human Development Report*, but not for all countries. The 1998 *Human Development Report* has the following statement:

The 1996 revision incorporates the demographic impact of HIV/AIDS in the population estimates and projections for developing countries where HIV seroprevalence had reached 2% in 1994 or where the absolute number of infected adults was large: Benin, Botswana, Brazil, Burkina Faso, Burundi, Cameroon, the Central African Republic, Chad, the Congo, Côte d'Ivoire, Democratic Republic of the Congo, Eritrea, Guinea-Bissau, Haiti,

India, Kenya, Lesotho, Malawi, Mozambique, Namibia, Rwanda, Sierra Leone, the United Republic of Tanzania, Thailand, Togo, Uganda, Zambia and Zimbabwe. (p. 127)

The 1999 *Human Development Report* added Cambodia, Ethiopia, Gabon, Liberia, Nigeria and South Africa.

The note was dropped from the 2000 *Human Development Report* so we must assume no new countries have been added. This means that Swaziland, with HIV prevalence at over 30%, has life expectancy indicated at over 60 years.

We don't know if or how AIDS is being considered in the World Bank's *World Development Report* – which does not give us data for all countries anyway. Up to 1998, the *World Development Report* contained a mass of statistics in its *World Development Indicators*. In 1998, the *World Development Report* changed and many statistics previously included were omitted, as indeed were a number of countries. The new document, *World Development Indicators*, purports to be comprehensive but the user guide states: 'Selected indicators for 58 other economies – small economies with populations of between 30,000 and 1 million, smaller economies if they are members of the World Bank, and larger economies for which data are not regularly reported are – shown in Table 1.6.' In other words detailed data on 58 countries are omitted. It is perhaps unsurprising that data are not provided for countries like Afghanistan, Liberia, and Somalia: it is a source of concern that the only data available for others like Bahrain, Swaziland and Fiji, are gross national product, life expectancy, adult illiteracy and carbon dioxide emissions.

The third and fourth social development goals relate to access to health care. The targets are 75% reduction in maternal mortality and access through the primary health care system to reproductive health services as soon as possible, and no later than the year 2015. How will AIDS affect these goals? We believe that access to health care will be more difficult due to increased demand and reduced supply. It is unlikely that these goals will be achieved.

Does it matter? Do people take any notice of goals and indicators? Do they notice how things are changing, and in the case of HIV/AIDS, for the worse? Certainly the authorities in Botswana sat up and responded as that country slipped down the UNDP's HDI rankings in the late 1990s.

HIV/AIDS and development: the real costs

In the absence of life, all other indicators are irrelevant. AIDS causes premature death and means that international, national, and personal development goals and aspirations are not achievable. These deaths appear at the aggregate level as decreased life expectancy and increased infant and child mortality. It is difficult to assess the degree to which the HIV/AIDS effect is felt beyond these limited indicators because:

• The indicators are based on the demographic event of death. AIDS deaths are preceded by a period of long, debilitating and unpleasant illness. This is not reflected in the gross indicators we have available
• The disease has unexpected and long-term consequences, for example, enrolment in primary education decreases because parents cannot afford to send children to school. Child labour is needed at home. Teachers are sick or have died so there is no school. This will affect human capital stocks, will increase child mortality in the next generation (mother's levels of education are a good predictor of this), and could maintain infection rates.

One way to assess the impact of AIDS other than through numbers of deaths is to look at the burden of disease[6] expressed as disability adjusted life years (DALYs). DALYs are calculated by estimating the years of life lost to a specific disease or to disease in aggregate. DALYs express loss to a disease as a unit of life and time, as a percentage of the total health burden, or in relation to total population. Apart from its complexity this approach has its own limitations. Health is a continuum. You can be located anywhere on it from mortally ill to sparklingly healthy. DALYS only measure life years and fail to capture the idea of 'quality of life'. Health economists have developed the idea of quality adjusted life years (QALYs), to try to measure both quantity and quality of life lost to specific diseases. DALYs and QALYs are still in development; their calculation is impenetrably complex for the non-specialist and probably inappropriate for use by policy makers.[7]

Although we are in the third decade of the epidemic, the international development community has not taken AIDS on board. There is little appreciation of what HIV/AIDS means for development targets. Those charged with measuring development have failed to respond. Their indicators do not pick up the impact of the disease, because they are based on historical data and take no account of current and future impact. Even with existing data it is not clear what is and is not included; and those who prepare the data do not compare with and without AIDS scenarios. This is a long-wave event. The impacts are complex and possibly self-reinforcing. Development targets need to be revised in the light of HIV/AIDS – along with the measures of 'development'.

National economic growth

Economic growth is necessary for national development. Growth creates wealth, increases employment opportunities, raises government revenue and improves material well-being. Will HIV/AIDS affect economic growth? Early in the epidemic people believed AIDS would slow growth. Showing that AIDS resulted in slower growth and smaller economic output was an argument for spending resources and mobilising political commitment to support prevention measures. In the 1980s a few economists were asking:

- Would national output grow more slowly or even decline because of AIDS?
- What would the effect be on per capita incomes?

The gross domestic product (GDP) and the gross national product (GNP) measure economic output. GNP is the total value of output from an economy; GNP is calculated by taking the GDP figures, subtracting outflows of wealth and adding any inflows. In some countries GNP is higher than GDP because of migrant remittances and inflows of foreign aid. For example, in the Philippines GNP is US$78.9 billion while GDP is US$65.1 billion.

GDP and GNP have limitations as indicators. Most obviously they are *economic* measures. Life and quality of life is about more than economics. Per capita indicators are crude averages. Output is simply divided by population. The measure does not consider how the wealth of a country is distributed among people. Chapter 5 argued that income distribution may be more important than overall level of income in determining how the epidemic spreads and how it is tackled.

The effect of the epidemic is felt through increased sickness (morbidity) and higher death rates (mortality). Understanding the macroeconomic impact of HIV/AIDS is not easy. The epidemic is a *long-wave event*, and so also are economic trends which reflect its impact. And economic policies take time to evolve and alter things. The macro-economic consequences of AIDS have to be understood through econometric models.

Modelling the economic impact of AIDS

A number of models have been developed to look at this problem. In 1992 Mead Over (1992) of the World Bank published one of the earliest. It looked at how AIDS affected economic growth in 30 African countries through its effect on the labour force, capital accumulation and other factors. The model projects economic growth rates with and without AIDS from 1990 to 2025 and suggests that:

- there are two key parameters: the distribution of infection and hence illness and death across the labour force; and the degree to which the illness will be funded from savings and hence limit investment
- under all scenarios AIDS meant economic growth rates would be 0.56–1.47% lower
- GDP per capita impact is less clear cut. If the costs of AIDS are not financed from savings and most illness is among lower skill levels then per capita income could rise by 0.17% across the 30 countries and 0.13% in the ten worst affected. If all the costs are met from savings and illness is concentrated among the highest skill levels then per capita income would fall by 0.35% across the 30 countries and 0.60% in the ten worst affected.

This work was done a decade ago but nonetheless most subsequent models have come up with similar figures.

✦ Most recent cross-country comparisons indicate that AIDS has had an impact. It is estimated to have reduced Africa's economic growth by 0.8% in the 1990s (Bonnel, 2000b). HIV/AIDS and malaria combined resulted in a 1.2 percentage point decrease in per capita growth between 1990 and 1995.[8]

There are two groups of country-specific studies: the first in the early to mid-1990s, followed by a flurry of studies in 2000. The models and their findings are summarised in Table 11.7.

The studies became more sophisticated, considering additional variables. These included work on Cameroon (Kambou et al., 1992) and Tanzania and Malawi (Cuddington, 1993a, 1993b; Cuddington and Hancock, 1994a, 1994b). Their results did not vary much: GDP grew more slowly with AIDS than it did without AIDS, and the per capita income effect was sensitive to assumptions – it could rise or fall. The macro-economic impact of AIDS was likely to be negative but small, even over a 25-year period.

Similar results come from the Futures Group International advocacy documents.[9] The advocacy packages and associated publications have been developed for Bénin, Ethiopia (and Addis Ababa City alone), Ghana, Haiti, Kenya, Madagascar, Mozambique, Zambia and Zimbabwe. The Futures Group has been influential in showing policy makers that AIDS is more than a health issue and has economic consequences. However professional economists, central banks, and Ministries of Finance remain, for the most part, unconvinced by all models. This is because very large-scale long-wave events are difficult for them to see, models are hard to understand, and there is a general denial of the problem.

However in 2000 there were signs of serious interest in macro-economic impact and a number of important papers appeared (Bonnel, 2000b; Nicholls et al., 2000b; Arndt and Lewis, 2000; BIDPA 2000b; Dixon et al., 2000; Quattek, 2000).[10] Why this renewed interest? The answer to this question shows that the impact of the epidemic is now inescapable. This was finally recognised by the world community at the UN General Assembly Special Session on HIV/AIDS held in New York in late June 2001.

It can no longer be denied as people see that:

- the scale and speed of the epidemic is worse than expected
- known demographic effects are now such that recognition of economic consequences is unavoidable
- there is evidence of impact at micro levels, making macro impacts credible
- The complexity of the disease and the scope of its consequences is better understood; for example, loss of key government workers means work is not done efficiently, investment is reduced and economic growth slows
- The development consequences of the disease are becoming apparent, in these circumstances there must be a macro-economic impact

The most recent publications come from South Africa (two papers) and Botswana (one). Why the focus on Southern Africa? This may be because here data are available, as is the capacity to carry out such

Table 11.7 Comparisons of macro-economic studies

Country/region	Predicted impact	Author	Forecast dates
Africa and sub-Saharan Africa	Annual GDP growth 0.56–1.47% lower than without AIDS Annual per capita growth will be between +0.17% and –0.6% compared to without AIDS	Over (1992)	1990–2025
Tanzania (a) Solow-type growth model	Annual GDP growth falls from 3.9% without AIDS to 2.8–3.3% Annual GDP per capita growth falls from 0.7% without AIDS to 0.2%–0.7%	Cuddington (1993a)	1985–2010
Tanzania (b) As above but introduces dual labour market	AIDS reduces real GDP by 11% to 28% over period Per capita income change rangesfrom rise of 3.6% to a decline of 16.1% over period	Cuddington (1993b)	1985–2010
Malawi (a) As for Tanzania (a)	Annual GDP growth ratesreduced by 0.2–1.5% Annual GDP per capita growth reduced by 0.1–0.3%	Cuddington and Hancock (1994a)	1985–2010
Malawi (b) As for Tanzania (b)	Annual GDP growth reduced by 3% to 9% Annual GDP per capita growth reduced by 0% to –3%	Cuddington and Hancock (1994b)	1985–2010
Botswana Production functions (takes Cobb-Douglas form)	Rate of GDP growth falls from 3.9% per annum without AIDS to 2.0–3.1% After 25 years, economy 24–38% smaller. In the best case per capita GDP rises from 1.5% to 1.9% a year, average incomes 9% higher after 25 years. In the worst case, GDP per capita growth will fall to 1% a year, and be 13% lower after 25 years	Botswana Institute for Development Policy Analysis (BIDPA) (2000b)	1996–2021

Table 11.7 Comparisons of macro-economic studies *cont.*

Country/region	Predicted impact	Author	Forecast dates
Sub-Saharan Africa Growth equations Ordinary Least Squares and Tuso Stage Least Squares	African economic growth hasbeen reduced by 0.8% in the 1990s Per capita growth was reduced by 1.2% per year 1990–95	Bonnel (2000b)	1990–97
South Africa Full supply-demand econometric model	Real GDP is 0.3% lower in AIDS as opposed to no AIDS scenario in 2001, 0.4% in 2006–10	Quatteck (2000)	2001–15 By year to 2005 then 2006–10 and 2011–15
South Africa CGE model	The difference in GDP growth is 2.6% in 2008, by 2010 the economy is 17% smaller than it would have been without AIDS. The per capita income is 8% smaller	Arndt and Lewis (2000)	1997–2010
Trinidad & Tobago (T&T) and Jamaica	GDP in 2005 is 4.2% lower in T&T and 6.4% lower in Jamaica than it would have been in the absence of AIDS	Nicholls et al. (2000b)	1997–2005 but results seem to be for 2005

analyses. Or perhaps the AIDS conference in Durban in July 2000 gave an impetus to these studies. It may also be that investors want this information and will pay for it.

Investment bank ING Barings (Quattek, 2000) published the first study using demographic data from models developed by the Actuarial Society of South Africa. Economic impact was modelled though incorporation in a macro-economic framework developed by the consultancy group WEFA. The results of the exercise are among the most comprehensive ever published. They predict the impact of AIDS on real GDP, real household disposable income and real consumption expenditure. In addition there are tables showing impact on demand components of GDP, government finances, components of domestic savings, trade and the current account, and financial variables and employment (the summary table, Table 11A.2, is included in the appendix to this chapter). AIDS will cause the economy to grow more slowly. GDP growth in 2001 will be 0.3% lower because of AIDS, and for 2006–10 it will be 0.4% lower each year. Household income and expenditure will decrease as will government revenue and domestic savings.

The second study of South Africa presents a *preliminary* analysis (Arndt and Lewis, 2000; original emphasis). In this the economy grows more slowly and by 2010 is 17% smaller than it would have been in the absence of AIDS; by 2010 GDP per capita will be 8% lower than it would have been. The main reason (accounting for 45% of the variance) is the shift in government spending towards health, which increases the budget deficit and reduces total investment. A further 34% of the variance is due to slower growth in productivity.

At the same time in Botswana, a report on the macro-economic impacts of HIV/AIDS was prepared for the Ministry of Finance and Development Planning (BIDPA, 2000b), one of a number of studies on HIV/AIDS impact. This focused on GDP growth and per capita incomes from 1996 to 2021 (the key results for the model are shown in Table 11A.1 in the appendix to this chapter). Botswana's epidemic is worse and further advanced than South Africa's. GDP growth will fall from 3.9% a year without AIDS to between 2.0% and 3.1% a year with AIDS. After 25 years the economy will be 24–38% smaller. Wages are expected to rise, and skilled wages will rise most, while underemployment will fall, reflecting labour shortages at some levels.

The most innovative work to appear in recent years is that of MacPherson et al. (2000). Their argument is that conventional economics misses the complexity and full significance of the epidemic. When the epidemic was in its early stages projections based on scenarios computed 'with AIDS' and 'without AIDS' were reasonable, but such comparisons are no longer valid.

> The impact of the disease cannot be treated as an 'exogenous' influence that can be 'tacked on' to models derived on the presumption that the work force is HIV-free. HIV/AIDS has become an 'endogenous' influence on most African countries that has adversely affected their potential for growth and development. In some cases, such as Zambia, Zimbabwe, and the region covering the former Zaire, the spread of HIV/AIDS may have already undermined their ability to recover economically. (Macpherson et al., 2000, p. 3)

Unfortunately although this conceptual framework is useful and the arguments are clearly made, the model is not fully developed.

The authors point out that rising prevalence of HIV/AIDS lowers worker efficiency, raises costs, and reduces individual savings and firms' profits.

> Individuals who are HIV-positive increase their consumption, in part to combat the effects of the disease and, in part, because the prospect of a premature death raises the opportunity cost of time. These changes lower the supply of investible resources, at both the individual and national levels, and reduce the efficiency with which the existing stock of productive assets is used. Those effects, in turn, lower the rate of growth of per capita incomes, setting off a further cycle of declining savings and investment. (Macpherson et al., 2000, p. 3).

The problem with economic decline is that once it begins it is not easy to halt. AIDS has the potential to push economies into decline and then keep them there. 'The reduction in savings and loss of efficiency associated with the spread of the disease is akin to "running Adam Smith in reverse"' (Macpherson et al., 2000, p. 11).

AIDS causes economies to grow more slowly, the predicted order of magnitude has remained consistently in the range of 0.5–1.0% lower per year than in the absence of the disease. In no case has it been predicted that economies will actually contract. The impact on per capita incomes is uncertain.

The implications and constraints of macro-economic modelling

There are a number of (acknowledged) problems with these models.

- The models assume economic growth in the absence of AIDS. On this basis an impact is predicted. Economic modelling is complex at the best of times, and there is no certainty that the 'without AIDS' predictions would have been accurate. Indeed it has been suggested that reductions in GDP and GDP per capita growth caused by AIDS are probably less than variations in growth rates resulting from changes in the broader economic policy – unless the full complexity is considered.
- Incorporating an HIV/AIDS scenario means that assumptions have to be made about the number of people infected, their skills and employment, the period from infection to illness, how care will be provided and funded, and how all these will change over time. If economic modelling is fraught with difficulty then the introduction of these uncertainties makes it even more difficult.
- Modelling involves simplification. It cannot reflect how economies actually operate. An example illustrates this. Foreign investment is crucial for many poor countries, but AIDS may influence potential investors, not because there is evidence that it will affect growth – but because of the investors' perceptions.
- Finally: 'It is worth stressing that the results presented here make no reference to the human suffering caused by HIV/AIDS. Even in the scenario where per-capita incomes are said to rise as a result of the epidemic, it must be stressed that they rise only for the *survivors'* (BIDPA, 2000b, p. 39).

Policy implications

Macro-economic modelling is esoteric but important for policy and advocacy. The impact on economies cannot now be averted. Too many people are infected, and will fall sick and die. However governments have time to introduce policies to counteract some of the macro-economic consequences. Four studies drawn on for this section conclude with proposals for action. (Arndt and Lewis, 2000; Bonnel, 2000b; Quattek, 2000; BIDPA, 2000b). Their recommendations are remarkably similar, differing in emphasis in relation to their intended audience.

Arndt and Lewis (2000) (an American academic and a World Bank economist respectively) conclude that:

> key policy decisions, such as financing for AIDS related government expenditures, are shown to be very important ... while the human

crisis appears to be practically unavoidable, appropriate economic policy measures have the potential to significantly palliate the negative economic effects of the epidemic ... For the policy-making process, the slow moving nature of the epidemic needs to be borne firmly in mind. The AIDS crisis does not require the snap policy decisions of, for example, the Asia financial crisis. Instead, deliberate speed, careful planning, and competent execution by government and other actors could substantially ameliorate the economic aspects of the AIDS crisis. (p. 884)

Bonnel (2000b) (of the World Bank) notes that 'HIV/AIDS affects economic growth because it erodes the institutions and policies that are crucial for long-term growth. These include sound macroeconomic policy, efficient regulation and a good legal framework.' He concludes that:

among the determinants of growth, macroeconomic policies have the largest impact on growth. In view of recent work showing that growth has a substantial impact on poverty, growth-enhancing measures may create a virtuous circle. Growth can provide the fiscal resources needed for governments to address on a sustainable basis the effects of the HIV/AIDS epidemic, which due to the long incubation period are likely to worsen during the next decade. (p. 14)

For Quattek (a private sector investment analyst, writing specifically in the South African context), the most important need is leadership and clear strategies to mitigate the destructive effect of the epidemic throughout economy and society. She argues for a clear AIDS strategy allowing funds to be channelled from domestic institutions and international development agencies; for providing the public with more up-to-date and complete data on the spreading of the epidemic; and allowing better responses from the private sector. She warns that foreign investors, in particular, will be deterred by uncertainties surrounding the effects of the disease on the economy.

The BIDPA (a think tank which is partly supported by the Government of Botswana) study suggests that the key areas are the supply of skilled labour, investment, and productivity growth. In particular, policy efforts should be devoted to maintaining investment, especially by the private sector. Factors to be addressed are:

- any increase in uncertainty – for instance, if firms did not know they would be able to obtain skilled workers (Batswana or foreign)

- rising levels of crime, the result of policy failure towards AIDS orphans
- reduced profit expectations, due to higher training, recruitment and salary costs for skilled workers (BIDPA, 2000b, p. 70).

This study suggests that government needs to maintain efficiency by sharing training costs, encouraging and supporting firms to plan ahead, providing backup for scarce skills, all to avoid disruption when skilled workers are lost to HIV and AIDS.

What are we to make of this? AIDS has an adverse macro-economic impact. The complexity and long-term interrelated nature of these impacts is beginning to be appreciated. Government and policy makers are not, and need not be, passive in the face of the epidemic. There are things they can do but they must be imaginative and act now. Policies will need to be innovative. Additional resources will have to be found and used in new ways. For example skill shortages probably cannot be met from local sources and additional education and training for nationals requires long-term investment. The answer may be imported labour, this requiring policies to speed up processing of work and residence permits: anathema to most governments. Welfare spending may have to be increased and directed at people who would not normally receive it. There is a larger role for government. That conclusion immediately confronts us with issues of government efficiency; the need for national human resource planning; and the political implications of this disease. It makes us rethink the view that government's role should be as small as possible. Consistency and sustainability will be fundamental to these responses; neither of these qualities is characteristic of the NGO sector where fashion and donor inclination often determine policy. The private sector is hardly likely to make a profit in many of these activities and countries and if it does consistency and sustainability cannot be guaranteed. Which leaves government with all its imperfections and limitations.

Appendix

Table 11A.1   Results of macro-economic projections for 10 scenarios in Botswana

Parameter values	No AIDS	Scenario									
		A	B	C	D	E	F	G	H	I	J
Skilled workers HIV rate (% overal rate)	–	100%	100%	150%	100%	150%	100%	100%	100%	150%	100%
Skilled workforce growth rate (cf. LF growth rate)	–	0%	0%	0%	-2%	-2%	0%	0%	0%	-2%	0%
Productivity loss of HIV+ workers	–	10%	20%	10%	10%	20%	10%	10%	10%	20%	20%
Investment rate (with AIDS)	–	25%	25%	25%	25%	25%	23%	20%	25%	23%	25%
Formal sector productivity growth w/AIDS	–	1.0050	1.0050	1.0050	1.0050	1.0050	1.0050	1.0050	1.0025	1.0025	1.0025
Results											
GDP growth (average)	3.9%	2.8%	2.8%	2.8%	2.7%	2.6%	2.4%	1.8%	2.5%	1.9%	2.4%
GDP/capita growth (average)	1.5%	1.9%	1.9%	1.9%	1.8%	1.7%	1.5%	0.9%	1.5%	1.0%	1.5%
Average wage growth	0.8%	1.4%	1.4%	1.4%	1.3%	1.3%	1.0%	0.5%	1.3%	0.9%	1.3%
Skilled wage growth	1.0%	1.9%	1.9%	1.9%	2.1%	2.2%	1.4%	0.7%	1.7%	1.5%	1.7%
Underemployment	36%	26%	26%	27%	30%	31%	32%	40%	28%	37%	28%
Results (compared to No AIDS)											
GDP	–	-22.9%	-24.7%	-23.5%	-25.3%	-28.2%	-30.2%	-40.2%	-29.8%	-38.1%	-31.3%
GDP/cap	–	8.9%	6.4%	8.1%	5.5%	1.5%	-1.4%	-15.6%	-0.8%	-12.6%	-3.0%
Skilled wage	–	20.2%	17.6%	19.2%	28.2%	23.1%	7.8%	-9.3%	16.0%	11.1%	13.4%
Average real wage	–	14.0%	11.2%	13.4%	11.3%	7.3%	4.9%	-7.7%	10.8%	-0.1%	8.2%
Capital-output ratio	–	12.0%	12.5%	12.3%	14.3%	15.5%	8.1%	2.3%	17.8%	16.2%	18.3%

Scenario Summaries

A - base case (most optimistic)
B - higher labour productivity loss due to AIDS
C - higher HIV prevalence amongst skilled workers
D - slower growth rate of skilled workforce
E - combination of B, C & D
F - lower investment - 23%
G - lower investment - 20%
H - lower TFP growth
I - combination of B, C, D, F & H (most pessimistic)
J - severe productivity impact, no other impact

Table 11A.2   Percentage point difference in growth rates between the AIDS and no-AIDS scenarios, South Africa

	2001	2002	2003	2004	2005	2006–10	2011–15
Real GDP	-0.3	-0.2	-0.2	-0.2	-0.3	-0.4	-0.3
Employment	-1.5	-2.1	-2.8	-3.7	-4.7	-8.3	-14.1
Unemployment	-0.3	-0.3	-0.4	-0.5	-0.8	-0.9	-1.2
Real household disposable income*	-1.3	-1.7	-2.1	-2.4	-2.8	-4.4	-5.8
Real PCE	-4.3	-0.4	-0.3	-0.4	-0.5	-0.8	-0.8
Real government consumption	0.1	0.1	0.1	0.1	0.1	-0.1	-0.2
Real DGFI	-0.1	0.1	0.2	0.2	0.1	-0.1	0.0
Real inventory investment (Rm difference)	-130	-698	-935	-852	-1116	-4014	-4675
Real exports	0.1	0.1	0.1	0.1	0.1	0.1	0.0
Real imports	0.4	-0.2	0.2	0.0	-0.1	-0.3	-0.5
Current account balance GDP**	-1.0	-1.2	-1.4	-1.7	-1.7	-2.4	-2.4
Trade weighted nominal exchange rate*	-0.7	-1.3	-1.4	-1.6	-2.1	-3.0	-3.9
Budget deficit GDP**	-0.3	-0.3	-0.4	-0.5	-0.6	-0.8	-0.9
CPI inflation rate	0.7	0.2	0.4	0.3	0.4	0.4	-0.1
Prime lending rate**	0.0	0.0	0.0	0.1	0.2	0.3	0.5

* Real % difference between AIDS and no-AIDS scenarios, not year-on-year growth rate differences
** % point difference
Source: WEFA

12
Government and Governance

A review of HIV prevalence shows that the worst sexually transmitted epidemics are in the 'new' nations of Africa and the Caribbean. In former Soviet countries and satellites, drug-driven epidemics are spiralling out of control. Those countries in Europe, Asia and Latin America with a history of nationhood have the lowest prevalence. The second half of the twentieth century saw two periods of state formation. Independence came to most African, Asian and Caribbean countries in the 1950s and 1960s. The last decade saw the breakup of the Soviet Union with the creation of 15 new countries including the Russian Federation. The former Yugoslavia spawned five countries, Czechoslovakia split into the Czech and Slovak Republics and in Africa Eritrea gained independence from Ethiopia. This process of 'Balkanisation' may continue in the Democratic Republic of Congo and Indonesia. This is not to suggest that there is any *simple* correlation between ideologies and histories of nationhood and low seroprevalence. It is worth noting, however, certain predictable relationships:

- 'old' European nations were also imperial powers and benefited from that in terms of wealth
- 'old' nations have strong and legitimate state ideologies which enable concerted social action – plus, in many cases, the resources and infrastructure with which to act
- in Latin America and the Philippines, churches are very powerful and there is a history of strong oligarchic control combined with unequal income distribution and overall low wealth.

States have governments of various types, ranging from consolidated democracies to autocracies and military regimes. In the final chapter we argue that states and governments are becoming less powerful, especially in the global context. But despite this, in much of the poor world government is the major producer, employer and provider of social and welfare services. Government expenditure accounts for 40.6% of GDP in Lesotho, for 25% in Panama, and for 30.5% in Bulgaria (World Bank, *World Development Report*, 2001, p. 300). In some cases its main *raison d'être* appears to be processing aid into government and government into social provision. Official development assistance accounts for 28.2% of GNP in Mozambique, 20.6% in Mongolia, 23% in Latvia, and 28.1% in Nicaragua (World Bank, *World Development Report*, 2000, p. 315). Government, however imperfect, may represent the only hope of betterment, development and improved life quality for many people.

Chapter 5 argued that the colonial and pre-colonial history of Africa did not provide a firm foundation for the establishment of legitimate states and governments: complex ethnic mixes, cross-border affiliations, Cold War rivalries, adverse terms of trade, economic incentives to massive corruption and the consequent creation of a 'kleptocracy', the baleful influence of the apartheid regime in South Africa – all meant the value of government was rarely established in the minds of the people after the initial euphoria of independence.

Africa has a longstanding crisis of legitimacy. Combined with geographical disadvantage (Bloom and Sachs, 1998), the huge debt burdens, and overextension of the state sector in many countries as part of an attempt to develop along 'socialist' lines (as in the USSR), have resulted in most African governments being perceived as illegitimate in the eyes of their people. Sometimes, as Hyden once remarked (1983), the state in Africa appeared to float like a balloon over civil society, only very occasionally contacted by messages from below sent by those who would use their familial, ethnic or business affiliations to penetrate its superior isolation. This pattern appears to be repeated in parts of Eastern Europe and the former Soviet states.

In such societies the impact of AIDS on government will be considerable. If we add the new pressures of shifting alliances characteristic of the post-Cold War world, the fluidity of global capitalism, the pressures from donors for privatisation, 'good governance' and opening of economies, then the impact on states is magnified and the possibilities of response are limited.

Yet HIV/AIDS is the major challenge to government in most poor countries. The previous chapter showed how AIDS is placing development in jeopardy and affecting growth prospects. In this chapter we argue that AIDS will affect governments' ability to deliver goods and services, its efficiency and, in extreme cases, its existence.

Reports of varying reliability suggest AIDS has caused deaths of politicians and civil servants throughout Africa over the past decades and numbers are increasing. For example Zimbabwe's president Robert Mugabe has revealed that at least three cabinet ministers and several chiefs have died of AIDS-related diseases (*Namibian*, 11 September 2000); and Malawi's parliamentary speaker, Sam Mpasu, indicated that some of the 29 deaths of MPs over the last five years were AIDS-related (*Business Day*, 11 August 2000).[1] These reports are faceless statistics, and to date the only confirmed AIDS-related death of a politician or civil servant in South Africa is Themba Khoza (Inkatha Freedom Party MP) who died of AIDS-related meningitis in May 2000 (Dispatch Online, 12 June 2000). Media reports suggesting that the recent death of President Thabo Mbeki's Press Officer, Parks Mankahklana (a former leading member of the ANC Youth League and SA Youth Congress), was AIDS-related have been denied by his family (*Business Day*, 2 November 2000).

These examples accurately illustrate just how unwilling politicians are to disclose their HIV status, despite pressure from media, AIDS activists and other politicians. In countries where lack of resources, low salaries and sometimes downright corruption have made states inefficient or incapable of governing, this illness and death has added momentum to an apparently endless downward spiral. How has AIDS contributed to the situations in Sierra Leone, Liberia, Democratic Republic of Congo, and Angola? Could it be a factor in pushing other states along that path? How do the interminable conflicts in these countries contribute to the spread of HIV?

For the most part governments have been extremely slow to react to the potential impacts of the epidemic. Early responses (Chapter 13) centred around prevention, and even here responses – under the tutelage of the WHO Global Programme on AIDS – were limited in scope and success. It has been impossible for governments to grasp the potential effects of the epidemic, much less to put responses in place.

The most extreme manifestation of government's inability to respond has been in South Africa. President Thabo Mbeki appeared transfixed by the looming catastrophe, despite initially recognising the epidemic in 1998 when he said:

the power to defeat the spread of HIV and AIDS lies in our Partnership: as youth, as women and men, as business people, as workers, as religious people, as parents and teachers, as students, as healers, as farmers and farm-workers, as the unemployed and the professionals, as the rich and the poor – in fact, all of us ... Every day, every night – wherever we are – we shall let our families, friends and peers know that they can save themselves and save the nation, by changing the way we live and how we love. We shall use every opportunity openly to discuss the issue of HIV/AIDS. (Mbeki, 1998)

By 2000 he was in denial, most floridly manifest in his contact with the 'AIDS dissidents' and the organisation of a panel comprising 'mainstream' and dissident scientists to discuss, among other things, the cause of the immune deficiency that leads to death from AIDS. In other words, the President of South Africa was asking whether HIV existed and if it caused AIDS. There was consensus that this debate was confusing and damaging to South Africa's response to AIDS. In October 2000, Mbeki acknowledged this.[2]

AIDS and government

Governments face special challenges from HIV/AIDS: greater calls on their resources and a disease that cuts away at financial and personnel capacity.

Few data exist about the impacts on government activities, but Figure 12.1 provides a perspective. Governments need to look at the disease dynamic from HIV to AIDS (the horizontal axis in the figure) and respond to its external and internal impact on government (the

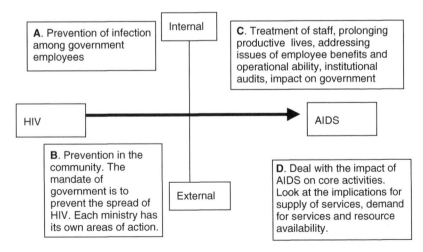

Figure 12.1   The impact of HIV/AIDS on government

vertical axis). Both the epidemic and people move along the line from HIV to AIDS. If the spread of HIV can be contained then there is less need to respond to AIDS. Where there is a serious AIDS epidemic, prevention remains a priority for the uninfected and those who are becoming sexually active.

Box A concerns internal government priorities with regard to HIV. Key is the prevention of infection among the staff. Examples of such responses include provision of education and condoms; less common is addressing how government works – for example, do they post spouses apart from each other?

Box B shows goverment's responsibility to its 'clients'. AIDS control is part of government's activities, but where there is a large epidemic each ministry or department should look at their activities and consider what they might do differently. For example, delays at borders due to slow customs and immigration procedures result in truck drivers spending days at border posts. Villages spring up to house, feed and entertain them. Prevention activities might include education and condoms for both the truckers and local women. Alternatively, government departments in charge of immigration and customs could work together to speed border crossings.

Box C asks what the impact of AIDS illness and death will be among government employees. The issues are similar to those discussed in Chapter 10 except that government has less flexibility than the private sector.

Box D examines the effect of AIDS on government's core business. What does the increase in deaths and illness mean for service provision such as education, the ability to supply that education and the demand for it?

What does AIDS do to governments?

This is not an under-researched area, it is one which has barely been touched at all. AIDS affects two key areas:

- government as a collector and spender of revenue and as a service provider
- governance: the style, manner and legitimacy of government.

Government expenditure

HIV and AIDS activities need financial and human resources. Government's first goal should be prevention. If prevention had worked there would be no AIDS cases to deal with. There are no recent data on expenditure on the epidemic. A study was carried out for UNAIDS in 1996/97 but has not been updated.[3] This obtained self-reported data from multilateral and bilateral agencies as well as from 64 countries. Selected data are presented in Table 12.1. The figures are for all spending on prevention, care and support and impact mitigation. These data are old, poor and cannot easily be interpreted. What is important is that there is no sense of the cost of the epidemic, either nationally or globally.

If prevention activities do not work then governments must plan for and deal with the impact of AIDS. There is always the 'do nothing' option but this undercuts the legitimacy of government and is politically or socially infeasible in all but a few countries.

However there is the question of what AIDS costs. It is alarming to find that there are few data on present costs and even fewer projections for the future. Health ministries don't have information about costs of care and are certainly not planning for increased demand. The few existing studies are based on estimates of current costs projected into the future and applied to modelled increases in cases.

South Africa (Quattek, 2000) provides the most detailed information about impact on the health sector. The current public sector cost of care per patient is between R3,000 (US$378) and R4,500 (US$567) per patient per annum, but 'it is important to note that there are no reliable estimates available' (Quattek, 2000, p. 42). The total cost of AIDS-related care to the government was R1,493 million (US$188 million) in 2000, rising to R4,077 million (US$514 million) in 2009. Arndt and

Table 12.1   Country-reported 1996 HIV/AIDS expenditure per HIV positive person (US$ at current prices and exchange rates)

Country	Adult prevalence rate 1996	Funds per HIV positive person	National funds per HIV positive person
Botswana	25.1	14.27	14.27
Cote d'Ivoire	10.06	10.85	1.62
Senegal	1.77	59.63	4.69
Thailand	2.23	100.65	94.95
Ukraine	0.43	1.5	0.00
Uganda	9.51	40.41	2.73
Zimbabwe	25.84	9.32	0.03

Source: UNAIDS (1999a).

Lewis (2000) estimate that AIDS means South Africa will require a real annual increase in government health expenditure of 6.9% per annum from 1997 to 2010 (p. 874).

Demand for increased government expenditure is felt beyond the health sector. Botswana's government undertook a comprehensive review of the consequence of AIDS for the budget. It concluded:

> AIDS is a development of such proportions that it will inevitably have an impact on government revenues and spending, and therefore on the budget balance and government saving or borrowing. AIDS will have direct effects on some key areas of government spending, most obviously the health budget, but there will also be a range of indirect effects as the ability to raise tax revenues is affected. (BIDPA, 2000a, p. 58)

The impact of AIDS expenditure is shown in Table 12.2.

The Government will have to spend between 7% and 18% more by 2010 because of AIDS, assuming that current levels of service are maintained. The greatest share of spending will go to health care, followed by poverty alleviation. Estimates for health expenditure do not allow for anti-retroviral therapy. At the time of the study, provision of double therapy to all those infected would have cost P3.9 billion (US$0.702 billion[5]) per annum, 17% of the total GDP and 56% of the recurrent budget.

Table 12.2 Botswana: estimates of impact on government recurrent expenditure after 10 years (%)

Budget categories	Low	Medium	High
health	3.0	7.5	12.0
poverty alleviation	3.0	3.5	4.0
employment	1.7	2.3	2.9
orphans allowance	0.3	0.6	1.2
recruitment/training	0.2	0.3	0.5
destitutes allowance	0.1	0.1	0.1
other	−0.4	−0.5	−0.6
pensions	−0.5	−0.6	−0.8
education	−0.6	−0.8	−0.9
Total	6.9	12.5	18.4

Source: BIDPA (2000a).

Even these figures underestimate demand for government resources because:

- there is no provision for increased numbers of hospital beds or health care facilities. It is assumed that services will be provided with the existing infrastructure
- it does not take into account increased poverty and loss of employment which means that as people exhaust their own resources or benefits so demand for public health care will increase.

Table 12.2 shows a number of other social benefits including an orphans' allowance, a destitutes' allowance and pensions. These welfare transfers do not feature in most poor countries' budgets. The only three that make these payments are Botswana, South Africa and Namibia. Botswana's grant to 'destitutes' and to orphans are P80 (US$14.4) and P216 (US$38.88) per month, respectively.

An AIDS literate forecast would show some savings; estimated in Table 12.2. Less is spent on pensions as fewer people reach pensionable age. Fewer births and higher infant and child mortality mean that fewer children require education. However this decrease is based on fewer pupils and does not consider that expenditure may have to increase to keep children in school. For example, orphans and AIDS-affected families may not be able to afford school fees, uniforms and books and will have to be assisted from the public purse.

Government revenue

As calls on government expenditure increase, revenue will decrease. This is shown for Botswana in Table 12.3. The country is fortunate, the bulk of government revenue derives from the Debswana Diamond Company (see Chapter 10) and is not expected to change much.

Table 12.3   Impact of HIV/AIDS on Botswana government revenue

Source	% of revenue	% Revenue reduction
Mineral revenue	49	0
Customs revenue	19	20
Tax revenue	19	20
Interest on reserves (BoB)	8	24
Other sources	6	0
Total revenue	100	9.6

Source: BIDPA (2000a)

The study of South Africa by ING Barings predicted that in 2000 government revenue was 0.7% lower than in the absence of AIDS and that by 2011 it would be 4.1% lower (Quattek, 2000).

Revenue is reduced because:

- GDP is lower. This has knock-on effects: companies making lower profits pay less company tax; fewer employed people means less personal tax; less economic activity reduces value added tax and customs revenues; reduced saving means less tax and stamp payments from financial institutions.
- where companies are not bound by minerals, other natural resources or markets, they may, if the epidemic and its impact are serious enough, move to other less affected locations; new investment and business may avoid affected areas.
- the revenue collection process itself may be affected. Morbidity and mortality hampers government operations and efficiency. For example, if border customs officers are absent or have died then revenue collection becomes less efficient.

Government costs and efficiency

Governments operate differently from the private sector. Government and its operations are more adversely affected than the private sector because of its employment practices and its constrained capacity to respond.

The civil service pays less than the private sector. The lower wages are compensated for in other ways; above all by security of employment – it is difficult to dismiss civil servants. Government officers' annual leave entitlements are usually greater, as are sick, compassionate and other special leave provisions. Poorer productivity is often tolerated. Pension benefits tend to be better. A government employee may retire after 20 or 25 years' service. In some African countries civil servants can retire at 45. Should government employees die in service or after retirement then their dependants will continue to receive the pension. Public service pensions are usually based on defined benefits rather than defined contributions. The latter are more expensive and more risky for the employee.

Government employees know that they cannot be easily dismissed. If they are ill they can take their generous paid and unpaid sick leave. If they take more leave, they cannot be dismissed without due process. This involves convening a 'medical board' to certify that their employment should be terminated with payment of benefits. A sick person can come to work and underperform but corrective action involves

---

Box 12.1   Benefits and contributions

Defined benefits: this means that a person's entitlement is set when he or she enters the service and the person will get this pension no matter what, provided he or she has have served long enough. For example a person may be guaranteed 60% of final salary after 30 years' employment. In this case the employer carries the cost.

Defined contributions: the amount paid into the pension fund by the employer and employee is set. The final pension is determined by the return on the capital sum accumulated when that person retires. It will therefore depend on the total invested and the performance of the investment. The *risk* is shifted from the employer to the employee.

---

long and complex procedures. The result is that as levels of illness and death rise, government departments, educational establishments and health facilities face situations where absenteeism increases, productivity falls and little can be done.

Table 12.4   A comparison of employee benefits in Swaziland

Benefits	Government	Private sector
Sick leave	6 months full pay, vacation leave, 6 months half-pay in three-year cycle	14 days full pay, 14 days half pay annually
Compassionate leave	Widow 28 days, widower 7 days, all entitled to 7 days on death of parent, sister, brother or child	3 days on death of spouse or close family member
Pensions	One year's salary on death in service, 50% of pension to spouse until their death or remarriage, children get 10% of pension (20% if no spouse) up to 5 children and to age 21 or 25 if in full-time education	Defined contributions but group life may experience increased claims if employees die in service

Source: Whiteside and Wood (1994)

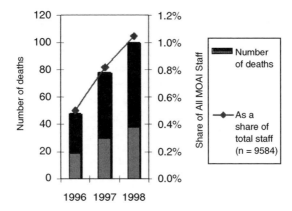

Figure 12.2　Deaths among Ministry of Agriculture and Industry Staff, Malawi
Source: Malindi and Roseberry (1998)

Many governments were overstaffed and could carry some level of absenteeism and inefficiency. Levels of illness and death were small and predictable. Mortality rates of about 0.4–0.5% per annum were expected and could be accommodated. AIDS means these rates have risen to 2–5% per annum, and this is all happening in an environment where the governments have been forced to 'structurally adjust', reducing staff complements. The result is frequently that posts will simply not be filled and work will not get done. Increased mortality in the Ministry of Agriculture in Malawi is illustrated in Figure 12.2; the consequences are described in Box 12.2.[6]

The private sector has a different culture and is able to be more responsive. The illness or death of an employee here will usually result in the person being replaced rapidly, especially if he or she is a key worker. The emphasis is on keeping the process going, and trades unions may be non-existent or weak.

Even allowing for the time and effort involved in replacing staff, government may confront additional difficulties in an AIDS epidemic. They are competing with the private sector and overseas demand for a dwindling pool of skilled people. If the supply of workers is scarce then wage rates increase, and the private sector is better able to respond.

Box 12.2   Decreasing staff levels in Mulanje, Malawi

The Mulanje Rural Development Project (RDP) covers the entire administrative district of Mulanje, segmented into five extension planning areas (EPAs). In Thuchila EPA, there were 16 field assistants at the beginning of 2000. In that year, four of these died, all of chronic illnesses. None have been replaced. A retired field assistant was recalled and allocated to one area temporarily, and some of the remaining field assistants have shared out the other vacant areas. This means that the overall workload has nearly doubled for each, but the field assistants have only the resources (bicycles) they were using for a single area.

Field assistants work with groups under the Training and Visit system. In principle, the system requires that the FA visit at least five fields following each group meeting. However with the increased workload, it is impossible for field assistants to visit individual families or fields, as they must bicycle to other areas for group meetings. The options are either to exclude some areas altogether or to visit others as groups. As a result, the RDP is not able to meet its targets.

Similar situations of understaffing occur in all EPAs. Another EPA further north should have eleven field assistants, but in fact has had only three for at least three years. This problem began around 1992–94, and is common all over Malawi. Other RDPs report deaths of field assistants, and young and middle-aged people are dying, not just elderly staff.

Finally, in many poor countries key functions are carried out by parastatals. These might include provision of power, water, transport, and of marketing and infrastructure development. These parastatals have the same culture and terms and conditions of employment as governments. The effects of this are apparent in Zambia, where unusually frequent powercuts in recent years are reportedly the result of illness and death among powerline maintenance engineers who are hard to replace.

We could identify only one published article on AIDS and government efficiency: it described a USAID-funded technical assistance project in the Ministry of Finance in Zambia (Hoover and MacPherson, 2000). The project's goal was to enhance the capacity of the Ministry to formulate and implement policies to foster growth and development. The authors noted that from the beginning of the project in 1992 there was evidence of growing impact of HIV/AIDS, but none of these problems had been anticipated during the formulation phase.

> The plan was to send overseas each year a small number of qualified individuals for long-term graduate training. Some officials would be sent for shorter courses abroad, within the sub-region, or to local training institutes. There would also be on-the-job training by the project's expatriate professionals.
>
> These plans unravelled as absenteeism, morbidity, opportunism, and death took their toll. There were five difficulties. First, given the prevalence of HIV/AIDS in Zambia and the expected long term losses of trained personnel, the effective cost of long-term training evaluated over a 5–7 year period doubled. Second, the loss of time and skilled personnel due to HIV/AIDS was having a major impact on the ability of the Ministry to function effectively. Third, the losses seriously eroded the Ministry's 'institutional memory'. Fourth, as the organization responsible for implementing Zambia's economic reform program, the Ministry was already overloaded without the difficulties created by losses from HIV/AIDS. And fifth, dealing with counter-productive behavior such as absenteeism and theft proved a challenge. (Hoover and MacPherson, 2000, p. 60)

The response was to cut back on long-term training and introduce short-term courses locally for all staff. This had the benefit of raising skill levels, minimising workflow disruption, showing the entire workforce they had a role to play in raising efficiency, and spreading the institutional memory. An unexpected benefit was that morale was boosted by showing staff that they were valued.

Case studies: health and education

The health sector

Globally, 5.5% of GDP is spent on health, 2.5% through public spending and 2.9 by the private sector. In low-income countries the relative percentages are 1.2% private and 2.8% public. In Africa the percentages are closer: 1.5% public and 1.8% private (World Bank, 2000b, table 2.14).

People use their own resources to visit health carers, including traditional healers. As these resources are exhausted people look to the public sector to provide care.

The health sector has a number of important roles that are public goods. These include:

- monitoring the epidemic and providing data
- assisting in design, implementation and evaluation of prevention programmes
- providing appropriate care and treatment
- mitigating the socio-economic impacts of HIV/AIDS.

Demand for services

People with HIV/AIDS have a range of health care needs. Most HIV-related conditions can be managed effectively at the primary-care level, and basic treatment and care can improve the quality and length of life. As the disease progresses, demand changes. Care is needed both for acute, treatable illnesses and terminal conditions. In settings where anti-retroviral drugs are available (such as Mexico and Brazil) new systems are required to manage complex therapies and ensure adherence to treatments.

Increased demand is from people who are not normally users of health care: young adults. In one relatively well-resourced South African province, projections indicate that HIV/AIDS alone will more than double the required number of hospital medical beds between 1997 and 2006.

The scale of this additional demand is particularly problematic. Health sectors already have difficulty in meeting basic medical care needs. If only a proportion of needs are met, HIV/AIDS will consume a substantial share of public health budgets. By 1995, HIV/AIDS care accounted for 27% of public health care spending in Zimbabwe and 66% in Rwanda. The World Bank estimated that the cost of care per person with HIV/AIDS was roughly 2.7 times per capita GDP for all countries (World Bank, 1997a). As the demand increases, so the human and financial resources decrease.

The challenge is to manage the burden on the formal public health care system without shifting an unsustainable burden on to individuals, families and communities. For example, home-based care may reduce the impact on public systems, but unless families are provided with adequate support they may be overwhelmed. Home-based care could then become home-based neglect (Foster, 1996, p. 83).

Capacity to deliver services

HIV/AIDS compromises capacity for health care through its direct and indirect impacts on employees. The following are of particular significance.

- Health workers are at risk of HIV infection. The greatest risk is through sexual exposure, although there is a small occupational risk. In Lusaka in 1991–92, HIV prevalence was 39% among mid-wives and 44% among nurses. In Kinshasa, hospital workers were shown to have levels of HIV infection similar to those of the general community (Mann et al., 1986). In two southern Zambian hospitals, mortality rates among nurses rose from 0.5% per annum in 1980 to 2.7% in 1991 due to HIV/AIDS (Buve et al., 1992). The death rate of Malawi health care workers was 3% in 1997, a sixfold increase on levels before the epidemic (Government of Malawi/World Bank, 1998). Increased absenteeism among nurses was already observable in Zambia in the early 1990s (Foster, 1996, pp. 94–6)
- Health workers risk other infections, particularly tuberculosis. This is most serious for those who are HIV positive. Annualised incidence of TB cases among health staff has increased fivefold over five years in certain high HIV prevalence areas, with up to 86% of tested cases being HIV infected (Harries et al., 1997)
- Impacts of HIV/AIDS on morale are particularly marked in the health sector. Workloads increase dramatically, stress and burn-out are exacerbated by factors such as high mortality among children, young adults and colleagues, and perceived risk of infection (Foster, 1996, p. 103).

The most detailed study of the impact of AIDS on a national hospital looked at Kenyatta hospital in Nairobi (Arthur et al., 2000). HIV prevalence among patients rose from 19% in 1988/89 to 39% in 1992 and 40% in 1997. Bed occupancy rose from 100% in 1988/89 to 190% in 1997. The stabilisation in demand between 1992 and 1997, although AIDS cases and deaths were rising, was attributed to a change in health-seeking behaviour by people with advanced illness. They did not go to the hospital. The reasons might have induded stigma, a belief and realisation that government hospitals can do little for the chronically sick, or actual or opportunity costs. This study concluded that 'an increased throughput of patients can be accommodated without seeming to compromise outcome and mortality ... [but] ... the sad fact is that twenty years into the HIV/AIDS epidemic there really are so few data about the impact on African health-care systems' (Arthur et al., 2000, p. 14).

The education sector

The largest cadre of government employees are those concerned with education, including teachers, administrators and ancillary staff. Education is crucial. It is argued that part of the East Asian miracle can be attributed to investment in human capital. The World Bank places great importance on education. In its publication *Can Africa Claim the 21st Century?* (World Bank, 2000a), four areas are identified as crucial: governance and leadership, investment in people (both health and education), reducing high costs and risks in the business environment, and reassessing the role of aid. The World Bank believes education to be 'the key to higher incomes, both for individuals and countries. But especially in an agriculture-based region, better health and nutrition are also likely to have major effects on labour productivity and income growth' (World Bank, 2000a, p. 86).

Education faces both supply and demand side impacts, as illustrated in Figure 12.3.

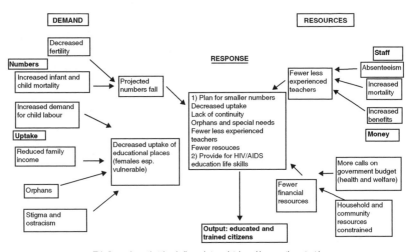

This figure shows that the challenge is to maintain and improve the output in the face of new pressures resulting from HIV/AIDS

Figure 12.3   The Impact of HIV/AIDS on education

Impacts on demand

Demographic impact results in smaller numbers of children needing education: fewer children are born and many HIV-infected infants do not survive to school age. In Swaziland by 2016, there will be a 30% reduction in the size of the primary school population for each grade, with somewhat lower, but still substantial, reductions in needs for secondary and tertiary education (Government of Swaziland/Ministry of Education, 1999). Enrolment may be further affected by household economic difficulties and the need for children's labour.

AIDS means that there are students at all levels with new special needs:

- orphans (this has been covered in Chapter 8)
- children exposed to infectious diseases and emotional trauma because they live with and care for family members with HIV/AIDS
- children who are discriminated against or isolated because they or their families are infected
- children in households where a parent is ill or has died, or where orphans have been taken in, who face difficulties.

The traditional roles of the education system in cultivating numeracy and literacy will have to be supplemented by supporting and nurturing large numbers of children in crisis, giving them life and survival skills from an early age.

Impact on supply

All teachers are at risk of HIV infection; there are some indications they may be at greater than average risk. Their status and income create opportunities for high-risk behaviour. Zambia's Ministry of Education reports that 2.2% of teachers died in 1996.

This was more than the number produced by all teacher training colleges. This death rate is expected to triple by 2005 (Kelly, 1998).

The methodology of the institutional audit (Chapter 10) can be applied to the education sector. However several specific aspects of impacts on education warrant further mention:

- death or absence of even a single teacher is particularly serious because it affects the education of between 20 and 50 children.
- loss of key individuals at leadership level, including planners, school inspectors and principals, may further compromise quality and efficiency of the education system. The average age and experience of teachers is expected to fall (see Figures 12.4 and 12.5).

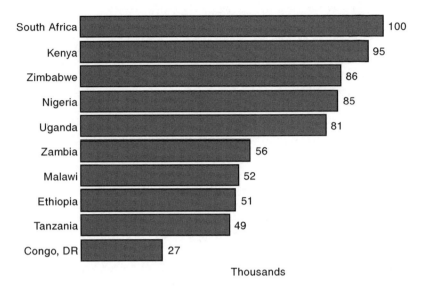

Figure 12.4   Primary schoolchildren who lost a teacher to AIDS
Source: Shell and Zeitlin (2000)

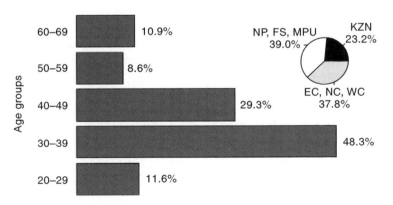

Key: NP = Northern Province, FS = Free State, MPU = Mpumalanga, KZN = Kwazulu-Natal, EC = Eastern Cape, NC = Northern Cape, WC = Western Cape

Figure 12.5   Deaths occurring in the teaching profession in South Africa, by age group, August 1999 to May 2000
Source: Shell and Zeitlin (2000)

Similar analyses can be made of any sector of government. The basic problem is that services are more difficult to supply and in some sectors demand increases. While government administration may be affected in these ways the effects on governance are even more corrosive.

The unmeasured impact: governance

The effects of AIDS on political and social stability and governance have been ignored. Between the extremes of highly regulated and controlled states such as Cuba and Myanmar; the *laissez-faire* economies of Botswana and the Philippines and the anarchic situation in Somalia, Afghanistan or Sierra Leone, there lie many different systems and traditions. Will AIDS have the same or similar impacts on all these countries? What impact will AIDS have on government, the ability to govern and the legitimacy of the state? Why have political scientists largely ignored the epidemic and its potential effects? As early as 1992 there were suggestions that AIDS might have economic, political and security implications (Whiteside and FitzSimons, 1992). Whiteside and FitzSimons noted that:

> Clearly more information is needed on the regional, national and local spread of the epidemic, to determine which groups are at risk and the attitude of society to those groups. Will limited resources be used to conserve a skilled elite, allowing AIDS to become entrenched as an endemic disease of the underclasses – like the poor, always with us? History warns that weak societies will be made weaker by the ravages of epidemics, heightening existing tensions. AIDS will be no exception. (1992, p. 34)

In 1996, the then US President, Bill Clinton, issued a Presidential Decision Directive calling for a more focused US policy on infectious diseases. This reflected the fact that the US State Department's Strategic Plan for International Affairs listed protecting human health and reducing the spread of infectious disease among its strategic goals. In 2000, HIV/AIDS was identified by the US National Intelligence Council as a new disease that

> will pose a rising global health threat and will complicate US and global security over the next 20 years. These diseases will endanger US citizens at home and abroad, threaten US armed forces deployed overseas, and exacerbate social and political instability in key countries in

which the United States has significant interests. (National Intelligence Council, 2000)

It is not solely sections of the American government and opinion formers who have constructed HIV/AIDS as a security threat. In January 2000, in an unprecedented event, the United Nations Security Council Session was devoted exclusively to the threat to Africa of HIV/AIDS. Meeting in Addis Ababa in December 2000, the African Development Forum attended by African political and business leaders, debated the HIV/AIDS epidemic in their meeting 'AIDS: the greatest leadership challenge'. Their consensus was that leadership is crucial at community, national and regional levels. They did not consider whether AIDS is a threat to government and stability. The issue was debated by the United Nations General Assembly in June 2001.

There are few fora of international leaders and organisations that do not, in some way, consider HIV/AIDS. They do not raise its political impact; perhaps the implications are too frightening. They should be considering:

- losses in production and taxes which result from deaths of people in their thirties and forties
- lost human capital
- lost leadership at all levels
- decreased numbers and efficiency in security forces as middle-ranking army officers, police and other security forces face increased illness and death
- the long-term challenge to stability and development of increased orphaning
- perceived political weakness because politicians are ignoring the greatest problem facing their citizens. The people are aware of increases in illness and death
- lack of leadership in times of crisis leads to blame and a sense of *anomie* in society. In societies already facing economic and political crisis, AIDS may cause instability
- infringement of human rights through discrimination against people with HIV/AIDS. These people have been excluded from employment, have been denied access to medical care, and have even been prevented from marrying. This cuts into the fabric of society and social cohesion
- government inefficiency

- declining experience among elected representatives – anecdotes from Zambia suggest more frequent local elections as local councillors die.

Less measurable consequences are decreased citizen 'support' and involvement in civil society and government. This is particularly significant for countries trying to move towards 'democracy', because:

- people who have a fatal disease, or believe they might have this disease, or who are burdened with caring for such people, are less likely to worry about how they are governed and have fewer incentives to participate in political life
- being sick or caring for those who are sick reduces the time, energy and financial resources available for participation in public life
- there may be pressure to try any form of government that purports to offer a solution, whether it is democratic or not
- people may be less compliant and willing to pay for public services if they believe they will die soon. Their goal may be to get as much as possible, as quickly as possible for minimum expenditure, whilst accumulating benefits for their families.

AIDS will erode the capacity of governments to govern. It may also change the environment in which they seek to exercise their authority. Of great concern is the impact that an AIDS epidemic may have on a nation. Civil society has been identified as a fundamental pillar of good government; declining life expectancy erodes the size and strength of leadership on which this is founded. There is some evidence from Uganda that responding to AIDS can build civil society. In most poor countries, however, AIDS threatens civil society and governments.

13
Responses

This chapter looks at responses to the HIV/AIDS epidemic, where priorities have been and where they should have been.

We argue that there should be a continuum of policy and practice spanning prevention and impact mitigation. Care is an important component of both of these. Prevention responses have been inadequate and generally ineffective. In the poor world the spread of HIV continues, requiring planning for increased care needs and other aspects of impact mitigation. There are few signs that this is happening.

Here we explore concepts that help understand the challenges of response.

Concept 1: timing and targeting

Responses and their targets depend on the stage of the epidemic. Early response should focus on prevention. If this fails and prevalence rises, impact must be considered. There are waves of spread and waves of impact.[1]

Table 13.1 shows six stages as an epidemic evolves. Although some countries have reached Stages 4 or 5, there is little evidence that any country has moved beyond that. At the sub-national level, some regions and communities that reached Stage 5 within the last decade may be approaching Stage 6. Anecdotal evidence exists at the sub-national, community, and enterprise level of Stage 5 and 6 impacts.

Concept 2: information, observation or instruction

For prevention to be successful, individuals must be able to make decisions to protect themselves, *and have the conditions and incentives that*

Table 13.1 The evolution of the HIV/AIDS epidemic and its consequences

Stage	Epidemiology and prevention	Impact and response
Stage 1: No one with AIDS identified; some HIV infections	HIV prevalence > 0.5% in high risk groups, targeted prevention	Planning only required
Stage 2: A few cases of AIDS seen by medical services; more people are infected with HIV	HIV prevalence < 5% in high risk groups, targeted prevention	Impact on medical demand and use of facilities: need to plan for this
Stage 3: Medical services see many with AIDS. Some policy makers aware of HIV infection and AIDS. The incidence of reported TB cases increases	Prevalence > 5% in high risk populations. Targeted prevention but general information	Impact still mainly medical but need to begin human resource planning and targeted mitigation especially for most vulnerable groups, institutions and sectors
Stage 4: AIDS cases threaten to overwhelm health services. Widespread general population awareness of HIV/AIDS	Prevalence > 5% in ANC women. Information available to all, continuing targeting of high risk groups	Impact now broader – need to start looking at education sector and all government activities. Private sector plans for impact
Stage 5: Unusual levels of severe illness and death in the 15–50 age group produce coping problems, large number of orphans, loss of key household and community members. TB is a major killer	Prevalence > 20% in ANC clinic attenders and has been so for 5 years. Full battery of prevention according to resources	Impact at all levels. Responses need to be equally diverse. They may include targeted relief or targeted ART
Stage 6: Loss of human resources in specialised roles in production and economic and social reproduction decreases the ability of households, communities, enterprises,and districts to govern, manage, and/or provision themselves effectively. Responses range from creative and innovative ways of coping to failure of social and economic entities	Prevalence > 15% in 15–49 age group and has been so for 5 years. Most now needs to be focused on key groups and interventions. Efforts to reach those below age 15 and for over-15s emphasis on voluntary counselling and testing	This impact requires massive intervention at all levels. The emphasis should be on children in crisis including orphans. Local programmes need to be scaled up and made sustainable perhaps with donor money

enable them to stick to those decisions. Effective impact mitigation requires understanding the effects that the epidemic will have and reacting to them, preferably in advance. There are three ways in which prevention and mitigation responses can be triggered:

- by information
- through observation
- via an instruction.

Information-based decisions are grounded on messages and the theory of reasoned action and planned behaviour (see Chapter 3) rather than experience or observation. People learn what is happening or may happen; they process this information and make decisions to change (or not change) their behaviour.

An observation-based decision is one where behaviour change is based on what people see or have personal experience of.

Instruction-based decisions are where people are told to do things, and do them. There may be disincentives for not following the instructions (in some countries you will be fined if you do not wear a seatbelt) or incentives for following them (tax cuts for having children). The instruction may come from various sources: religious leaders with moral authority or dictators with powers to coerce. Such instructions may smack of desperation and unreality. In July 2001, in a speech to the Kenyan Pharmaceutical Society, President Daniel Arap Moi said that he was reluctant to spend money on importing condoms to Kenya and that 'As president, I am shy that I am spending millions of shillings importing those things': it was better for Kenyans to refrain from sex 'even for only two years' and this was the best way to curb the epidemic (*Mercury*, KwaZulu Natal, 13 July 2001, p. 1).

In most settings responses cannot be based on observation because:

- HIV spreads invisibly and AIDS follows on some years later
- it is hard to ascertain causality
- cases and impact are diffuse (see Table 13.1).

The relative roles of information, observation and instruction are important for HIV/AIDS prevention programmes, their design and understanding why they have succeeded or failed. For example, the gay community in the US based much of its response on information and observation. The first indication that something was wrong was when men started falling ill and dying. This led to demand for knowledge and the process is documented in *And the Band Played On* (Shilts, 1987). This community asked: 'What is killing our colleagues, friends and lovers? Where did it come from? What can we do about it?' These questions arose from observation and required information. As this became available, so it shaped the response. Once the potential for transmission through sexual intercourse became apparent, the bathhouses were closed and safe-sex practices encouraged. Behaviour change was proposed and adopted before the HIV epidemic reached its 'natural' peak.

By contrast, in much of southern and eastern Africa, information about HIV/AIDS, how it is transmitted and how people may protect themselves has been around for more than a decade, and yet HIV prevalence continues to climb. Knowledge and observation have not translated into action. In South Africa one of the recent anti-AIDS campaigns was called 'Beyond Awareness'. Recent realisation of the scale of the problem in this region is partly due to the dramatic increase in mortality rates and the inescapable personal observations which go with these levels of illness and death. Here behaviour change is observation-based, although information is a prerequisite. It should also be noted that it is by no means certain that the 'right' behaviour change will occur – there may be a feeling of helplessness, disempowerment and fatalism. Among young men in South Africa, 'Contracting the HIV/AIDS virus was seen more or less as a new part of growing up, surely not something to be eagerly anticipated, but accepted nonetheless as an almost inevitable consequence of being an adult, a status which presupposes being sexually active' (Leclerc-Madlala, 1997). In addition the 'instruction' option does not work unless the authorities have legitimacy and sanction.

Uganda has steered a middle course. Here government, communal and individual response was based on a mixture of information, observation and instruction. However the information and in particular its source was crucial for acceptance of the message and subsequent action. This has been illustrated by Low-Beer et al. (2000). They compared epidemic patterns in Uganda with Zambia, Malawi and Kenya. The most important behavioural changes in Uganda related to lower percentages of 15–19-year-olds having sex, a higher percentage of people delaying sex until after marriage, and fewer non-regular partners. Condom use was similar across countries and condom usage at levels of 40–50% with non-regular partners was not in itself sufficient to substantially reduce HIV incidence.

Despite limited options and resources, Ugandans developed personal behavioural strategies which dramatically reduced HIV prevalence.

These changes were related to and driven by personal communication networks through which knowledge about AIDS was acquired. The main communication channel was discussions among friends and family. While 90% of Ugandans were having these discussions, less than 35% of South Africans were. In Uganda, 82% acquired AIDS knowledge through personal networks; in the other four countries the figure was 40–65%. In Uganda, personal networks have been crucial, rather than institutional or mass channels which dominate in other countries. The effective content of AIDS messages is only brought home after being communicated among family and friends.

Analysis of communication networks shows that even limited increases in 'openness', defined as discussing AIDS and AIDS status with 20% of close contacts, can result in most people knowing someone with AIDS at an early stage in the epidemic when HIV prevalence is less than 10%. In southern Africa, this wave of communication and identification of personal risk may only occur after HIV incidence has peaked. In Uganda, AIDS responses have been at family/friendship level, people developed personal solutions with dramatic impact on the epidemic.

These findings have important implications for prevention programmes, one of which is that the context must be right. A key feature of Uganda's response was leadership. This ensured that AIDS was consistently on agendas and people were not stigmatised. It began with President Museveni talking openly and frankly about AIDS as early as 1986 (Kaleeba et al., 2000). He insisted that AIDS be put on the political agenda at all levels, and set up the National AIDS Prevention and Control Committee – which was subsequently replaced by the better known Uganda AIDS Commission (UAC). Religious leaders – Protestant, Catholic and Muslim – were brought into the process and played an important role in prevention activities (the UAC has been chaired by Protestant and Catholic bishops). Of course the other ingredient arising from involvement of political and religious leaders is instruction: the population was being told what to do by a leadership – with legitimacy.

Information requires:

- the appropriate medium
- the ability of the target audience to access it
- the conceptual framework to understand it and translate it into action
- legitimacy and a framework for it to be processed.

None of the above are likely in a risk environment. Here resistance to prevention messages is high. Giving messages to change behaviour is not rocket science; advertisers try to do it all the time. From the point of view of the HIV/AIDS epidemic these distinctions are significant. Indeed the differences between information and observation may go some way to explaining the differences in the epidemic profiles in the rich and poor worlds. In the wealthy world, populations not only have the ability to receive the information, but can process it and relate abstract concepts to their lives and behaviours. Thus gay men were bombarded with information through the media, pamphlets and posters. They had the knowledge to relate this to the concept of a virus which allowed a range of diseases to develop, but could lie dormant for many years and which could be transmitted through sexual intercourse, although disease did not manifest itself in the genital area.

Poor people in any society have constrained decision horizons and little knowledge of scientific ideas about disease. Knowledge and experience of HIV/AIDS is related to their own cultural-conceptual frameworks and to their material circumstances. Television or newspaper advertisements can't reach populations who can't read and who do not have access to electricity. Disease can't be explained in terms of germ theory in cultures where this concept has no meaning.

Impact planning looks to the future. Information is not available so responses are based on models rather than hard data – although these will come as the epidemic evolves. Herein lies one of the paradoxes of the epidemic. If you plan for impact and avert it, then how do you justify what you did, to show that your planning and use of resources was necessary? To plan effectively for impact should turn out to be a self-defeating prophecy: what is prophesied does not happen. The paradox is further deepened when it becomes apparent that to educate people about potential impacts of the epidemic may be part of prevention.

Concept 3: advocacy and ownership

Three stages of response are identified here.

- *Identification of the disease*. People need to understand that there is an organism that causes illness
- *Ownership*. People have to recognise that the illness has implications for them and their societies
- *Empowerment*. People have to believe that there is something that can be done and they can be part of it.

This can be illustrated by reference to another global issue – climate change. Few would argue that our weather patterns are unchanged: floods, heat waves and droughts seem increasingly common and severe. Many suspect that human activity contributes to global warming and believe that something should be done, but don't know what they can do. The problem has to be recognised, owned and acted upon.

Advocacy is necessary to ensure that people are aware of the problem and are prepared to act on it. There is, however, no point in people being aware if they do not feel that it is their problem and that they can do something about it.

Concept 4: process versus product

In HIV/AIDS prevention or impact mitigation, while there may be a distinction between process and product, in some cases the process is the product.

Process can be setting up a national AIDS control plan or carrying out a study of the impact of the disease on supply and demand in the education sector. The product is the resulting study or plan which, in an ideal world, leads to implementation. Over the years it has become apparent that process is sometimes more important than product. Most of the studies of potential sectoral HIV/AIDS impact have been published and forgotten. Saying to a Minister of Education that AIDS will be an issue is not enough – he or she needs his or her own study to show that this is the case in his or her country. It does not help that the neighbouring country or province has done such a study and the results are applicable in that country's situation. The minister needs this study to be done for his or her country, for what is perceived to be that country's unique circumstances.

Uganda: a multisectoral response

The initial response established a National AIDS Control Programme NACP in the Ministry of Health. This dealt with issues of epidemiology, surveillance, education and prevention and blood transfusion services. The NACP was charged with co-ordination between and within other departments of government. This meant that HIV/AIDS was and continued to be seen as a medical problem. Other bodies, both within and outside government, felt that HIV/AIDS was not their concern or responsibility.

In 1990 a task force on AIDS was charged with developing a multi-sectoral response to AIDS control. Participants included all government ministries, local and international NGOs and the major international agencies. The process had strong support from President Museveni, and resulted in the establishment of the 24-member Uganda AIDS Commission. This Commission was required to:

- oversee, plan and coordinate AIDS control programmes
- be a reference point for the formulation of plans, policies and national guidelines for HIV/AIDS control programmes and activities.

None of this appears very innovative. But it was. Neighbouring Kenya only established similar processes in 1999. The key to the Ugandan response was that it:

- encouraged active participation of everyone in reducing transmission and spread of HIV/AIDS
- provided strategies for prevention and impact mitigation
- advocated for capacity building at the community, sub-national and national levels (Uganda AIDS Commission, 1993, p. 17).

This definition turned away from exclusively medical models of response, included epidemic consequences, and recognised that all sectors and levels of Ugandan society had to be involved.

The multisectoral response took years and involved wide dialogue and discussion within Ugandan society. A portfolio of over 50 interventions was identified. Through these Ugandan society set out to engage with the HIV/AIDS epidemic. Not all the interventions were successful; not all the goals were or could be achieved. The country- and community-wide debate and discussion which took place as part of the process of multisectoral response was undoubtedly an important factor in Uganda's success in responding to the epidemic.

In responding to the epidemic, process is as important as product, indeed process may be product! This may be frustrating for those who are aware of the magnitude and urgency of the crisis, but in the long run although sometimes slow it is the best way forward.

Concept 5: scaling up and sustainability

There are examples of remarkable AIDS interventions run by committed and concerned people. These include prevention, care and dealing

---

Box 13.1   Ownership, product and process

No ownership
In 1989 the British Overseas Development Administration commissioned a study of the impact of AIDS on rural life in Uganda. The fieldwork was carried out, the report presented and a book written. At no time in the next decade were the findings reflected in British Agricultural or Rural Development aid policy. *Ownership but no tools* In 1993 the Government of Swaziland carried out a National Development Strategy Process, reviewing the 25 years since independence and looking ahead to the next 25. An issues paper on the impact of HIV/AIDS and its implications was commissioned. The report 'Socio-economic Impact of HIV/AIDS in Swaziland' was written with maximum Swazi involvement. A steering committee was established to guide the work and provide input, the draft was discussed at a workshop. Despite these efforts local ownership was not sufficient to ensure integration of the recommendations into government activities. There were no clear and identifiable actions. The report was shelved.

Ownership and action
Debswana Diamond Company carried out the institutional audit described in Chapter 10. The study began with a consultative workshop for the staff of the company. This established the goals of the project, information needs and how analysis would be carried out. Data collection and much of the analysis was done by the employees. The results were presented and discussed in a two-day workshop. This ensured consensus on both the findings and the way forward. The actions were largely agreed in the workshop. The challenges are of implementation rather than substance or direction.

---

with impact through theatre groups, orphan care and income- generating projects. However these have neither stopped the epidemic nor alleviated much of the misery associated with it. The reason is that they are small-scale and localised.

Prevention has to be done at this level – after all it is individual behaviours that must be changed in a community context. A multitude of small-scale programmes across a country is needed. These will make a difference. By contrast, care and impact responses need to be scaled up because the numbers are large. While it is important to provide education for orphans in one area or home-based care through a particular church, these responses must be expanded. The difficulty is to achieve large-scale responses and remain sensitive to geographical and cultural variation – all when resources are limited.

The epidemic raises important questions about sustainability. People understand sustainability to mean that when the core funding, be it government or donor, runs out, the local community or administration will be able to continue the project using its own resources. This may be a laudable target for many projects. It makes sense that communities should be asked to cover the recurrent cost of providing clean water and should manage this themselves. Micro-credit projects take pride in being self-sustaining. However AIDS changes things and this is especially true for projects designed to assist people impacted by the disease.

Sustainability may not be achievable. 'Sustainability', like 'coping' (see below) is often another way of asking people to do more with less. A concrete example: a project designed to help orphans may be sustainable in a community where the number of orphans is constant and the community is becoming better off – or at least no worse off. In an AIDS-affected area, numbers of orphans will be rising and the community's resources – human, physical and financial – will be contracting as adults fall ill and die.

Sustainability is not a blanket criterion that can be used to judge the viability of projects in AIDS-affected areas. There are two main reasons for this. The first, alluded to above, is that the epidemic means that resources are being lost in communities and nations at the same time as demand rises. The second is the time-frame for support. The most extreme example is where young children are orphaned. They will need care and support at least until they are 16 years old, and possibly longer. Donors need to look at long-term assistance – something most cannot do because they have neither the time-frame nor the budget to make this sort of commitment.

Concept 6: the myth of coping

Like sustainability, the idea and language of 'coping' has to be questioned in relation to HIV/AIDS and its impacts. Yes, people 'cope': the alternative – not coping – means households dissolving or people dying. But it is odd and indeed offensive for the wealthy to suggest the poor should 'cope' and the rich will show them how to do it. The idea of 'coping' originates from the unwillingness of the rich to do anything more than apply sticking plaster to the wounds of global inequality when what has been required for a very long time is expensive surgery. This surgery requires major transplantation and reorganisation of resources.

Rugalema (2000) argues that coping is often a myth, because:

- many households affected by HIV/AIDS do not cope. On the contrary, they break up and their members – orphans, widows and the elderly – join other households
- it is not households that cope – rather it is individuals within them who manage to *survive*
- there may be precious little in the way of 'strategies' about how people manage crises. Rather the decisions made by household members may merely reflect efforts to survive in the very short term
- short-term solutions to crises – sale of household assets, withdrawal of young girls from school to help with domestic and farm work – have long-term effects and costs. These may include lower or no educational achievement, poor diet with associated stunting or wasting, lack of care and poor socialisation
- the impact of a large-scale event such as an HIV/AIDS epidemic has effects on wider social, economic and even environmental systems. For example, in a community or region that is hard hit, there are changes and costs at the levels of the farming system, social infrastructure and the maintenance of physical infrastructure. These all point to general impoverishment in many dimensions
- the effects of 'coping' are shouldered unequally between poorer and better off households, men and women, generations, and different social groups and geographical regions.

Why use the term 'coping'? It originates in literature about individuals and how they cope with stress (McCubbin, 1979; McCubbin et al., 1980). It has been used to discuss famines (Watts, 1983; Corbett, 1988; De Waal, 1989; Devereux, 1993). Other roots lie in ideas from social work and child care. Here the notion of 'good enough' care (Winnicott, 1965) emerged in the 1960s. It was an attempt to sensitise social workers to the idea that, while their clients' standards of care might appear inadequate by their own social and cultural standards, the clients' was 'good enough' as long as everyone was 'coping'.

In relation to HIV/AIDS, the story of coping mechanisms is really a part of the wider story of structural adjustment policies – before they began to be offered 'with a human face' (Mehrotra and Jolly, 1997).

Rugalema hits the nail on the head when he says that the concept of coping strategies is rooted in the neo-liberal worldview of the 1970s and 1980s. Non-intervention by governments and freedom or autonomy of economic agents to participate in the market were fundamental points of departure. As this worldview dominated that period, not least due to the influence of Reaganomics in the US and Thatcherism in the UK, so the concept of coping strategies gained credence (Rugalema, 2000, p. 5).

Throughout this book we have underlined the social roots of the HIV/AIDS epidemic and the social and cultural filters through which its impacts manifest themselves. Coping is about dealing with risk. Risk is not equally distributed. It is constructed for individuals and socio-economic groups through complex processes of economic, social and cultural relations. The constant struggles to survive that characterise the livelihoods of so many do not leave room for coping in the 'extra-ordinary' (in fact, for them, all too ordinary) circumstances in which many poor people live. That is what they do every day of every year. That is the nature of poverty. And when the big crisis hits them they do not cope. Thus, to talk of such poor people 'coping' is to cross the line between technical appreciation of what is possible and barely dis-guised cynicism and clear acceptance that different groups of human beings can only be offered second-, third- (or worst) best options. It is to accept the unjust structures of distribution in the world. A term such as 'coping' may be a way of escaping from the challenge of confronting how people's capabilities are stunted, how their entitlements are blocked and their abilities to function as full human beings with choices and self-definitions are frustrated.

Responding to the epidemic: prevention

Preventing new infections remains a primary goal. Key messages about prevention are:

- Even in Botswana (the worst affected country), where more than one-third of adults are infected, two-thirds are not.
- Where HIV prevalence is comparatively low, the challenge is to keep it so.
- Each year a new cohort of young people reaches adulthood and becomes sexually active. They can, and should, be kept HIV-free.

Identifying prevention as a goal is easy. It is more difficult to decide what to do. In earlier chapters two key ideas were introduced: differential susceptibility and differential vulnerability to the disease. Failure to think in this way accounts for limited success in prevention efforts. Figure 13.1, 'The Whole Story' shows where interventions have taken place to date.

Most interventions have been biomedical and behavioural. The biomedical interventions are obvious. Provision of safe blood and blood products are universal goals. Testing all donated blood and anti-selection – discouraging people in high-risk groups from donating – should largely accomplish this. Where this is done, including in the poor world, blood becomes much safer. Indeed wealth is not the only determinant: Zimbabwe was one of the first countries to introduce screening.

Determinants	Distal determinants $\longrightarrow$			Proximal determinants
	Macro environment	**Micro environment**	**Behaviour**	**Biology**
	Wealth	Mobility	Rate of partner change	Virus sub-types
	Income distribution	Urbanisation	Prevalence of concurrent partners	Stage of infection
	Culture	Access to health care	Sexual mixing patterns	Presence of other STDs
	Religion	Levels of violence	Sexual practices and condom use	Gender
	Governance	Women's rights and status	Breast feeding	Circumcision
Interventions	Social policy – redistribution	Social Policy Economic Policy	Behaviour change communication	STD treatment
	Legal Reform – Human Rights	Legal Reform Employment legislation	Condom promotion and marketing	Blood safety
	Taxation Debt relief		Voluntary counselling and testing	Anti-retroviral therapy during pregnancy
	Terms of Trade		IVDU harm reduction	Vaccines and microbicides (when developed)

Figure 13.1   The whole story
Source: Barnett et al. (2000)

Treatment of sexually transmitted infections

STIs enhance HIV transmission by increasing both susceptibility of HIV negative individuals and the infectiousness of HIV positive individuals. Treatment of STIs should assist control of HIV spread. However the first two trials of this strategy gave apparently contradictory results (Grosskurth et al., 2000). In the early 1990s randomised controlled trials of STI treatment for the prevention of HIV-1 infection were conducted.

- The Mwanza trial, conducted between November 1991 and December 1994 in Tanzania, involved *case management* of STIs
- The Ugandan trial in Rakai (south-western Uganda) involved *mass treatment* of STIs (Wawer et al., 1999).

The Mwanza study suggested that reduction in HIV incidence by 38% in a rural population over a two-year period could be achieved by improving syndromic[2] STI treatment services. In this study only symptomatic STIs were treated, and therefore it was expected that the results would underestimate the proportion of HIV infections attributable to STI infections.

The Rakai trial involved parallel cohorts of HIV negative individuals enrolled in control and intervention groups, respectively, with each group exhibiting similar STI prevalence rates. At the 20-month follow-up the intervention group displayed significantly lower incidence of syphilis and trichomoniasis, but the incidence of HIV infection was 1.5 per 100 person-years in both groups. The study concluded that STI intervention had no effect on incidence of HIV infection (*AIDS Scan*, 1999, 2000).

A possible interpretation of these results is that the HIV epidemic in Rakai had reached saturation with prevalence stable at 16%. Therefore a large proportion of new HIV infections was in individuals who did not fall into high-risk groups for contracting STIs. The Mwanza trial was conducted when the epidemic was immature. Interventions designed to treat symptomatic STI promptly and effectively can achieve a substantial reduction in HIV incidence in the general population (Orroth et al., 2000, p. 1,436), but treating STIs to reduce the incidence of HIV is likely to be most effective at earlier stages of the epidemic.

These trials provide clinical evidence to support what observational studies had long indicated, that STIs act as co-factors to enhance transmission of HIV and that improved STI treatment services can have a population-level effect on epidemics. This effect is most notable in areas where HIV prevalence is not high (Dallabetta, 1996; Grosskurth et al., 2000).

Mother-to-child transmission

Prevention of mother-to-child transmission has been widely researched. Relatively simple and inexpensive interventions can greatly reduce the chance of transmission (Gray, 1998). In the absence of intervention, between 15% and 45% of children born to infected mothers will themselves be infected. These children can be infected before birth (in vitro), during delivery or through breastfeeding after birth. Infection at delivery is most common. Anti-retroviral drugs decrease the mother's viral load and inhibit viral replication in the infant, thus decreasing the risk of MTCT. The US Center for Disease Control sponsored a trial of short-course AZT in Thailand. This involved AZT for the last four weeks of pregnancy. The result was a 50% reduction in transmission. Similarly, the PETRA (Perinatal Transmission) study in five urban settings in South Africa, Uganda and Tanzania showed transmission reductions of between 37% and 50%, depending on whether children were breastfed or not. In Uganda, trials of short-course doses of Nevirapine also produced a 50% reduction in MTCT (Whiteside and Sunter, 2000, p. 148).

The cost of the Thai and PETRA regimens was around US$89 for the drugs. The cost of Nevirapine for each treatment in the Ugandan regimen was US$4 (Marseille et al., 1999). However the patent holder of Nevirapine (Boehringer Ingelheim) 'recently stated that the company will make the product available for MTCT free of charge to the least developed and low income developing countries with specific programmes for the prevention of MTCT' (UNICEF et al., 2001, p. 11). However drugs are not the only cost. Counselling and testing as well as six months' formula feed at US$60 per infant will be required (Kinghorn, 1998).

Microbicides

It is strange that there has been so little research on microbicides. A microbicide is a substance (gel or foam) that a woman can insert into her vagina prior to intercourse, to kill viruses and bacteria. Microbicide could provide women with more control over their own protection in sexual encounters. Development of microbicides has been incomprehensibly slow, almost certainly because these preparations would have their main markets among poor women in poor countries – a market sector not renowned for it spending power!

Vaccines

Many believe the best hope for controlling the epidemic is a vaccine. Such a vaccine seems a long way off and even if one were developed it would need a high level of efficacy. The danger is that a vaccine might give people a false sense of security and actually increase the spread of HIV.

Vaccine development is resource intensive and most research is in the rich world. Such vaccines may not be appropriate or affordable for the poor world. The challenge is to find a solution that is acceptable, effective, affordable and deliverable. It has been necessary to persuade major pharmaceutical companies to pursue vaccine development with the enthusiasm they have devoted to anti-retroviral development. There is after all more profit in treatment which is repeated for life than in a vaccine which could be a one-time shot (Thomas, 2001).

Uncertainties associated with development of suitable vaccines include:

- The difficulty of establishing levels of immune response without human efficacy trials
- The existence of sub-types of HIV
- High risk behaviours associated with HIV infection are practised over an extended period. Any vaccine would need to induce a long-lasting immune response or involve regular boosters
- The lack of trained specialists and adequate infrastructure in poor countries for trials. Additionally, few countries will participate in trials unless they have access to the final, successful vaccine (HIV Vaccine Development Status Report, 2000 and Cullinan, 2001).

Despite the difficulties a number of countries are involved in trials. These are summarised in Table 13.2 below. International partnerships form an important component of vaccine development, as do public–private sector collaborations.

Behaviour

The second set of interventions is behavioural. Much has been written about these and there are numerous Knowledge, Attitude, Practice and Behaviour (KAPB) studies. It is increasingly recognised that knowledge is not enough. Most people are aware of AIDS and HIV. The problem is they do not see *themselves* as at risk. The need is to move beyond individual awareness to appreciation of the importance of risk environments. For example, condoms provide a biological barrier to infection but their use requires behavioural change. This change can only take place in the right context. A woman sex worker may be offered more money for sex without a condom by a man who believes his semen, left in a condom, could later be used for witchcraft.

Table 13.2 African AIDS vaccine research and development

Location	Main collaborators	Sponsors	Vaccine	Comments[1]
Kampala, Uganda	Makerere Univ., Case Western Reserve Uni.	NIAID[2]	Aventis Pasteur Canarypox	Ongoing Phase 1
Nairobi, Kenya	Univ. of Nairobi, Oxford Univ., IDT[3], Cobra Pharmaceuticals	IAVI[4]	Modified Vaccinia Anakara and DNA	December start
Hlabisa, South Africa	Univ. of Natal, Alpha Vax, Univ. of Cape Town	IAVI, NIAID, U.S Army	Venezuelan equine encephalitis	2002?
Kampala, Uganda	Johns Hopkins Univ., Makerere Univ.	NIAID	Canarypox and gp 120	For breast-fed infants
Uganda	Institute of Human Virology, Ministry of Health	IAVI	Salmonella and DNA	Team announced in May
Rakai, Uganda		U.S Army, NIAID	Canarypox Clade A	Under consideration
South Africa	Univ. of Cape Town, Univ. of Stellenbosch, Nat'l Inst. Virol.	SAAVI[5]	BCG, Modified Vaccinia Anakara, DNA, and fungal vectors	Pre-clinical
Tanzania	Muhimbili Univ., Swedish Inst. For Infect. Disease Control	Swedish Int'l Dev. & Coop. Agency		Cohort preparation
Addis Ababa, Ethiopia	Ethio-Netherlands AIDS Research Project	Neth. Ministry for Dev. & Coop.		Cohort preparation
Cote d'Ivoire	French cooperation	ANRS[6]		Cohort preparation

Source: AIDS Scan (2000b), p. 12.
[1] Dates as appear directly from the source
[2] NIAID: National Institute of Allergy and Infections Diseases
[3] IDT: Independent Development Trust
[4] IAVI: International AIDS Vaccine Initiative
[5] SAAVI: South Africa AIDS Vaccine Initiative
[6] ANRS: Agence Nationale de Rechérches sur le Sida

Voluntary counselling and testing is increasingly seen as an important component of prevention. The idea is to provide people with access to rapid testing in an environment where they will receive pre- and post-test counselling. If they are negative then they have an incentive to stay that way. If infected, the message is positive living. Such an intervention only works in a supportive environment – or one where levels of stigma are not high – and ideally where people can access some form of care.

Intravenous drug users

In areas where the epidemic is primarily among intravenous drug users, harm-reduction interventions are needed. These involve needle-exchange programmes, teaching addicts to clean their injecting equipment and trying to reduce the levels of drug abuse. Once again, context is important. In countries where drug possession is a capital crime, harm-reduction policies raise issues around criminality.

Upstream interventions

The argument is that policy makers and activists *do not* look beyond biomedical and behavioural interventions. They do not see the importance of factors that determine susceptibility to infection, that frame the behaviours that put people at risk. Responses must take account of determinants of the epidemic and address them. They must put in place 'upstream' interventions. The goal is to empower people to make decisions that reduce risks of infection, or to stick to existing behaviours that have the same effect. Although specific susceptibilities will vary from country to country, priorities might include:

- migrant labour systems (migrant miners in South Africa and commercial sex workers in Thailand and India) which fuel the epidemic in many parts of the world. Workers might be targeted with prevention messages (which is an individual approach), or alternatives to migration might be explored (a social and economic policy approach)
- enhancing the status of women. Actions range from training women and providing capital to assist them to become entrepreneurs, to tougher laws on rape, sexual harassment and protection of inheritance rights
- children, and particularly orphans, are vulnerable to sexual molestation. This subject must be discussed openly, and children must be placed in caring and protective environments

- Home ownership and electrification are potentially beneficial. Home-owners in some African settings are less likely to be infected because they have a long-term perspective and avoid risky behaviour. Electrification raises people's standard of living and gives them access to a range of recreational activities in addition to sex
- Displaced persons: these people can be given individual messages – probably inappropriate at times of extreme stress – or camps can be designed with HIV/AIDS in mind (Barnett, 1997).

What works?

This book argues for the importance of changing the risk environment as part of prevention. Focus on the individual can only be part of the strategy. Many of the simple individual behavioural interventions have been tried in various parts of the world. However in most settings, HIV prevalence has risen. What has worked and what lessons can be drawn? (World Bank, 2000).

National leadership and political commitment at all levels

Where the epidemic has been controlled at the national level there has been consistent and high-level leadership. President Museveni's response in 1986 has been described above. This initiative was not without political risk because at that stage AIDS was primarily identified with Western homosexual men.

In Thailand, in the late 1980s, fear that the public discussion of the epidemic might affect tourism meant that it was muted. Indeed an 'AIDS bill' proposed in 1990 would, among things, have required all newly discovered cases to be reported within 24 hours and the compulsory testing of people in 'high-risk' groups. In 1991/92, under the unelected government of Prime Minister Anand Panyarachun, HIV prevention and control became top priority. This was possible because leaders saw the scale of the potential problem and were willing to address it. The response was to:

- place AIDS policy under the co-ordination of the Office of the Prime Minister with a multisectoral National AIDS Prevention and Control Committee chaired by the prime minister. This signalled the high level of political commitment and encouraged sectors other than health to become involved. In particular, NGOs began to participate in the policy process
- a massive public information campaign was launched under the leadership of a well-known cabinet minister, Mechai Viravaidya

- the '100% condom programme' was adopted and promoted condom use in all commercial sex establishments all the time. Sex workers were screened weekly or biweekly at government STD clinics and were issued with free condoms. Contacts of male STD patients presenting at clinics were checked and if the patient had been infected in a brothel it was assumed to be a sign of non-compliance and the establishment could be closed.

There are two countries – Senegal and the Philippines – where the epidemic has not taken off and there is evidence of interventions that have helped (UNAIDS, 1999b).[3] Once again, leadership has been crucial. Obviously there are countries where there is no evidence of the epidemic having taken off. In some cases this does not mean that it has not or will not. We just do not have the data at present.

In Senegal, AIDS was first reported in 1986. A National AIDS Programme was rapidly established and had strong political support. In a country where 93% of the population is Muslim and 5% Christian, religious leaders played a crucial role. As early as 1989 the Islamic organisation JAMRA began talking with the national programme about its role in prevention activities. In March 1995 a conference of senior Islamic leaders gave clear support to AIDS-prevention activities. Christian leaders echoed this in January 1996 (UNAIDS, 1999b).

The Philippines saw its first AIDS case in 1984 and established the multisectoral Philippine National AIDS Council in 1992 (Philippines National AIDS Council, 2000). As in Senegal, high-level leadership resulted in destigmatisation and openness about the epidemic. This is seen most clearly in the Philippines AIDS Prevention and Control Act 1998 (Whiteside, 1998). This far-reaching legislation was debated extensively in both houses of parliament and created the framework for continued openness. For example, people could not be prevented from entering the country because they were HIV positive.

A necessary, but not sufficient, criterion for preventing spread of HIV or turning the epidemic round is political leadership. This must begin at the highest levels if there is to be national success. South Africa provides an example where absence of clear and decisive leadership damaged prevention activity.

Targeted interventions make public health and economic sense

Too often the response to the epidemic produces plans that list endless interventions. Most countries facing AIDS epidemics are poor financially and in administrative and human resources. Furthermore AIDS is not the only problem they face. Mozambique has a GNP per capita of only US$230 per year. Only 40% of children are in primary school and 22% in secondary schooling. Less than one-third of the population has access to clean water, and 37% live on less than US$1 per day. Health spending is a modest 2.1% of GDP, and has to cover all diseases – TB, malaria and annual cholera outbreaks, as well as HIV/AIDS. The country experienced years of civil wars, and in 2000 and 2001 devastating and widespread floods covered large areas and destroyed infrastructure. In this setting it is hard to prioritise AIDS, which is after all not yet visible.

Ainsworth and Teokul (2000, pp. 55–60) note that 'government AIDS control strategy documents typically embrace everything that might be done to fight AIDS'. These strategies are reinforced by technical best practices on specific interventions and by international donors, which may be able to support only interventions that address their institutional mandates. Objectives are expressed in terms of programme components, not outcome. The programme elements are typically not ranked in terms of their effectiveness in preventing the overall epidemic, given their costs. The result is that many activities and pilot projects are launched by government, donors and NGOs, but very few are implemented on a scale that would register an effect on the overall epidemics and the activities selected are not necessarily those that would yield the greatest impact. Furthermore, in the absence of any sense of priority, the activities that tend to get done are those with political support and those that are the least controversial. Those likely to have the largest impact on the epidemic – prevention among those most likely to pass HIV to others – are the lowest on the political agenda. Failure to prioritise has resulted in a lack of focus on specific objectives and a lack of results.

Countries that have prioritised show success. Thailand's concentration on public information and the 100% condom campaign was immediately effective. In Uganda, the leadership's support for behaviour change together with a multitude of small initiatives made the difference. In Senegal, leadership, information and massive promotion of condoms kept infection levels down. This may also be the key to the Philippines' success.

A multisectoral approach

A common feature of these countries is that they adopted a 'multisectoral response'. At the end of the 1990s this became an international buzzword, although it meant different things to different people. What seems to have worked is commitment across a society, from political leaders at all levels through to religious leaders, NGOs, the private sector and, where appropriate, traditional leaders. Ministries of Health had to relinquish ownership of the disease. This is seen in the location of AIDS leadership outside the health sector – in the Prime Minister's Office in Thailand and Uganda. In countries where health has jealously guarded its interests, success has either been slower or non-existent.

Multisectoral means looking beyond prevention to the whole epidemic. This includes treatment, policies and programmes to mitigate the impact of AIDS, and policies that will change the societal factors that influence long-run susceptibility and vulnerability to HIV/AIDS. In government each ministry has to ask what HIV and AIDS means for its core businesses and what it should be doing differently. Multisectoral response recognises the role of social and contextual factors conditioning individual decisions.

Good STD services are important

In Senegal and Thailand public STD services have been in place for many years. The Thai STD network was not sufficient to prevent the epidemic – an important point – but its existence was critical to monitoring the success of the 100% condom use campaign. In Senegal the STD service provided health checks and clearances for commercial sex workers and played a crucial role in information and condom distribution programmes.

The lesson seems to be that while STD services cannot prevent the spread of HIV, they are an important part of the portfolio of responses. Furthermore, the longer they have been around, the more likely they are to be accepted and respected.

Sexual practices

Are there common sexual practices that have helped to prevent the spread of HIV? There are two examples. Male circumcision is one, and is common in Senegal, the Philippines, Islamic countries and parts of Uganda. The results of two studies [4] in Uganda suggest that pre-pubertal male circumcision may reduce male HIV acquisition (Serwadda et al., 2000a). Similarly a study conducted in Kenya, Zambia, Cameroon and Benin (Buve et al., 2000[5]) concluded that there is strong enough evidence of the protective effect of male circumcision to start considering researching its feasibility as a preventative intervention. However, Serwadda et al. (2000a) caution that in the study in Uganda, male circumcision is associated with Islam and therefore any assumptions on the effectiveness of circumcision as a method to reduce acquisition of HIV may be influenced by other behavioural differences.

The second is attitudes to sex work. In Senegal sex work is licensed and controlled and women are required to have health clearance. While not legal in Thailand, the government recognises that sex work takes place and that it is regulated by a legal framework. A similar situation applies in the Philippines. There is not the gross exploitation of sex workers found in many other countries: sex workers have status, legal protection and their activities and health can be controlled. Recognition of the 'oldest profession' is realistic and a major requirement for addressing the epidemic. Hypocrisy, evasion and denial have no place in the control of sexually transmitted infection.

The role of treatment[6]

People who are infected with HIV require treatment. Prior to treatment is 'positive living' where people are encouraged to eat healthy balanced diets, avoid stress, give up harmful substances such as drugs and alcohol and lead more balanced lives. When their immune systems begin to fail they contract opportunistic infections such as TB, diarrhoea and thrush. Most of these can be treated or in some cases prevented by the judicious use of drugs which cost only a few dollars per patient per year. As the immune system deteriorates, patients can be provided with anti-retroviral therapy.

Since 1996, in the US, Western Europe and Brazil, highly active anti-retroviral therapy (HAART) has dramatically reduced death rates from AIDS and hospital admissions for AIDS complications. People have been able to return to full functioning (Beyrer, 2000). Additional benefits are that treatment with ARTs reduces viral load so people are less infectious (if they practise unsafe sex), experience fewer opportunistic infections and require less treatment.

When these treatments were first introduced they were extremely expensive – the drugs cost more than US$10,000 per patient per year. The disproportion between treatment cost and per capita health budgets was risible: US$5 per year for all health care as against US$10,000 per year for ARTs drugs alone. In addition, every dollar spent on drugs has to be matched with at least three more spent on adequate health infrastructure (Kallings and Vella, 2001).

Recent court cases and negotiations show that drug prices can be substantially reduced – to as little as US$300 per patient per year for a

Box 13.2   Anti-retroviral therapy (ART)

ART suppresses HIV, maintaining the integrity of the immune system and postponing development of opportunistic infections. First introduced in 1986, ART has evolved from mono (single)-drug therapy (AZT or Zidovudine) to dual-drug regimens (including AZT plus ddI, or AZT and/or ddI with d4T and 3TC) to triple-drug therapy, usually adding a protease inhibitor, in 1996. Single-drug therapy has been shown to have little effect on morbidity and mortality and is no longer used for treatment. Dual-drug regimens are only moderately effective in reducing morbidity, add less than one year of disease-free survival and have no real beneficial effect on length of life (Concorde, 1994). Effective ART generally requires a minimum of three agents used in combination to show real benefits in disease-free survival times and quality of life. HAART includes combinations of three and as many as five drugs, usually from one to three different classes of drugs, multiple regimens and combinations, and intensive monitoring of patients for resistance. HAART is an individualised treatment that evolves over time as patients develop resistance or side-effects that cannot be tolerated, requiring alternative drug combinations. ART must be taken for life, and requires high physician and patient compliance to be effective. For those who can comply with the therapy, it can greatly enhance the length and quality of life.

triple-drug combination. There are a number of important issues with regard to drugs, and not only ARTs. First is the issue of intellectual property and patent rights in medicines; second is the question of profit; third is the question of how practicable it is to provide these treatments in poor countries.

The Trade-Related Aspects of Intellectual Property Rights agreement (TRIPS), signed in 1994, is supposed to be included in the laws of all signatory nations by 2005. It is important for the availability of medicines in some of the world's poorest countries. These include treatments for conditions such as malaria, sleeping sickness and bilharzia, as well as HIV and AIDS. The TRIPS agreement makes it difficult for countries to purchase generic medications. In 2001, the

South African government was taken to court by a group of 39 pharmaceutical companies led by Merck and GlaxoSmithKline. These companies argued that for countries such as South Africa to obtain drugs cheaper than the major pharmaceutical companies were willing to sell them was to threaten profitability and ability to continue expensive research and development. The Treatment Action Campaign, an AIDS campaigning organisation, showed by means of sworn evidence from industry insiders that 'a third of all life saving drugs developed in the United States received federal aid to the tune of hundreds of millions of dollars' (*Observer*, 22 April 2001, p. 3). This evidence showed that profitability and levels of research and development were not as intimately related as the companies had claimed. The companies subsequently withdrew from the action, and this in turn meant that generic forms of patent-expired drugs could now, in principle, be freely purchased. However, combination ARTs will still have to be purchased at market prices because they are not yet patent-expired.

Countries can circumvent the TRIPS constraints if they declare that they face a 'national emergency' and that the drugs are necessary. However, so far even the South African government, with 4.5 million people HIV positive, has not seen fit to use this tactic, so the precise definition of a national emergency remains unclear. Indeed immediately after the court case the South African Minister of Health made it clear that the Department of Health had no intention of buying or distributing ARTs through the state facilities. She said: 'There is ... growing pressure for the use of anti-retrovirals on a much wider scale in SA. Our position on this matter is clear: at current prices we simply cannot afford to give anti-retroviral therapy in the public sector' (*Business Day*, 30 March 2001).

However, the story does not end with the pharmaceutical companies. Even if the drugs were available, they could not and cannot be ladled out like aspirin. These are complex treatment regimes which need to be monitored by laboratory tests and be adapted to individual patient needs over time. Medications may have to be taken at certain times of day, sometimes on an empty stomach, sometimes on a full stomach. And the full stomach may be a problem in many cases. Once again HIV/AIDS leads back to poverty. These drugs are less effective if patients do not have appropriate lifestyles and a good diet, and if the treatment is not monitored. Such conditions are untenable in poor countries where public medical services provide only the most basic treatments.

According to guidelines from UNAIDS, WHO and the International AIDS Society, 'due to the high cost of antiretroviral drugs, the complexity of regimens and the need for careful monitoring, specific services and facilities must be in place before considering the introduction of ART into any setting'. These include assured access to voluntary counselling and a test before and after treatment is initiated, capacity to recognise and manage common HIV-related illnesses; reliable laboratory monitoring services, assurance of adequate supply of quality drugs; identification of resources to pay for drugs on a long-term basis, information and training on safe and effective use of ART, and establishment of reliable regulatory mechanisms against misuse of the drugs. Once again, the guidelines emphasise the need for adequate nutrition and supportive environments (WHO, 2001, p. 16).

In many countries, counselling and testing services to identify clients, laboratory services to identify and monitor the disease stage and progress in treatment and sustained drug access do not exist. Use of public funds to provide ART for the small number of mainly urban, educated and comparatively wealthy people who can access these services would shift health resources from the poor to those who are not poor. Access to ART must therefore be improved together with the delivery of adequate, reliable health services for the poor. Such basic services are not yet secured, even for the treatment of common opportunistic infections.

There are other issues:

- the social and economic context of treatment. The need for correct diet is a prime example
- patient adherence to complicated treatment regimes
- to be effective, drugs must be taken every day for life in the prescribed manner
- resistance of HIV to anti-viral drugs. Resistance is most frequent for single or dual-drug therapy but is emerging with other treatment regimes and is a major cause of treatment failure. Inconsistent or incorrect use of the drugs speeds the development of resistant strains. In a study in the US, the majority of patients on HAART developed resistance (Ross et al., 2000). Some patients never achieve good control of HIV viral levels on ART or HAART, and the longer a patient takes these drugs, the less likely they are to be effective. In the EuroSIDA study, 12–15% of patients never responded to HAART, and 25% were no longer responding after 48 weeks on treatment (Mocroft et al., 2000)

- Adverse side-effects. Common side-effects, which can be debilitating and life-threatening, include anaemia, inflammation of the pancreas (pancreatitis), inflammation and pain of the nerves in the hands and feet (peripheral neuropathy), adult onset diabetes, elevated blood lipids (hyperlipidemia), heart attacks (myocardial disease), sharply elevated cholesterol levels (hypercholesterolemia), marked changes in body fat distribution (lipodistrophy syndrome), death of bone without infection (aseptic necrosis of bone), and kidney stones (nephrolithiasis)
- complexity of regimens for health care providers. Providers who treat patients on HAART need training and access to current data on this evolving therapy.

In other words, ARTs, even at much lower prices, are not 'the answer'. They are part of an answer, which must include head-on confrontation with the conditions that contribute to the epidemic in the first place. Those conditions are poverty-related risk. Access to affordable treatment and adequate health services has become one of the single most important differentiating factors between HIV-related survival in rich and poor countries and communities. As drug prices are reduced it will become more apparent that the critical constraints are health service provisioning and households' abilities to gain access to resources.

The poor world's best response is to recognise the role of appropriate treatment in prevention and mitigation. In particular there should be specific measures to strengthen primary-care levels of health systems and reduce barriers to access in low-income groups. At the end of the day the issue of relative poverty is crucial.

Responding to the epidemic: impact

If prevention does not work we do have to deal with the impact. A major problem is that we have not yet seen impact. In the UNAIDS *Guidelines for Studies of the Social and Economic Impact of HIV/AIDS* (Barnett and Whiteside, 2000), we concluded: 'One of the most important messages of this document is that, if consultants and researchers want to see the socio-economic impact of HIV/AIDS, *they have to look for it*. It is particularly hard to detect impact that is not measured by existing and conventional economic instruments.' Responding to impact involves planning; for example, provision of extra hospital beds and increasing health budgets, but if there is no evidence of impacts either within a country or from similar settings, then it is hard to persuade anyone to do anything. Response to impact is the greatest challenge.

The first reaction of a country reaching Stage 3 in epidemic impact evolution is to commission impact studies. The arguments are that if there is a measurable or predictable impact, then people can be convinced of the problem. Showing impact becomes an important tool for advocacy, as much for prevention as in relation to impact. It is necessary to know its location, scale, and form, and to begin planning for mitigation of impact.

Impact studies have a dual purpose. They provide the rationale for prevention and for mitigation. For countries in the early stages of the epidemic there is a paradox: if advocacy is successful, prevention may be more effective and reduce impact, and people may then regard these warnings as mere scare tactics – as HIV/AIDS is inevitably tied into broader political debates and competitions. Impact studies should be able to accommodate this tendency and not produce alarmist scenarios. In countries with more advanced epidemics, there is no doubt that there will be an impact; the challenge is to predict and mitigate it.

In Uganda and Thailand, the 'success story' countries, impact studies were not carried out. But these countries had data on the scale and extent of the epidemics. Uganda was the first African country to collect such data, no matter how imperfect. In Thailand early surveillance was extensive and convincing. Ainsworth and Teokul note that 'The implementation of the national "sentinel" surveillance system to monitor HIV infection in key population groups in 1989 and the public dissemination of results made it difficult to maintain an official position of denial and helped initiate the change in social norms necessary to change behaviour' (2000, p. 8).

There is no prescription for dealing with impact. There has been no national or regional plan that addresses this in a holistic manner. Experience shows that there exists a sparse range of responses. These are listed in Table 13.3.

In contrast, impact mitigation must start from the following principles.

Start with the numbers: predict impact

To assess the likely impact of HIV/AIDS, it is necessary to have an idea of the future course of the epidemic and of how many people will fall ill and die. It is important to keep in mind that models are simply tools that may be used to guide decision making.

Set priorities

Responses should follow the epidemic development curves outlined in Chapter 2. They should be informed and guided by the scale and stage of the epidemic, although given timelags and political resistance, for

Table 13.3   Responses

	Examples of targets	Responses	Examples
Group specific	Orphans in an area People living with AIDS	Care for orphans Home based care	NGOs, e.g. FXB, World Vision International agencies, e.g. UNICEF Various national NGOs Many national NGOs
Ministry specific	Revenue and expenditure Education	Plan for changes Changed demand and supply	Ministry of Finance Ministry of Education
Industry specific	Labour supply Employee benefits	Plan for labour shortages Reduce benefits	Various companies
National	Human resources Welfare benefits	Plan for changing populations and welfare transfers	There are none as yet

practical purposes planning should begin simultaneously in as many areas as possible.

Health care

The number of people needing care begins to rise. The public sector has to provide appropriate treatment within the constraints of a limited budget. HIV/AIDS will be the single biggest health care issue in many countries, including Asia and Latin America for years to come. Resource limitations and massively increased demand mean HIV/AIDS must be fully integrated into all aspects of health care and welfare planning. Failure to abide by this principle results in injustice to people with HIV/AIDS as well as to people with other health needs.

The private sector will not provide this care unless it is paid to do so or, as in the case of some companies, it is clearly in its interests. The public sector has to ask:

- Can money be switched from other areas of government to augment health care expenditure?
- Is it possible to develop a health care delivery system which meets HIV/AIDS needs in affordable, socially and politically acceptable and cost-effective ways?

The latter exercise cannot be left to doctors who are formally bound to seek the best care for patients regardless of cost. It requires inputs from professionals who are used to balancing patient needs against available public funds.

Government employees and capacity

Government conditions of service are generous. Government employees are not immune to infection. No government services, however poor, can be provided if staff are falling ill, and are dying and not being replaced.

Children

Of particular concern is the impact of AIDS on children. We must 'take full cognisance of the consequences of a rapidly increasing orphan population ... it is, however, both dangerous and wrong to exclude the very real needs and rights of other children, all of whom will be affected by the pandemic' (Morgan, 2000, p. 3). Amongst the most threatened are children from 'infected' households who are affected both before and after the deaths of their parents.

The consequences of *not* caring for affected children will be felt throughout society for generations. To avert this social disaster calls for urgent, imaginative responses from both the public and private sectors.

Box 13.3   One way to care for orphans

A suggestion is to train foster/adoptive parents selected by communities and church groups in conjunction with local authorities. Orphans (and here no distinction should be drawn between AIDS and non-AIDS orphans) will either be housed with these 'parents' or left in the family home under their supervision. The parents would be paid a small salary for supervision and provided with sufficient funds to cover food, clothing and incidental expenses. Such provision would require monitoring. NGOs might be appropriate bodies to do this. The aggregate costs of implementing such a proposal may be high, but the costs of not doing it – and producing a generation of neglected young men and women – will be even higher. Moreover, it highlights the point that the extra resources required to cope with the AIDS epidemic are not just monetary. Human resources are needed as well; the epidemic's impact affects socially reproductive labour. The terrible irony is that these resources will be depleted by the epidemic at the very time they are most needed. (See also Table 8.3.)

The private sector

Once the private sector perceives a threat it will respond to it. This response will prioritise corporate well-being rather than the interests of the nation or the population. Here the HIV/AIDS epidemic raises a recurring theme in this book – the boundaries between public and private where health is concerned and the closely related issues of corporate responsibility and accountability.

Response to HIV/AIDS has been inadequate. In most settings prevention has not worked, HIV prevalence continues to rise. Prevention strategies must relate to risk environments and not focus on behaviours. Few plan for impact. The rise in AIDS cases threatens to overwhelm health care systems, destroy families and impoverish communities. No response can be effective if it does not take into account the gross global inequalities that exist and are continuing to evolve.

14
Globalisation, Inequality, HIV/AIDS and the Intimacies of Self

In every possible way the essential public health trusts between authorities, science, medicine and the global populace were violated during the 1994 plague outbreak in India.

(Garret, 2000, p. 48).

Even the most natural action of all – the inhaling of clean air – ultimately presupposes a revolution in the industrial world order.

(Beck, 2000b, p. 168)

The HIV/AIDS epidemic has deep historical roots. Its impacts indicate a long, history-changing trajectory. The epidemic must be seen against this broad background. In contrast to previous generations, and from the vantage point of the twenty-first century, we can think about the epidemic in its full waveform. We can discern some of its deepest origins and reflect on its distant effects. There are lessons to be learned, not just about this disease, but about health, well-being and development as well. It is the first global epidemic of which we have been commonly conscious. It *may* be the epidemic that enables us to respond to the need for a common global public health. The epidemic makes us think how to bend global forces to provide more 'goods' for more human beings, and in areas beyond what is usually thought of as 'health'.

Health and well-being are not individual concerns: they are global issues. Paradoxically, there is a good to be gained, a lesson to be learned, from the HIV/AIDS epidemic. That lesson is neither straightforward nor will it be easy to understand because there is much resistance. It is the following: we need, at the beginning of the twenty-first century, to wake up to the emergency of global public health. We can

347

no longer depend on a view of disease, illness and disease control which is essentially medieval in conception and understanding. We must turn away from the excessive individualism of the final decades of the twentieth century to a *re-cognition*, literally a rethinking, of the ways in which our individuality depends upon common undertakings for the common good. Health and well-being are human rights; they are also public goods.

Rights can be protected and deepened through legal instruments and international agreements; public goods must be protected by collective action and organisation. But first of all a change of consciousness is required. It is necessary to recognise health and well-being as public goods, like the road networks, clean air and clean water (Yach and Bettcher, 1998). Right now this in not the case. President Franklin Roosevelt said: 'We have always known that heedless self-interest was bad morals; we now know that it is also bad economics.' One would now have to add 'and poor public health' (cited in Navarro, 1998, p. 743). Individualistic attitudes to health and well-being lead naturally to a defensive stance towards public health, a view that it is a last ditch stand against disease. This is a primitive stance which has its origins in the Middle Ages and before, in a more parochial and local period of our history.

A medieval approach to disease

Laurie Garrett's Pulitzer Prize-winning documentation of emerging diseases and their implications in *The Coming Plague* (1995), contains startling accounts of brave scientists from the US, Belgium, UK or somewhere else in the rich world, travelling to the Congo, Uganda, Bolivia or wherever to identify, confront and contain local outbreaks of terrifying disease. These people *are* committed and courageous; Garrett's account sometimes reads like a thriller. But the theories underlying the need for such adventures are a hangover from, and an extension to, medieval thinking. Instead of quarantining the infected households into the lazar house of a medieval town or village, we now send out the viral emergency SWAT squad to quarantine and contain the threat that may emerge from some remote neighbourhood of our global village. In the process we also save lives.

This is done in the interests of the rich – they want disease contained. It also has an air of charity about it. And what is wrong with charity? What is wrong with charity is its personal, fickle nature; its air of the dependence of the weak and poor on the will and disposition of the rich and powerful. What is wrong with charity is that it is subject to the vagaries of short-term funding. What is wrong with charity is that it should be a complement to, not a substitute for, concerted social, economic and political commitment and action for common welfare. What is wrong with charity is that personal moral agendas can be smuggled into action and remain unexposed to public examination and debate.

Right now, we try to contain infectious disease in the poorer neighbourhoods of the world as we have always tried to keep them in the poorer parts of our cities and whole societies. This was a sensible risk-avoiding response in a small village or town. It will not work in a global society. The flux of the globalised world of the twenty-first century is too porous, too flexible, too changeable and capricious to permit us to avoid risk. We live in a world of global risks; disease is only one of them: 'Distant happenings impinge on both local events as well as on ... the "intimacies of self"' (Caplan, 2000). The very large scale – what happens a world away – has serious and often immediate implications for the workings of our bodies, our intimate selves. Epidemics are societal events: disease is individual, corporeal distress; sexually transmitted diseases are intimate in the extreme. And, as we have found with HIV/AIDS, the construction and fulfilment of our intimate desires has implications for our common good. We need to think differently about health and well-being.

An outdated view of medicine, health, well-being

'Health' appears to be a quality of the body. That is where we feel unwell, where the symptoms of disease are experienced. It appears 'natural' that we should see health, or its opposite, sickness, as an individual, isolated experience for which we take individual responsibility. The underlying metaphor is of a machine that we either maintain or neglect. Such ideas link with broader notions in Western thought concerning the importance of the individual and his or her responsibility for his or her actions. This is not the only way to see the issue. Consider the following two problems:

- Is health really the issue or is there something broader called 'well-being' which questions the purely individual and bodily nature of 'health' and places more emphasis on the social and economic origins of 'ill-being'?
- Do we need to understand the idea of 'the individual' differently? This is not to suggest that individuals do not exist or have

significance; rather, it is to point out that the centrality of the individual as an acting and responsible entity is a product of Western history and experience. Others, elsewhere, see things differently, placing the social nature of the individual centre stage.

Amartya Sen[1] is an important commentator on these issues. He is deeply steeped in both Western and Eastern philosophical traditions. His approach to problems of poverty and well-being starts from the use which people get from their lives, how they are able to express and/or present themselves in the world. To understand the injustice of inequality, we need to see how economic, social, institutional and cultural structures stunt people's abilities to gain access to the resources which enable them to function as full human beings.

Cameron summarises Sen's account of this stunting and limiting process as follows:

- ... from sets of commodities available to an individual, to the individual's potential absolute capabilities, there will be limitations arising from particular advantage or disadvantages which they encounter in comparison with others consequent upon their historical, economic, cultural and social environment
- the actual capabilities that an individual achieves in their life means that they have a particular set of abilities to function
- the next step is to note that these abilities to function – 'functionings' in Sen's language – are the direct source of a particular individual's particular level of well-being. (Cameron, 2000b)

Sen's 'capability' approach focuses on the *opportunities* for choice open to people, rather than on the final outcomes they achieve. Potentially, this approach offers a way of limiting the need for contestable judgements about the nature of well-being as it notes that there can be a variety of limits to opportunity, different from one society to another. In this book we have seen many ways in which economy, society and culture may limit opportunity. We have also seen – in the case of Uganda – that a perception of a better future, that there is a future to plan for, may be a factor in enabling people to change their behaviour (Low-Beer et al., 2000).

These ideas are important because they move away from the dominant Western account of health and poverty as aspects of the individual. They involve a much broader perspective that spans cultures.

Sen's is a cross-cultural perspective. It allows a variety of interpretations of what it means to be a person and to have an identity. It engages with issues beyond the Western cultural tradition and conflicts with the currently dominant emphasis on 'the market' and 'the private' in considering the provision of public goods and services. These ideas were foreshadowed in the work of Karl Polanyi (1945). Polanyi's view was that in past societies the market mechanism was closely integrated with other aspects of social relations. But in 'the West' it became separated, 'disembedded', and thus uncontrolled and unmoderated by considerations of values other than price. In its most extreme manifestation, 'the market' is today held up by many politicians and philosophers as the best and only 'rational' way to decide on the allocation of goods and services, including health and welfare.

Polanyi's perspective engages with a question that takes us beyond the conventional perspective of the 'individual'. While the Western medical tradition deals with 'individuals' and even dissects individual's complaints into 'specialisms', this question locates individuals in their social field. It asks whether social relations can be considered as ends as well as means. In other words, whether social relations should themselves be considered as part of well-being. If this were to be the case, then the social relations of making a living, living with other people and rearing children, would have to be taken seriously as components of 'well-being' in ways which are not currently the case in the 'health' industry.

We live our lives in our minds but also through and in our bodies. We guard and worry about our health. *Our* health, *our* individual body, *our* well-being or *our* ill-being. Medical doctors deal with our individual health. We pay them or make public provision for them to be paid. But is this really what health, well-being and ill-being are about? These questions confront us with the necessity to consider how we relate to each other in this new world which we all share.

These social relations are all important aspects of public health inasmuch as the perspective which identifies 'health' with 'medicine' implies a much more individualistic version of a 'person' than does that which identifies 'health' with 'public health'. In the process, of course, the issue of whether or not social relations can be considered ends as well as means links once again to the notions of social cohesion, solidarity and public goods and their location and guardianship in a globalised world.

Social relations contribute to well-being.[2] They may be:

- 'relational goods' (Gui, 2000)
- goods which have characteristics of being 'public' or 'common' like, for example, transport infrastructure.

It may not be possible to supply the former category of good through markets, depending on whether a relationship, which is the good, is provided through a market. For example, a foster parent provides care and support, a parent provides love as well. Can money buy love? Can you cost a cuddle? The latter is not supplied or is under-supplied by markets because individuals and corporations have little incentive to supply those goods. Relational goods can be final consumption goods (that is, valued for themselves) and/or intermediate goods (for example, certain social relations may facilitate co-operation and trust). Social relations can be a source of value in themselves (Sugden, 2000; Bruni and Sugden, 2000). Social capital, social cohesion (as described in Chapters 3 and 4) or community connectedness make a huge difference to many facets of human life. Putnam (2000, p. 290) argues that 'social capital makes us smarter, healthier, safer, richer and better able to govern a just and stable democracy'.

Such ideas are rich in their implications for thinking about public health. Public health should be seen as a communal process that has elements of both a public good and a *relational good*: the good is consumed and enjoyed but the relationships through which it is provided are in themselves a 'good'. This 'good' is one which demonstrates care for others, an aspect of living with others. The problem is to develop an institutional locus for provision of such goods. These ideas about public health, health, medicine and the individual confront us with both challenges and opportunities in an era of 'globalisation'.

What is globalisation?

Globalisation means many things: the unleashing of market forces; the triumph of capitalism; the dominance of the 'truth' of neo-liberal economic theory; the market as the arbiter of welfare; the death of Keynesian intervention; minimisation of the role of the state; concern with economic growth at the expense of growing inequality; the assumption of individualism as the wellspring of human endeavour. In practice it means greater integration of the world's economies and formation of large trading blocs such as the European Union and the North American Free Trade Area. These organisations are remote from democratic control. The multinational companies that do most of the business are by definition not democratic. They answer to their shareholders. In these circumstances, many of our most important relationships are remote from democratic control or popular participation other than through the clumsy operation of markets and

Byzantine bureaucracies whose operation remains opaque to ordinary people.

Globalisation: upsides and downsides

There are profound disagreements about globalisation. Some argue that it must lead to greater inequality, more poverty, more exploitation on a global scale (Went, 2000). The result would be increasing exclusion and marginalisation of all those areas lying outside of the Triad (see Chapter 1) – the EU, Japan and US – where 15% of the world's population lives. Others believe that such dramatic developments offer opportunities for greater assistance to the world's poor; innovative and creative use of the new interdependence and interconnectedness of the modern world. In this view, globalisation means better communication, more sharing of ideas and information, decreased cost of international transactions, more perfect markets and thus better distribution of goods and services, the spread of norms and values and the proliferation of global agreements on things such as human rights. The new wealth so created could be managed wisely to provide opportunities and better levels of life for more people (HM Government UK, 2000).

But globalisation is not about markets and economics alone. It is about cultural and political change. There was a time when locality was of the greatest importance and reputation mattered. That has been less the case since the growth of industrial society. Our relationships are mediated through an often distant market. Those processes have moved even further ahead in the past 20 years with the development of electronic communications, of branding (Klein, 1999), marketing and a global culture. Some of us can move beyond the local and maintain quite complex and close relationships across timezones and cultures.

What does globalisation do for the distribution of 'goods' and 'bads' in the world? This question must be considered as we think about the impact of HIV/AIDS and its implications. Globalisation is not a neutral process of closer and faster linkages between diverse areas of the world. It is an asymmetrical process. It does not affect all areas of the world equally or in the same way. Certain relationships, for example, capital transactions, are highly integrated, while others, movements of people and access to technology, are governed by restrictive regulations – as, for example, with regard to anti-retrovirals and other pharmaceuticals. The result is that certain regions of the world – notably sub-Saharan Africa – 'remain on the periphery of these trends towards progress and economic dynamism' (Alonso, 2001, p. 87), except where skilled labour is imported or the poor world provides a dumping ground for toxic waste and a location for hazardous and arduous work.

This global process has local effects. Highly qualified Filipinos work as nurses and teachers and even as house servants in Europe and America. Britain imports doctors and nurses for its 'national' health service because it does not invest sufficiently in training. Harsh immigration and asylum laws are waived for 'useful' refugees who can contribute to British economic growth. In each case 'local' talent, trained with the resources and within the constraints of a poor country, moves across the world to make its contribution in another locality. One locality bears the cost, another reaps the return.

Investment, cost, productivity and realisation of profit are spread across a whole world of space through complex networks of finance and organisation, and through decades of time. Cause and effect are often so widely separated in space and time that it is difficult or impossible to locate responsibility. The same is true of losses and costs associated with the impact of HIV/AIDS. With an epidemic affecting the whole world we must think about how much it is costing whom and when and over what period. This question is not simple and it has social, economic and ethical dimensions.

There is another argument. This recognises that the globalised world is replete with risk and hazard. The risks arise from the complex interactions which occur when, for example, uncontrolled industrial production results in pollution and environmental damage, when inadequately controlled animal feed processing resulting in prions jumping species and the 'mad cow'/nvCJD epidemic saga erupts in Europe. Or when new processes, genetically modified organisms for example, are introduced and the only real 'test' of their safety is their mass marketing and use. At this stage, 'risk' becomes an *inappropriate* word, with its implications of calculability and scientifically based knowledge (Beck, 2000b, pp. 50–1). It has to be replaced by another word: 'hazard'. Hazards are uninsurable because the risk is incalculable and the 'experiment' to ascertain the degree of risk is in effect carried out on the world at large. However, these new risks and previously unperceived hazards may, paradoxically, offer opportunities. They are no longer controllable by the nation state and thus they require an alternative form of organisation if they are to be brought under control and contained.

For the past 200 years human beings have found it useful – even 'natural' – to live in nation states and for nationality to be their primary identity along with sexuality, gender, language and belief. This process has gone further in some parts of the world than in others. In Europe there are now strong but contested moves away from nationality towards 'super-nationality', the European Union. In other parts of the world, ethnicity competes with and contests nationality as in multiethnic states like Indonesia where the construction of nationality remains incomplete and maybe unachievable (Leith, 2001). Nationality is one of the great 'imagined communities' within which we live our live – but it is imagined and therefore changeable.

Few politicians seriously argue that national governments can control and manage the economies of individual nation states. Many large international companies have turnover and reserves far larger than many nation states.[3] Indeed, there are several individuals whose total wealth far exceeds that of a swathe of the world's states. The power of large multinational corporations suggests that nation states may no longer be the right, appropriate or effective mechanism for dealing with the risks and hazards created by such powerful entities. There is a disjuncture between personal identity as a member of a nation and this realisation.

The limitations of the nation state should be obvious to us all. Indeed, one of the key functions of the idea of the nation state – in the hands of contemporary politicians, at least – now seems to be to explain why it is *not* possible to do things that citizens may wish to have done on their behalf. There is some justifiable concern about the potential and future of nation states. There is a real issue: nation states may in fact be fossils from an earlier period of political evolution, inappropriate mechanisms for the challenges that we now face. The difficulty is that those who govern and administer them have an interest in their maintenance. For the rest of us it is hard to see viable alternatives.

In the absence of effective nation states and in a world of multinational corporations, who are the agents and actors in the drama and how are they to exercise and make manifest their agency and action? The answer is just discernible. The agents are networks and movements of actors in different nation states, focused on issues, pursuing common and sometimes conflicting strategies. At times these strategic alliances may consist of combinations of nation states, international agencies, national non-governmental organisations, international non-governmental organisations, UN agencies, and so on. This is a complex game. While the world of nation states may be akin to chess, this new world is akin to multidimensional chess played across cyberspace without a board. The nature of that game cannot be more poignantly evident than in the terrible events of 11 September 2001 in the US and their equally terrible sequelae, as nation states try to engage with a threat which does not originate in a nation state. Nowhere more than in these events and in the HIV/AIDS epidemic can we see the need to begin creating a 'global civil society'[4] and the inadequacies of our existing arrangements.

In fact, though, this is not only a hope for the future: it is the way that the fight against HIV/AIDS has been and is being pursued. It is paradoxical and part of the contradictions of globalisation that the mechanisms for intervention are often so remote from the lives of those, particularly the very poor, who are acutely affected. Indeed, the mechanisms of the internet and the email which permit effective strategic co-ordination are distant from these lives. International email and internet discussion and information groups are far from the sick person in a Nairobi slum or an orphaned child on the streets of Calcutta. But they can and do influence those lives.

It is significant that UNAIDS was established in a way which was and remains different from other United Nations agencies. It contrasts with the feudal fiefs of the UN's older and bigger agencies. These – the Food and Agriculture Organisation, based in Rome, or the International Labour Office and the World Health Organisation, both in Geneva, or the United Nations Development Programme and the United Nations Children's Fund, both based in New York – are quite autonomous bodies with a high degree of independence from the central UN organisation. In contrast, UNAIDS struggles to be a coalition-building, inter-agency co-ordinating body. In addition to its work with the NGO and corporate sectors, UNAIDS works with some of the major actors on the AIDS scene, a veritable spaghetti soup of acronyms: the World Bank, the European Union, the United Nations Development Programme, the United Nations Children's Fund, the United Nations Population Fund, the United Nations International Drug Control Programmes, the United Nations Educational, Scientific and Cultural Organisation, the World Health Organisation.

HIV/AIDS is a problem that is not handled easily by the mechanisms and methods of the nation state. It has drawn out from the world community a response that depends on fluidity rather than extreme bureaucracy – although UNAIDS is inevitably affected by these features of the international administrative culture.

It is in this fluid coalition of agencies, old traditions, new technologies, new links and alliances between private, public and 'third sector' (NGO) funding and action, 'client' and 'activist' groups, that early forms of an effective engagement with this first globally perceived epidemic are visible. This could go far beyond HIV/AIDS towards an engagement with global public health.

There are opportunities for innovation and for more 'goods' but there is only a glimmer of hope. We must think about areas of immediate and medium-term action that may make for the wider availability of the 'goods' which the global systems could and ought to provide. These are:

- global intersectoral action through transnational co-operation and partnerships between public health and trade and finance sectors
- an enhanced role for international legal instruments, standard setting and global norms with regard to entitlements to health and well-being
- comprehensive global vigilance, research, monitoring and assessment to provide information about comparative health status and global determinants of health and well-being
- research programmes that concentrate on developing cost-effective technologies to improve the status of the poor
- development of international agreements regulating prices of medications in different markets
- recognition that management of health and well-being is a common human project and that the for-profit sector can only have limited incentives to meet those needs (Alonso, 2001).

But while they are desirable, pursuit of these goals is difficult. There are many obstacles. First, we have to persuade people of the true cost of HIV/AIDS. Second, business has a role to play, but the business of business is profit not welfare. Perhaps that is also an assumption that must be challenged. In the same way that HIV/AIDS is about more than health, so business has responsibilities beyond profit.

In every society, processes of distribution and social co-ordination combine three complementary mechanisms:

- the market – distribution through competitive pricing
- hierarchy – distribution through organisation processes
- values – distribution as a response to accepted ethical principles (Alonso, 2001, 91).

Globalisation is an ideology that suggests distribution through the market is the best and only way, to the exclusion of the other two. The challenge is to find arrangements whereby the production and distribution of international public goods such as primary health care and public health provision may be managed within a multilateral system. UNAIDS is a precursor of how this might be achieved. And it is perhaps also a signifier of the forces against such change and the conservatism of the institutional fossils of the UN system that efforts are apparently afoot to reabsorb UNAIDS back into the World Health Organisation![5]

Responsibility in a global economy

The impact of the HIV/AIDS epidemic affects the poor, local and already risk-burdened more than it does the rich and the cosmopolitan. Of course it affects individuals, and that pain is never to be discounted just because they are rich. But the impact of the epidemic causes more than individual pain among the poor. Indeed this book argues repeatedly that the epidemic has very far-reaching consequences.

There is an issue of remoteness: How far do you track the process of cost-bearing? Anybody who has had an inconsiderate neighbour hold a noisy party knows the cost of the neighbour's enjoyment is paid through others' loss of sleep and bad mood the following day. With a long-wave epidemic of infectious disease, the question of downstream costs – impacts – is very complex. So also is the question of upstream responsibilities – the roots of the epidemic in social and economic events. We have examined this is detail in Chapters 3, 4 and 5. And with those questions arise also the possibility of demands for compensation from those who are paying today and tomorrow for events which happened long ago. Of course such responsibilities cannot be clearly identified, causal chains will be debated, and arguments as to legal liability and compensation would enrich many lawyers. But the idea that such things could be possible should make us more careful about current neglect of those who do not live in the Triad countries. The decidedly minority interests in saving threatened species and environments of 50 years ago are becoming mainstream global political issues, demands for apology and compensation for the abuses of the north Atlantic slave trade are seriously – if unproductively – debated in international fora.

We think of costs as associated with identifiable units, individuals, households, communities, companies and nations. These entities have legal statuses and can be held responsible because they are subject to legislation and due legal process. At least in principle. The problem is that it is just this perspective of legally responsible entities, bounded by identifiable spatial spheres of assumed influence and effect of their actions that may limit consideration of *responsibility*. It is quite possible for an irresponsible group of producers in the same industry to cause general hazard to the environment and yet escape individual responsibility. This is because in a world of legal entities, individual contributions to the hazard cannot be precisely identified through any legal process. Many activities undertaken in the pursuit of 'wealth', 'economic growth' and 'development' involve transferring the costs to another place which is geographically remote, or to another time (as with disposal of highly radioactive waste). Economists describe the idea of a project's cost being paid elsewhere as an 'externality'. We have seen cases of this in Chapter 5. In the late nineteenth and early twentieth centuries, availability of impermeable rainwear and motor tyres in the rich world were rooted in the brutalities associated with wild rubber supplies in King Leopold's Congo. Ironically, this was true also of the rubber condoms that facilitated the birth control revolution in Western Europe and North America (Banks and Banks, 1954), the mechanism for the famous Western 'demographic transition'.

While the world's wealthy and comparatively wealthy create problems for the poor, the poor create problems for themselves as they endeavour to survive. The poor are very likely to inhabit or move within a series of overlapping risk environments. On most measures, chances of encountering a hazard are high. If you are very poor, a recent migrant to a city, with accommodation hard to find, then a riverbank shanty settlement may be the only option, despite the flies, the slant of the floor and the density of people. More people, more sanitation problems, more marginal areas of the riverbank are colonised. The riverbank is undermined and then, in addition to the costs in illness and death associated with poor sanitation and drinking water, the next flood brings death, destruction and environmental change as the riverbank is swept away. As Michael Zurn puts it:

Whereas many wealth-driven ecological threats stem from the *externalisation of production costs*, in the case of poverty-driven ecological destruction it is *the poor who destroy themselves* with side effects for the rich. In other words, wealth-driven environmental destruction is distributed evenly around the globe, whereas poverty-driven environmental destruction strikes at particular spots and becomes international only in the form of side-effects appearing over the medium term. (quoted in Beck, 2000b, p. 35)

The conditions whereby the poor destroy themselves are another aspect of the local risk environment, that aspect of abnormal normality that has been described in Chapter 5. The long history of disruption in Africa described there represents just one aspect of the way that large-scale events and processes associated with economic growth in some parts of the world have resulted in impoverishment and local damage – of which the HIV/AIDS epidemic is but one manifestation.

So what does it cost for a Filipino woman with a college degree to leave her home and work as a maid in Los Angeles? What does it cost for a trained teacher to leave rural Uganda to seek work in a town in Europe? What does it cost if a woman teacher dies of AIDS in Tanzania, Thailand or South Africa? The movement of a migrant, the loss of a person to illness; both of these impact upon the individual concerned of course. But they also affect and change the lives of those who are left behind and on the lives of people beyond the immediately identifiable domestic unit where the obvious burden of cost is concentrated. However, the optic of globalisation should ensure that we no longer fall into the trap of thinking that anything is any longer 'local'.

What has HIV/AIDS to do with corporations?

Large corporations operating in a global economy can plan their way out of the AIDS epidemic just as they avoid most other local constraints on their activities. By the 1990s some large corporations operating in Africa had completed AIDS-related risk analyses. For reasons of commercial and political sensitivity, these studies remained confidential. These actions have to be understood against a background of how business is done in a world of intimate global links and increasingly centralised and concentrated corporate structures and finance.

In the last 40 years, business has changed fundamentally. The first industrial revolution of the eighteenth and nineteenth centuries depended on large, underpaid and initially non-unionised workforces and involved cheap labour, mass production methods and the satisfaction of home markets followed by expansion overseas. Such highly integrated factory-based organisations were profitable and expanded against a background of regular fluctuations in the trade and production cycles. These corporations were a clear target for workers' organisations. During the twentieth century, workers gained better wages and working conditions. They made *political* bargains assuring additional social wages in the form of health care provision, pensions and education, and government intervention to create better lives and reduce individual risk.

By the mid-1960s this was changing. The limits of mass production, with its inflexibility, fixed capacity and inability to respond to trade and production cycles, had been reached. Some economists and politicians saw the social wage as unsustainable. This was the beginning of the 'new international division of labour', a period of peripheral industrialisation when production capacity and plant was relocated to low wage regions of the globe. These countries offered cheap labour and weak workers' organisations, often associated with 'strong', undemocratic governments which did not respect human rights. This was an important point in the process that has come to be called globalisation. A recurring theme throughout has been the search for co-ordination and control. The electronic and communications revolution of the past 50 years has made this easy and instantaneous.

In the past three decades, many companies have endeavoured to free themselves from fixed plant and large workforces with complex needs through becoming increasingly virtual organisations. In principle, a modern corporation might be located in a small suite of offices in an anonymous city block anywhere in the world. From there it would make contracts with subcontractors and other suppliers, with assembly plants and packaging and logistic specialists. E-commerce is the end-state of the globalised multinational corporation. In such systems of production and distribution, a company is immune to many risks, including those of the AIDS epidemic. It has insignificant numbers of employees, holds little in the way of stock, and has no long-term commitment to a workforce. Therefore it can and will move its production requirements to wherever they can be fulfilled at the cheapest price available. Or it can move its capital assets to the market with the best yield. Only if the epidemic hits sales do modern corporations have to take HIV/AIDS on board. Even then they have little incentive to deal directly with the immediate or long-term effects of the epidemic. They could simply withdraw from that market.

Few corporations have achieved quite this degree of elevated virtuality – a kind of corporate other-worldliness.

> By shifting more and more of their production to contractors, companies can distance themselves from potential charges of labour rights abuses and other illegal behaviour and keep labour costs low by forcing contractors to compete for business with an ever smaller number of giant purchasers. The giant firms also have more freedom to hire and fire contractors to meet shifting demand. (Anderson and Cavanagh, 2000, p. 5)

Firms can avoid cost-incurring risks associated with employing a labour force. They can at the same time avoid any involvement with or concern about what, viewed from within the Triad, looks like a 'local' HIV/AIDS epidemic.

Some companies do consider HIV/AIDS and are prepared to bear the costs, as in the case of Debswana (Chapter 10). This company is special. The corporation is part of a major multinational (De Beers) but is co-owned by the Government of Botswana. It has decided to care for its workforce and their spouses. This decision was taken after consideration of the complex balance between legality, morality and profitability that involved tough decisions and tough negotiations within the company. In some respects, a mining company is exceptional because the mineral deposit is fixed. This means that the company cannot move to a less expensive and risk-laden environment.

Other companies are tied to particular geographical regions and will have to take the potential costs and liabilities on board. In particular smaller companies perhaps more tightly tied into local or regional economies will not be in that position at all. Indeed, the further down the chain of value a company is, the more likely it is to be a subcontractor to a contractor to one of the virtual corporations at the top of the chain. In effect, it is these third- or fourth-order local companies which will be bearing the burden of HIV/AIDS risk locally while the larger international corporations will be able to avoid those direct costs which attack the bottom line. The statistics for the degree to which major multinationals avoid employing people directly are arresting. The sales of the top 200 corporations world wide are the equivalent of 27.5% of world economic activity, yet they employ only 0.78% of the world's workforce. At the same time, between 1983 and 1999, the profits of the top 200 firms grew 362.4%, while the numbers of people they employed grew by only 14.4% (Anderson and Cavanagh, 2000, p. 1).

As pressure for cost reduction is passed down the chain, so the final squeeze is applied to labour which must either be substituted for by capital or persuaded to accept lower wages and/or less favourable working conditions. The local effects of this downward pressure are in low wages, poor conditions, occasionally coerced working conditions and ultimately the creation of urban and rural risk environments in which infectious diseases, among them HIV, are more easily transmitted. This applies as much to the rural producers of high-value horticultural products and cut flowers in Kenya, Nicaragua or Malawi as it does to the factory workers in Thailand, Cote d'Ivoire or China. Only through a sustained campaign to get businesses and governments to sign up to ethical policies and legal provisions in relation to the rights of their workers, will we be able to intervene to stop businesses from burden shifting and thus creating the risk environments which facilitate an epidemic such as HIV/AIDS. In the absence of this the costs will devolve to government and ultimately households.

Inequality, susceptibility and outcomes

Whether a person contracts HIV depends on his or her social and economic position. Social class, gender, ethnicity, market position all combine to create particular ways of making a living. Livelihood opportunities determine entitlements. Together these are the major influence on sexual networks. Farmer commented, in relation to Haiti, that:

> conjugal unions with non peasants (salaried soldiers and truck drivers who are paid on a daily basis) reflect women's quest for some measure of economic security. In the setting of a worsening economic crisis, the gap between the hungry peasant class and the relatively well-off soldiers and truck drivers became the salient local inequality. In this manner, truck drivers and soldiers have served as a 'bridge' from the city to the rural population, just as North American tourists seemed to have served as a bridge to the urban Haitian population. (Farmer, 1999, p. 135)

This is a microcosm of the global situation. Some of us inhabit a world where we can be spatially – if not sexually – polygamous; others are stuck in their locality, but the world comes to them. We should not be surprised that the initial distribution of this epidemic was among the rich and more cosmopolitan in Africa and elsewhere. They could travel and become infected. They had easy sexual access to 'local' people, people who were neither cosmopolitan nor wealthy. Hence the later and continuing epidemic among the poor. This is the effect of globalisation as a creator and distributor of 'bads'.

Initial states of individual health, nourishment, parental and grandparental nutritional status, degree of physical exhaustion, mental state, work conditions, residential location all influence susceptibility to infections (Farmer, 1996; Cohen et al., 1997; Cohen et al., 1999). With specific relation to HIV/AIDS, how the disease progresses, its outcome, is also an expression of social and economic inequality (Chaisson et al., 1995). Life expectancy after HIV infection is associated with diet, environment, state of mind, housing and a host of other factors that are usually associated with income. With the introduction of ARTs the difference in outcome between the rich and the poor has become even more stark.

Treatment is not really the starting point of the problem; it is the end-state. To always think about treatment is to remain distanced from the social and economic origins of illness and ill-being. Illness and ill-being are not only or most importantly about individual risk. Rather they are 'systematic events, which are accordingly in need of general political regulation. Through the statistical description of risks ... the blinkers of individualisation drop off' (Beck, 2000b, p. 51). We have adopted this perspective in our discussion of susceptibility and vulnerability in Chapter 3. It is important. Risks appear as systematic events, common events, when they are described and measured. Otherwise they appear as local or even individual events. We only see aggregates through measurement and abstraction. When we are aware of these aggregate events we can then respond. But response requires that we can enable 'the blinkers of individualisation' to drop off and see what is common. For the moment, we tend to see 'risk' in very local terms, either geographically or the individual. These blinkered perceptions are no longer appropriate, but they are part of a process of denial.

All human groups know how to insure by spreading and thus sharing risk. This is not because they are motivated by altruism or are natural socialists. Rather it has to do with the need to survive. Risk spreading and sharing may range from very simple and humane interactions – the care that we give each other in the domestic group, the intergenerational bargains which extend that care over time, the immediate care found in the domestic bonds of childrearing. In a globalised world, risks are amplified and the opportunities for risk differentiation are greatly augmented as the number of risk niches increases. Advances in data collection and analysis enable those with power to identify and avoid these risks. However, the possibilities and mechanisms for risk sharing among the poor barely exist. There are few structures and little willingness beyond the ideologies of charity and self-interest. Public health is a way of pooling risk. And in the contemporary world we have to put risk in a perspective that is wider than the individual.

A broader implication of the HIV/AIDS epidemic is that we must examine and reflect upon the ideas of 'health' and 'well-being' critically and anew. We cannot act as though we were inhabitants of a medieval city state and exclude those who are sick and/or poor. There is no longer any quarantine, we cannot avoid contagion. This is a vital task for the first decade of the twenty-first century. Debates about and understandings of poverty have moved from 'absolute' poverty to relative deprivation, inequality and the multidimensional nature of deprivation: so too must our understanding of well-being.

But we must go further. Human beings must and will continue to interact. Will we build just and cohesive societies both within and beyond national borders? Or will we continue to isolate and defend ourselves in islands of prosperity, in Europe, North America and then in city blocks and rural refuges within those regions, or within elite enclaves in the capital cities of the poor world, while remaining surrounded by an increasingly hostile, desperate and suspicious world?

Human beings have rights. We began this book with an African woman pleading that 'people are dying', '*Abantu Abaafa*'; we end by taking her plea further: to recognise the importance of '*ubuntu*', an African idea, that we are only people because of other people. We are all human and the HIV/AIDS epidemic affects us all in the end.

Notes

1 Disease, Change, Consciousness and Denial

1 This is the title of a PhD thesis about HIV/AIDS and the elderly in Uganda by Alun Williams (1998).
2 <www.undpp.org.ws/HIV/aidsfacts.htm>
3 This may seem paradoxical, but there are undoubtedly some winners, for example those who are uninfected and inherit property.
4 Updated information may be obtained from the UNAIDS website <http://www.unaids.org>
5 Data are taken from the UNAIDS website <http://unaids.org>
6 Authors' fieldnotes, 1989.
7 Ibid.

2 The Disease and its Epidemiology

1 <http://news.bbc.co.uk/hi/english/events/newsnight/newsid_1274000/1274831.stm>
2 <www.sirius.com>
3 Phylogeny is the classification of organisms in terms of their distance from each other as measured by particular characteristics. In the case of HIV this classification is done in relation to the presence or absence of different proteins on the coat of the virus. Different systems of classification will suggest differences in relatedness, both contemporary and evolutionary.
4 Van der Vliet. She quotes a report from B. Korber 2000. 'Timing the Origin of the HIV-1 Pandemic'. Unpublished paper, Seventh Annual Conference on Retroviruses and Opportunistic Infections, San Francisco, 30 January–2 February 2000.
5 Cohen and Mitchell, 1998.
6 Most of the data on TB is taken from the Health Systems Trust, 1999.
7 <http://www.unaids.org/hivaidsinfo/statistics/june00/fact_sheets>
8 These may be accessed on line at <www.census.gov/ipc/www> or on CD #623510.
9 Although if misused they could form the basis of an entirely new dating culture in richer societies where their cost is by no means prohibitive – about US$20 a test – and the result can be known in 20 minutes (OraQuick®, Epitope, Inc.).
10 UNAIDS and UNICEF have models for the calculation and estimation of number of orphans on their websites.
11 These types of projection may be done with Spectrum software available from the Futures Group.

3 Epidemic Roots

1 This has long been well-known in a vernacular sense. It was not until McNeil (1976) wrote his work on the subject that the view was explored in any great detail.
2 There are also some diseases which are caused by a different class of organisms, prions.
3 Life Years – this is used to refer to the Disability Adjusted Life Years (DALYs) which is a measure of the burden of disease in a population. For more information and explanation see World Bank, *World Development Report* 1993, 27 and WHO, 2000, pp. 27–9.
4 Summarised from a box by Richard Rothenberg in Mann et al., 1993, pp. 176–7. More detailed discussion of this work may be found in Hethcote and Yorke (1984) and in Anderson and May.
5 Author's field work.
6 Personal communication, Prof. Jim Kiernen, Department of Social Anthropology, University of Natal.
7 For a critical discussion of this perspective, see Le Blanc, et al. 1991. See also a number of articles in the *Journal of Southern African Studies*, 27(2) 2001 edited by Deborah Potts and Shula Marks. These argue that in a number of countries of southern and eastern Africa fertility levels have been falling, in some cases for 20 or 30 years. We are grateful to Shula Marks for drawing this material to our attention.
8 Extract from internet discussion about HIV/AIDS and youth in Africa as preparing for meeting of the African Development Forum special session on HIV/AIDS 2000, author James Okee-Obong (PhD). Ludwig Boltzmann Institute for Sociology of Health and Medicine, University of Vienna, Austria. Text as presented on internet side.
9 These ideas are discussed further in Chapter 5 and in Manderson and Jolly, 1997.
10 See for example Fransen and Whiteside, 1995 and Filmer, 1996.
11 Such as South Africa's *Immorality Act* (Republic of South Africa, 1927)
12 There is a large and growing literature on these relationships. See for example Egolf et al. 1992, Fiscella and Franks, 1997, Gravelle, 1998, Gregorio et al. 1997, van Doorslaer et al. 1997, Kaplan et al. 1996, Kawachi and Kennedy, 1997a, 1997b, Kawachi et al., 1997, Wilkinson, 1997, 1999a, 1999b, Wilkinson et al. 1998.

4 Cases

1 The Bank's income divisions were, in 1999: low income US$755 or less; lower-middle-income US$756–$2,995; upper-middle-income US$2,996–$9,265; high income above US$9,266. The UNDP has a geographical division similar to but not exactly the same as the Bank's, an incomes classification based on those of the Bank, and two different ones: a 'world classification' and a division according to Human Development Index (HDI) level. The world classification is: industrialised countries; all developing countries; and Eastern Europe and the CIS. There are three clusters of HDI level: high human

development, HDI of 0.800 and above; medium HDI of 0.500–0.799; and low HDI of below 0.499.

2   In our previous publications developing these concepts, this was referred to as the 'Jaipur Paradigm'. It was first developed, together with the South Asian participants, in a policy research workshop in Jaipur, Rajasthan; see Barnett et al., 2000a.

3   Data for this section are taken from *AIDS/HIV Quarterly Surveillance Tables no. 36, 97/2*, August 1997 and from the PHLS website <http://www.phls.co.uk> in February 2000.

4   The definition used in the PHLS AIDS and STD Centre tables is 'individuals from abroad and individuals from the UK who have visited abroad, for whom there is no evidence of "high risk" partners'.

5   It has been impossible to identify any research to support this assertion. However, personal communications from individuals at the PHLS suggest that this has indeed been the case.

6   This may be an important issue in many countries where there is a market in blood and blood products. We have recent but unsubstantiated reports of seroprevalence in a rural part of western China reaching 20%, probably as a result of blood collectors using the same needles in a population where intravenous drug use is common.

7   Barnett (1995, 1998).

8   NACO (2001).

9   The social and cultural nuances of migration in India are complex. For a detailed discussion of this we are grateful to Ben Rogaly (Rogaly et al., 2001; Rogaly and Coppard, 2001). These complexities result in a wide range of 'risk environments' and susceptibilities which are worthy of extended research if we are to understand the social and economic roots of the Indian epidemic.

10   Information for this section is based on interviews conducted in India in 1997 and on more recent data collected in 2000 and in 2001. Statistical data were collected from Manipuri informants and have not been checked for consistency with published sources.

11   Authors' fieldwork.

12   The data for this section are taken from the report *The Social and Economic Impact of HIV/AIDS in Ukraine*, Barnett and Whiteside, 1997. This report was prepared in close co-operation with Lev Khodakevich, Yuri Kruglov and Valentyna Steshenko. The report is available on the website of the British Council, Kyiv. See also Barnett et al. 2000b. Further data collection was undertaken in 2001 as this book was being finished.

13   This total may seem unlikely but there is evidence that such a programme was completed.

5   Why Africa?

1   Authors' fieldwork.

2   The following description is based on Kjekshus (1997).

3   Personal communication from Philip Setel.

4   Thanks to Martin Wallis for his assistance with this section.

5 Although these figures may give an impression of spurious accuracy, incredibly detailed records were kept by the Department of Co-operation and Development. (For additional information see Whiteside 1986.)

6 This view is based on Mills (2000) plus official reports to which we have had access. These suggest that the South African army has HIV levels of over 50%.

6 Introduction to Impact

1 For some countries, a third source of data is available, the Demographic and Health Surveys conducted by Macro International Inc. of Calverton, Maryland, USA. These surveys have been carried out and repeated in a number of countries.

2 For the most recent and complete review of the thinking on this topic see Carael and Schwartlander (1998).

3 Personal communication from John Stover, the Futures Group.

4 Infant mortality measures death below one year while child mortality measures all deaths below five – and includes infant mortality.

5 United Nations, *Human Development Report* (1996, 1997, 1998, 1999, 2000).

7 Individuals, Households and Communities

1 Asian Women Facing Greater Risks, <www.hain.org/aidsaction5/women.html>

2 The study was done as a four-round panel survey between 1990 and 1994. The survey looked at the impact of adult mortality and a total of 913 households were interviewed at least once with 759 households completing all four waves. The study was funded by USAID, Danida and the World Bank Research Committee. The findings have unfortunately been neither fully analysed nor published, although some have been presented in various fora including international conferences. The most accessible account can be found in World Bank (1997a). Some further findings are discussed in Lundberg and Over (2000).

3 The first lost generation is considered by Shell (2000) to be those children who grew up in the last years of apartheid.

4 We were unable to take into account the excellent thesis by Kongsin (2001) which was completed as this book was going to press. This study of HIV/AIDS morbidity in some northern Thai communities will be an important source on this underresearched subject.

5 AIDS-affected was defined as a family in which one or both parents and/or major breadwinner died due to AIDS in the five-year period from January 1991 to December 1995.

6 According to the 2000 United Nations *Human Development Report*, 32.7% of the populations of both sub-Saharan Africa and South Asia are urban.

8 Dependants: Orphans and the Elderly

1 This otherwise measured report by UNAIDS is marred by the use of terms such as 'skyrocketed' and 'astounding', because the data are not adequate to support such dramatic language – that is not to underestimate the seriousness of the situation.

2 In many countries fees are only part of the costs of attending school. There are book fees, building fees, Parent Teacher Association fees, uniforms and, of course, the opportunity costs of time and labour forgone.

3 This section has benefited from discussions with Marguerite Daniel and from an unpublished paper by Divya Rajaraman (Rajaraman, 2001).

4 Botswana became a signatory to the United Nations Convention on the Rights of the Child in 1995.

5 Personal communication from Veena Lakhumalani.

6 A visit to a Ukrainian orphanage in 2001 made the implications of this painfully clear. Children who have spent their childhood in an institutional regime that is simultaneously underfunded and deriving from the Soviet tradition cannot make a satisfactory transition to the world outside at age 16. This is particularly so when the Soviet support services of health care, employment and housing have disappeared. The Deputy-Director of the orphanage was close to tears when describing the trauma for staff and orphans of pushing the latter out of the institution when they reach 16. 'In winter', she said, 'they try to creep back into the orphanage so that they can at least sleep somewhere warm.'

7 The Convention on the Rights of the Child was unanimously adopted by the UN General Assembly in 1989 to form a legally binding international instrument containing a set of universally agreed (only two states, the US and Somalia, have not ratified the treaty), non-negotiable standards and obligations. All the human rights (civil, political, economic, social and cultural rights) are bought together for the first time in this convention spelling out the right of every child

- to survival
- to develop to the fullest
- to protection from harmful influences, abuse and exploitation
- to participate fully in family, cultural and social life.

All of which are deemed necessary to the human dignity and development of every child.

Every country that ratifies the Convention is obliged to bring its national legislation in line with the standards set by the Convention. However, in order for the Convention to be effective, the guiding principles advocated within the Convention must be respected not only by governments but also by all members (institutions and individuals) of society. Civil Society is described as having a critical role in ensuring that the Rights of the Child as outlined in the Convention are not open to free and arbitrary interpretation, but are accepted as clear values that are inherent to the human dignity of all people.

The Convention consists of 54 Articles and has been supplemented by two optional protocols since May 2000. The first 41 Articles outline the requirements that need to be met to achieve the fundamental aims of the protocol as outlined by the four guiding principles. Briefly, these guiding principles are: non-discrimination, best interests of the child, survival and development and participation. Articles 42–45 cover the implementation, monitoring and progress towards the realisation of the Rights of the Child. Articles 46–54 deal specifically with the ratification process. For the purposes of this Convention, children are defined as all humans under the age of 18 years, unless relevant national laws recognise an earlier age of majority.

8 'Developed countries' comprise all nations in Europe and North America, plus Japan, Australia and New Zealand.

9 'Oldest-old' is defined by Velkoff and Lawson (1998) to be aged 80 and older.

10 We arrive at this conclusion through a careful literature search which turned up fewer than ten articles, theses or books. Only Williams (1998) presents extensive and detailed data.

11 This section is based on fieldwork by Barnett and Blaikie in the late 1980s. It describes a situation that has not altered very much, if at all, and which is now more widespread in Africa and elsewhere than when these notes were first made.

12 Williams (1998), p. 216.

9 Subsistence Agriculture and Rural Livelihoods

1 This concept is explored and has been researched in some depth in relation to the fresh fruit and vegetable industries by Catherine Dolan and John Humphrey (Dolan 2000; Dolan and Humphrey, 2000).

2 Authors' fieldwork, 1991.

3 The sources for data in this table are the FAO's Geographical Information Early Warning System (FAO/GIEWS) available on <http://www.fao.org/WAICENT/faoinfo/economic/giews/english/fs/fs0011/FS0011.htm>; US Census Bureau, International Programs Center, Health Studies Branch, HIV/AIDS Surveillance Data Base CD # 623510.

4 Barnett, unpublished fieldwork, Bihar, 1993.

5 This figure derives from personal communications with people having local contacts in rural China.

6 Authors' fieldwork, 1998.

7 PIN stands for Product Index Number, a unique identifier used for each crop in the FAO system. For further information see: <http://apps.fao.org/lim500/nph-wrap.pl?Crops.Primary&Domain=PIN&servlet=1>

8 This section is informed by discussion on the World Bank website on climate change at: <http://worldbank.org/html/extdr/climchng/afrclim.htm> and also on the website of Climate Network Africa at: <http://www.igc/.org/climate/E3/Africa.html>

9 Polity means the entire sphere of political life, not only government.

10 We do not give detailed references for the points made in this section as they are derived from an overlapping literature. Sources include Abel et al., (1988), Gillespie (1989), Barnett and Blaikie (1990, 1992), Barnett (1995), Rugalema (1999), Barnett and Rugalema (2001).

11 This section is based on observation and discussion with key informants and farmers in Uganda and Tanzania in 1993.

12 <http://www.fao.org/WAICENT/OIS/PRESS_NE/PRESSENG/2000/pren0037.htm>

10　HIV/AIDS and 'For Profit' Enterprise

1　<http://www.tata.com/tata_fin/releases/20001030fin.htm>
2　This view was expressed to Whiteside at the International AIDS Conference in Vancouver in 1996.
3　Resource-based means the operation has to be in that location to exploit a natural resource, for example a mine or plantation. Market-based means the firm is selling to the local market.
4　This table is based on ideas developed by Dennis Bailey at a Social and Economic Impact Policy Research Workshop in Durban, South Africa in 1999.
5　MIS – management information system – a *system* of data *collection* and *organisation* designed to provide management with information that will answer key strategic questions. For example: how many people and at what levels are taking sick leave, early retirement, compassionate leave? Which grades of employee are taking what periods of sick leave or early retirement and what are the causes of these absences and retirements? At current rates of sickness, early retirement and death in service, how many years of work might be expected from each year of training or unit cost of training? At which points in the organisational process is it clear that unexpected absence, early retirement or death in service will affect the smooth operation of the enterprise?
6　This audit was assisted by the authors in 1997.
7　This study was assisted by the authors from 1999 to 2000.

11　AIDS, Development and Economic Growth

1　For some debate, see *European Journal of Development Research*, 11(1) (June 1999) with four articles: Peter W. Preston, 'Development Theory: Learning the Lessons and Moving On', pp. 1–29; Ray Kiely, 'The Last Refuge of the Noble Savage? A Critical Assessment of Post-Development Theory', pp. 30–55; Ronaldo Munck, 'Dependency and Imperialism in the New Times: A Latin American Perspective', pp. 56–74; Jan Nederveen Pieterse, 'Critical Holism and the Tao of Development', pp. 75–100.
2　These goals were revisited and reissued by the UN following the Millennium Summit of the United Nations on the theme 'The role of the United Nations in the Twenty-First Century', New York, from 6–8 September 2000.
3　In industrialised countries the HPI includes a measure of social exclusion – the long-term unemployment rate (UNDP, *Human Development Report*, 2000).
4　Extensive data are provided in the appendix to Chapter 6.
5　The full table is given in the appendix to Chapter 6.
6　This was well-described in the 1993 World Bank *World Development Report*.
7　Just how complex is illustrated in the tables at the back of the 2000 *World Health Report* (WHO, 2000).
8　Recent work by the Liverpool School of Tropical Medicine suggests that the interactions between malaria and AIDS may be marked. Rates of malaria fever rise sharply with falling CD4 cell counts. The data suggest that with worsening

immunosuppression caused by HIV/AIDS, protective immune responses to malaria in adults are progessively lost. (Personal Communication, Gilks, 2002).
9 Available from <www.tfgi.com> or <www.policyproject.com>.
10 Several of these papers have subsequently been published. They are given in both unpublished and published form in the bibliography.

12 Government and Governance

1 <www.bday.co.za>.
2 A Brief report appeared in the electronic *Weekly Mail and Guardian* website (15 October 2000) <www.mg.co.za> 'President Thabo Mbeki has withdrawn from the public debate on the causes of Aids after admitting he had created confusion, but has not backed down from his controversial stance which questions the orthodox scientific view that HIV is the cause of Aids.'
3 This study took a huge amount of work and its limitations reflect problems with data not the researchers.
4 Figures calculated using the exchange rate of US$1 = R7.93.
5 Exchange rate used P1.00 = US$0.18.
6 The data for Figure 12.2 were kindly provided by Wendy Roseberry of the World Bank; those for Box 12.2 by Dan Mullins of Oxfam.

13 Responses

1 This has been portrayed in various ways. The UNDP presented it diagrammatically in an early paper by Desmond Cohen. The World Bank has characterised the epidemic as having three broad stages: nascent, concentrated and generalised. The example in this book is from Barnett and Whiteside (2000). The point is not the naming of the stages but recognising that they exist and that different stages require different response.
2 The syndromic approach to STI treatment is based on diagnosing STIs using a set of easily observed symptoms such as genital discharge. These are treated with a broad spectrum of drugs aimed at treating all the infections that could potentially account for these symptoms.
3 Joint UNICEF–UNAIDS Secretariat–WHO/HTP–MSF Project, 2001: *Sources and prices of selected drugs and diagnostics for people living with HIV/AIDS*, May 2001.
4 'HIV incidence associated with male circumcision in a population-based cohort, and HIV acquisition/transmission associated with circumcision and viral load in discordant couples: Rakai, Uganda'. R. Gray, M.J. Wawer, N.K. Sewakambo, D. Serwadda, N. Kiwanuka, F. Wabwire Mangen, C. Li, T. Lutalo, T.C Quinn. Paper presented at the XIII International AIDS Conference, Durban South Africa, 9–14 July 2000 (MoOrC193). Potential efficacy of male circumcision for HIV prevention in Rakai, Uganda. D. Serwadda, R. Gray, N. Kiwanuka, N. Sewnkambo, R. Kelly, M.Wawer. Paper presented at the XIII International AIDS Conference, Durban South Africa, 9–14 July 2000. (MoOrC194)
5 'Male Circumcision and HIV spread in sub-Saharan Africa'. A. Buve, B. Auvert, E. Lagarde, M. Kahindo, R. Hayes, M. Carael. Paper presented at the XIII

International AIDS Conference, Durban South Africa, 9–14 July 2000. (MoOrC192)
6 The technical information in this section is largely drawn from Beyrer (2000).

14 Globalisation, Inequality, HIV/AIDS and the Intimacies of Self

1 These ideas have been developed in a variety of publications over the past 25 years – see for example Sen (1985, 1997); Sen and Sengupta (1983); Drèze and Sen (1989). Many of the arguments and ideas are usefully reviewed in Cameron (2000a).
2 We are grateful to Richard Palmer-Jones, Cecile Jackson and Robert Sugden for their helpful discussion of these ideas in an unpublished document circulated in the School of Development Studies.
3 'Of the 100 largest economies in the world, 51 are corporations; only 49 are countries (based on a comparison of corporate sales and country GDPs)', and 'The Top 200 corporations' combined sales are bigger than the combined economies of all countries minus the biggest 10' (Anderson and Cavanagh, 2000, p. 1).
4 This idea has wide resonances: see Kaldor (2001).
5 Personal communications from several senior UNAIDS officials.

Bibliography

Abel, N., Barnett, T., Bell, S., Blaikie, P.M. and Cross, J.S.W. (1988) 'The Impact of AIDS on Food Production Systems in East and Central Africa over the Next Ten Years: a programmatic paper', in Fleming, A. et al. *The Global Impact of AIDS*, (New York: Alan R. Liss Inc.) pp. 145–54.

Adams, B. (1998) *Timescapes of Modernity: The Environment and Invisible Hazards* (London and New York: Routledge).

Adetunji, J.A. (1997) 'Assessing the Mortality Impact of HIV/AIDS Relative to Other Causes of Adult Deaths in Sub-Saharan Africa'. The Socio-Demographic Impact of AIDS in Africa Conference, International Union for the Scientific Study of Population and the University of Natal, Durban, February.

AIDS Analysis Africa (1990) Southern African edition, vol. 1(1) (June/July).

AIDS Control Programme/Ministry of Health (Uganda) <http://www.aidsuganda.org/>

AIDS/HIV Quarterly Surveillance Tables (1997) No. 36 (97/2) (August).

AIDS Scan (1999) 'Community-level Control of STIs in Uganda Did Not Affect HIV Prevalence in the Targeted Community', vol. 11(2) (June).

AIDS Scan (2000) 'Lessons from African STI Trials and their Impact on HIV Infection', vol. 12(3) (October/November).

Ainsworth, M. and Semali, I. (2000) 'The Impact of Adult Death on Children's Health in Northwestern Tanzania'. Policy Research Working Paper No. 2266 (January) (Washington, DC: World Bank, Development Research Group, Poverty and Human Resources).

Ainsworth, M., Fransen, L. and Over, M. (eds) (1998) *Confronting AIDS: Evidence from the Developing World, Selected Background Papers for World Bank Policy Research Report, 'Confronting AIDS: Public Priorities in a Global Epidemic'* (Brussels: European Commission).

Ainsworth, M. and Teokul, W. (2000) 'Breaking the Silence: Setting Realistic Priorities for AIDS Control in Developing Countries', *Lancet*, 356: 55–60.

Ali, A.A.G. and Elbadawi, I. (1999) 'Inequality and the Dynamics of Poverty and Growth'. CID Working Paper No. 32 (Cambridge, MA: Harvard Center for International Development, Harvard University).

Alonso, J.A. (2001) 'Globalisation, Civil Society, and the Multilateral System', in D. Eade and E. Ligteringen (eds) *Debating Development* (Oxford: Oxfam GB), pp. 86–103.

Anderson, R.M. (1996) 'The Spread of HIV and Sexual Mixing Patterns', in J. Mann and D. Tarantola (eds) *AIDS in the World II* (Oxford and New York: Oxford University Press).

Anderson, R.M. (1999) 'Transmission Dynamics of Sexually Transmitted Infections', in K.K. Holmes, P.F. Sparling, P.A. Mardha, S.M. Lemon, P. Piot and J.M. Wasserheit (eds) *Sexually Transmitted Disease* (New York: McGraw-Hill), pp. 25–38.

Anderson, R.M. and May, R.M. (1992) *Infectious Diseases of Humans: Dynamics and Control* (Oxford, New York and Tokyo: Oxford University Press).

376 *Bibliography*

Anderson R.M., May, R.M., Boily, M.C., Garnett, G.P. and Rowley, J.T. (1991) 'The Spread of HIV-1 in Africa: Sexual Contact Patterns and the Predicted Demographic Impact of AIDS', *Nature*, 352: 581–9.

Anderson, S. and Cavanagh, J. (2000) 'Top 200: The Rise of Corporate Global Power'. (Washington, DC: Institute of Policy Studies) <http://www.ips-dc.org/downloads/Top_200.pdf > p. 5.

Apt, N. (1996) *Coping with Old Age in a Changing Africa: Social Change and the Elderly* (Aldershot: Avebury).

Apt, N. (1997) *Ageing in Africa* (Geneva: WHO).

Arndt, C. and Lewis, J.D. (2000) 'The Macro Implications of HIV/AIDS in South Africa: A Preliminary Assessment', *Journal of South African Economics*, 68(5): 856–87.

Arndt, C. and Lewis, J.D. (2001) 'The HIV/AIDS Pandemic in South Africa: Sectoral Impacts and Unemployment', *Journal of International Development*, 13(4): 427–49.

Arthur, G., Bhatt, S.M. and Gilks, C. (2000) 'The Impact of HIV/AIDS on Hospital Services in Developing Countries – Will Service Breakdown Ensue?', *AIDS Analysis Africa*, 10(6).

Aventin, L. and Huard, P. (1997) 'HIV/AIDS and Manufacturing in Abidjan', *AIDS Analysis Africa*, 7(3) (June).

Awusabo-Asare, K. et al. (1999) '"All Die be Die": Obstacles to Change in the Face of HIV Infection in Ghana', in J.C. Caldwell et al. (eds) *Resistances to Behavioural Change to Reduce HIV/AIDS Infection* (Canberra: Health Transition Centre, Australian National University), pp. 125–34.

Azjen, I. (1985) 'From Intentions to Action: A Theory of Planned Behavior', in J. Khul and J. Beckman (eds) *Action-Control: From Cognition to Behaviour* (Englewood Cliffs, NJ: Prentice Hall).

Azjen, I. and Fishbein, M. (1980) *Understanding Attitudes and Predicting Social Behavior* (Englewood Cliffs, NJ: Prentice Hall).

Backlund, E., Sorlie, P.D. and Johnson, N.J. (1996) 'The Shape of the Relationship between Income and Mortality in the United States: Evidence from the National Longitudinal Mortality Study', *Annals of Epidemiology*, 6: 12–20.

Baggeley, R., Chilangwa, D., Godfrey-Faussett, P., Porter, J. (1993) 'Impact of AIDS on Zambian Business' (Abstract WRT0031). VII International Conference on AIDS in Africa/VIII African Conference on Sexually Transmitted Diseases, Marrakech, December.

Balakireva, O., Federenko, O., Galustian, Y. et al. (2001) *The Social and Economic Impact of HIV/AIDS in Ukraine* (December) (Kyiv: Ukrainian Institute of Social Research and the British Council).

Banks, J. and Banks O. (1954) *Prosperity and Parenthood* (London: Routledge and Kegan Paul).

Barfield, T. (ed.) (1997) *The Dictionary of Anthropology* (Oxford: Blackwell).

Barnett, T. (1995) 'HIV/AIDS Impact on Some Communities in Rajasthan, India: Some Observations from Experience in Affected Countries in Africa'. UNDP Regional HIV/AIDS Programme, Delhi, June.

Barnett, T. (1997) 'Un cadre pour l'analyse de la situation des camps de réfugiés en termes de sensibilité et vulnérabilité', in A. Desclaux and C. Raynaut (eds) *Urgence, Précarité et Lutte contre le vih/sida en Afrique* (Paris and Montreal: L'Harmattan, Inc.).

Barnett, T. (1998) 'The Epidemic in Rural Communities: The Relevance of the African Experience for India', in P. Godwin (ed.) *The Looming Epidemic: The Impact of HIV/AIDS in India* (Delhi: Mosaic Press; London: Hirst & Co.), pp. 150–70.

Barnett, T. (2001) 'Development', *International Encyclopaedia of Political Economy* (London: Routledge).

Barnett. T. and Blaikie, P. (1992) *AIDS in Africa: Its Present and Future Impact* (London: John Wiley; New York: Guilford Press).

Barnett, T. and Blaikie, P.M., with Obbo, C. (1990) *Community Coping Mechanisms in Circumstances of Exceptional Demographic Change, Final Report to the Overseas Development Administration on Community Coping Mechanisms in Circumstances of Exceptional Demographic Change*, Vol. 1, *Executive Summary*; Vol. 2, *Main Report* (London: ODA; Norwich: University of East Anglia).

Barnett, T. and Haslwimmer, M. (1993) *The Impact of HIV/AIDS on Rural Livelihoods and Farming Systems in Eastern Africa* (Rome: United Nations FAO).

Barnett, T. and Rugalema, G., (2001) 'HIV.AIDS: A Critical Health and Development Issue', in P. Pinstrup-Andersen and R. Pandya-Lorch, *The Unfinished Agenda: Perspectives on Overcoming Hunger, Poverty and Environmental Degradation* (Washington DC, International Food Policy Research Institute) pp. 43–7.

Barnett, T. and Whiteside, A. (1997) *The Social and Economic Impact of HIV/AIDS in the Ukraine* (Kyiv: British Council).

Barnett, T. and Whiteside, A. (2000) *Guidelines for Studies of the Social and Economic Impact of AIDS* (Geneva: UNAIDS).

Barnett, T., Whiteside, A. and Decosas, J. (2000a) 'The Jaipur Paradigm: A Conceptual Framework for Understanding Social Susceptibility and Vulnerability to HIV', *Journal of the South African Medical Association*, 90: 1,098–101.

Barnett, T., Whiteside, A., Khodakevich, L., Kruglov, Y. and Steshenko, V. (2000b) 'The Social and Economic Impact of HIV/AIDS in Ukraine', *Social Science and Medicine*, 51(9): 1,387–403.

Barratt Brown, M. (1995) *Africa's Choices After Thirty Years of the World Bank* (London: Penguin).

Barrett, H.R. and Browne, A.W. (2000) 'Children's Value in Sub-Saharan Africa: The Impact of Environmental and Social Change in Zambia'. African Studies Centre, Occasional Papers Series No. 6, Coventry University.

Bassett, M. and Mhloyi, M. (1991): 'Women and AIDS in Zimbabwe: The Making of an Epidemic', *International Journal of Health Services*, 21(1): 143–56.

Bayley, A. (1984) 'Aggressive Kaposi's Sarcoma in Zambia', *Lancet*, April to June, 1(2) (April/June): 1318–20.

<www.bday.co.za>

Beck, U. (2000a) *World Risk Society* (Cambridge: Polity Press).

Beck, U. (2000b) 'Living Your Own Life in a Runaway World', in W. Hutton and A. Giddens (eds) *On the Edge: Living with Global Capitalism* (London: Jonathan Cape).

Beisel, W. (1996) 'Nutrition and Immune Function: Overview', *Journal of Nutrition*, 126: S2611–15.

Beyrer, C. (2000) (MD, Johns Hopkins University School of Public Health, October) 'Issues from International Experience with Combination Anti-retroviral Therapy: Background Note' for *Thailand's Response to AIDS: 'Building on Success, Confronting the Future'* (Bangkok: World Bank, November) <www.worldbank.or.th/social/index.html>

Bijlmakers, L., Bassett, M. and Sanders, D. (1998) 'Socio-economic Stress, Health and Child Nutritional Status in Zimbabwe at a Time of Economic Structural Adjustment'. Research Report No. 105.

Blaxter, M. (1990) *Health and Lifestyles* (London: Routledge).

Bloom, D.E. and Sachs, J.D. (1998) 'Geography, Demography and Economic Growth in Africa'. Brookings Papers on Economic Activity 2 (Washington, DC: Brookings Institution).

Boerma, J.T., Ngalula, J., Isingo, R., Urassa, M., Senkoro, K., Gabone, R. and Mkumbo, E.N. (1997) 'Levels and Causes of Adult Mortality in Rural Tanzania with Special Reference to HIV/AIDS'. The Socio-Demographic Impact of AIDS in Africa Conference, International Union for the Scientific Study of Population and the University of Natal, Durban, February.

Bond, G.C. and Vincent, J. (1990) 'Living on the Edge of Structural Adjustment in the Context of AIDS', in H.B. Hansen and M. Twaddle (eds) *Uganda: Structural Adjustment and Change* (London: James Curry).

Bonnel, R. (2000a) 'HIV AIDS: Does it Increase or Decrease Growth? What Makes an Economy HIV-resistant?' International AIDS Economics Network Symposium, Durban, 8 July.

Bonnel, R. (2000b) 'HIV/AIDS and Economic Growth: A Global Perspective', *Journal of South African Economics*, 68(5): 820–55.

Botswana Institute for Development Policy Analysis (BIDPA) (2000a) *Macroeconomic Impact of HIV/AIDS in Botswana. Report* (February/March) (Gaberone: BIDPA).

Botswana Institute for Development Policy Analysis (2000b) *Macroeconomic Impacts of the HIV/AIDS Epidemic in Botswana. Final Report* (May)(Gaberone: BIDPA).

Bourdieu, P. (1980) 'Le capital social, Actes de la récherche', *Sciences Sociales*, 21 : 2–3.

Bourdieu, P. (1986) 'The Forms of Capital', in J.G. Richardson (ed.), *Handbook on Theory and Research for the Sociology of Education* (New York: Greenwood Press), pp. 241–58.

Bourdieu, P. and Wacquant, J.D. (1992) *An Invitation to Reflexive Sociology* (Chicago, IL: University of Chicago Press).

Brett, R. and McCallan, M. (1998) *Children: The Invisible Soldiers* (Stockholm: Radda Barnen/Save the Children).

Brookmeyer, R. and Gail, M. (1994) *AIDS Epidemiology: A Quantitative Approach* (Oxford: Oxford University Press).

Bruni, L. and Sugden, R. (2000) 'Moral Canals: Trust and Social Capital in the Work of Hume, Smith and Genovesi', *Economics and Philosophy*, 16: 21–45.

Bryant, A.T. (1949) *The Zulu People* (Pietermaritzburg: Shuter and Shooter).

Bryson, Y.J. (1996) 'Perinatal HIV-1 Transmission: Recent Advances and Therapeutic Iinterventions', *AIDS*, 10 (Supplement 3): S33–42.

Bujra, J. (2000a) 'Masculinity in Africa'. Lecture in the series 'HIV/AIDS: The First Epidemic of Globalisation', School of Development Studies, University of East Anglia, Norwich, May.

Bujra, J. (2000b) 'Targeting Men for Change: AIDS Discourse and Activism in Africa', Agenda No. 44, Durban, South Africa, <www.agenda.org.za/#search> pp. 6–23.

Business Day (2001) 30 March.

Buve, A. et al. (1992) 'Mortality Among Female Nurses in the Face of the HIV/AIDS Epidemic: A Pilot Study in the Southern Province of Zambia', *AIDS*, 8: 396.

Buve, A. et al. (1999) 'Differences in HIV Spread in Four Sub-Saharan African Cities' (Geneva: UNAIDS) <www.unaids.org/lusaka99Buve.htm>

Buve, B. Auvert, Lagarde, E., Kahindo, M., Hayes, R. and Carael, M. (2000), 'Male Circumcision and HIV spread in sub-Saharan Africa'. Paper presented at the XIII International AIDS Conference, Durban South Africa, 9–14 July, 2000. (MoOrC192)

Caldwell, J.C. and Caldwell, P. (1990) 'High Fertility in Sub-Saharan Africa', *Scientific American* (May): 82–9.

Caldwell, J.C., Caldwell, P. and Quiggin, P. (1989) 'The Social Context of AIDS in Sub-Saharan Africa', *Population and Development Review*, 15(2): 185–234.

Cameron, J. (2000a) 'Amartya Sen on Economic Inequality: The Need for an Explicit Critique of Opulence', *Journal of International Development*, 12(7): 1,031–45.

Cameron, Mr Justice Edwin (2000b) (High Court of South Africa, Johannesburg) First Jonathan Mann Memorial Lecture: 'The Deafening Silence of AIDS'. XIII International AIDS Conference, Durban, 7–14 July.

Campbell, C. (1997) 'Migrancy, Masculine Identities and AIDS: The Psychosocial Context of HIV Transmission on the South African Gold Mines', *Social Science and Medicine*, 45(2): 273–81.

Caplan, P. (ed.) (2000) *Risk Revisited* (London: Pluto Press).

Carael, M. and Schwartlander, B. (eds) (1998) 'Demographic Impact of AIDS', *AIDS*, 12 (Supplement 1).

Carmichael, F. and Charles, S. (1999) 'Caring for the Sick And Elderly – An Intergenerational Bargain that Could Break Down'. Paper presented at the Development Studies Association Conference, University of Bath, 12–14 September.

Carpenter, L.M., Nakiyingi, J.S., Ruberantwari, A., Malamba, S., Kamali, A. and Whitworth, J.A.G. (1997) 'Estimates of the Impact of HIV-1 Infection on Fertility in a Rural Ugandan Cohort'. The Socio-Demographic Impact of AIDS in Africa Conference, International Union for the Scientific Study of Population and the University of Natal, Durban, February.

Carswell, J.W. (ed.) (1986) 'AIDS in Uganda: A Review', *Health Information Quarterly* (Uganda: Ministry of Health), 2(4): 22–43.

Chaisson, R., Keruly, J. and Moore, R. (1995) 'Race, Sex Drug Use and Progression of Human Immunodeficiency Virus Disease', *New England Journal of Medicine*, 333(12): 751–6.

Chandra, R.K. (1997) 'Nutrition and the Immune System: An Introduction', *American Journal of Clinical Nutrition*, 66: S460–3.

Chinnock, P. (1996) 'Breast is Best, but what if the Mother is HIV-positive?', *AIDS Analysis Africa*, 6(5) (October).

Chong, S.F. (1999) 'A Critical Review of Household Survey Methodology: Assessing the Cost Effectiveness of Household Responses to the Economic Impact of HIV/AIDS'. MA thesis, School of Development Studies, University of East Anglia, Norwich.

Clancy, P. (1998) Impact of HIV/AIDS on Organisations in Tanzania'. MA thesis, School of Development Studies, UEA, Norwich.

Climate Network Africa <http://www.igc.org/climate/E3/Africa.html>

Cohen, D. (1999) 'Poverty and HIV/AIDS in Sub-Saharan Africa'. Issues Paper No. 27, HIV and Development Programme (New York: UNDP).

Cohen. S., Doyle, W.J. and Skoner, D.P. (1999) 'Psychological Stress, Cytokine Production, and Severity of Upper Respiratory Iillness', *Psychosomatic Medicine*, 61: 175–80.

Cohen, S., Doyle, W.J., Skoner, D.P., Rabin, B.S. and Gwaltney, J.M. (1997) 'Social Ties and Susceptibility to the Common Cold', *Journal of the American Medical Association*, 277: 1,940–4.

Cohen, P. and Mitchell, K. (1998) 'Practical Guide to Primary Care of Patients with HIV Infection' HIV InSite Knowledge Base chapter. P.T. Cohen MD PhD, Washington University, St. Louis; Mitchell H. Katz MD, San Francisco Department of Public Health (June) <http://hivinsite.ucsf.edu/InSite.jsp?page=kb-03&doc=kb-03-01-05>

Coleman, J.S. (1987) 'Norms as Social Capital', in G. Radnizky and P. Bernholz (eds) *Economic Imperialism: The Economic Method Applied Outside the Field of Economics* (New York: Paragon), pp. 133–56.

Coleman, J.S. (1988) 'Social Capital in the Creation of Human Capital', *American Journal of Sociology*, 94 (Supplement): 95–120, reprinted in R. Swedberg (ed.) *Economic Sociology* (Cheltenham: Edward Elgar), pp. 319–44.

Coleman, J.S. (1990) *Foundations of Social Theory* (Cambridge, MA: Harvard University Press/Belknap Press).

Collard, D. (1999) 'The Generational Bargain'. Paper presented at the Development Studies Association Conference, University of Bath, 12–14 September.

Collins, J. and Rau, B. (2000) 'AIDS in the Context of Development'. Paper prepared for UNRISD (June).

Colvin, M. (2000) 'Sexually Transmitted Infections in Southern Africa: A Public Health Crisis', *South African Journal of Science*, 96 (June): 335–9.

Concorde Coordinating Committee (1994) 'Concorde: MRC/ANRS Randomised Double-blind Controlled Trial of Immediate and Deferred Zidovudine in Symptom-free HIV Infection', *Lancet*, 343(8,092): 871–81.

Conroy, R., Tompkin, A., Landsdown, R. and Elmore-Meegan, M. (2001) 'AIDS Orphans: An Emerging Problem – A Study of 5,206 Orphaned Children in Kenya and Tanzania, January'. Paper in PowerPoint Format of a study funded by the Elton John AIDS Foundation; Government of Japan; Mercury Trust; ICROSS Canada; Elizabeth Taylor; ICROSS Ireland.

Cook, N.D. (1999) 'Smallpox in the New World and the Old from *Epidemics and History*' [review of S. Watts (1999) *Epidemics and History: Disease, Power and Imperialism* (new edn) (New York and New Haven, CT: Yale University Press)], *Journal of World History*, 10(2): 434–6 <http://muse.jhu.edu/journals/jwh/>

Corbett, J. (1988) 'Famine and Household Coping Strategies', *World Development*, 16(9): 1,099–112.

Corbridge, S. and Harriss, J. (2000) *Reinventing India* (Cambridge: Polity Press).

Cornia, G., Jolly, R. and Stewart, F. (eds) (1988) *Adjustment with a Human Face: Vol. II, Country Case Studies* (Oxford: Clarendon Press).

Coutinho, A.G. (2000) 'An Assessment of the Economic Impact of HIV/AIDS on the Royal Swaziland Sugar Corporation'. MA research report, Department of Community Health, University of Witwatersrand, Johannesburg (August).

Cuddington, J. (1993a) 'Modeling the Macroeconomic Effects of AIDS, with an Application to Tanzania', *World Bank Economic Review*, 7(2): 173–89.

Cuddington, J. (1993b) 'Further Results on the Macroeconomic Effects of AIDS: The Dualistic Labour-Surplus Economy', *World Bank Economic Review*, 7(3): 403–17.

Cuddington, J. and Hancock, J. (1994a) 'Assessing the Impact of AIDS on the Growth Path of the Malawian Economy', *Journal of Development Economics*, 43: 363–8.

Cuddington, J. and Hancock, J. (1994b) 'The Macroeconomic Impact of AIDS in Malawi: A Dualistic Labour-Surplus Economy', *Journal of African Economies*, 4(1): 1–28.

Cullinan, K. (2001) 'South Africa to Start Testing AIDS Vaccine', *Mercury* (KwaZulu-Natal), 7 March.

Dallabetta, G. (1996) 'The STI–HIV Link', *AIDScaptions*, 3(1) (May).

Davies, R. and Sanders, D. (1988) 'Adjustment Policies and the Welfare of Children: Zimbabwe, 1980–1985', in G. Cornia, R. Jolly and F. Stewart (eds) *Adjustment with a Human Face: Vol. II, Country Case Studies* (Oxford: Clarendon Press), pp. 272–99.

De Cock, K.M. and Brun-Vézinet, F. (1996) 'HIV-2 Infection: Current Knowledge and Uncertainties', in J.M. Mann and D. Tarantola (eds) *AIDS in the World II* (Oxford and New York: Oxford University Press).

Deininger, K. and Squire, L. (1996) 'A New Data Set Measuring Income Inequality', *World Bank Economic Review*, 10 (September): 595–91.

Demery, L. and Squire, L. (1996) 'Macroeconomic Adjustment and Poverty in Africa: An Emerging Picture', *World Bank Research Observer*, 11(1): 35–59.

Department for International Development (DfID) (1997) *Eliminating World Poverty: A Challenge for the 21st Century*. White Paper on International Development (November).

Desowitz, R.S. (1997) *Tropical Diseases from 50,000 BC to 2500 AD* (London: HarperCollins).

Deutsche Securities (2000) 'ABI Limited Living with HIV/AIDS: Positioned for Growth', 22 November.

Devereux, S. (1993) 'Goats before Ploughs: Dilemmas of Household Response Sequencing during Food Shortages', *IDS Bulletin*, 24(4): 52–9.

De Waal, A. (1989) *Famine That Kills* (Oxford: Clarendon Press).

Dorrington, R. and Johnson, L. (2001) *The Ingredients and Impact of the HIV/AIDS Epidemic in South Africa and its Provinces* (Pretoria: UNICEF).

Diamond, J. (1998) *Guns, Germs and Steel: A Short History of Everybody for the Last 13,000 Years* (London: Vintage).

Diamond, J. (1999) *Guns, Germs and Steel: The Fates of Human Societies* (New York: W.W. Norton).

Dixon, S., McDonald, S. and Roberts, J. (2000) 'AIDS and Economic Growth: A Panel Data Analysis'. Sheffield Health Economics Group, Discussion Paper Series (August).

Dolan, C. (2000) Unpublished paper on the relationship between contracted French bean production and conflict over rights, obligations and resources in Meru District, Kenya. School of Development Studies, UEA Norwich.

Dolan, C. and Humphrey, J. (2000) 'Governance and Trade in Fresh Vegetables: The Impact of UK Supermarkets on the African Horticulture Industry'.

Unpublished paper, School of Development Studies, UEA, Norwich, and Institute of Development Studies, University of Sussex, Brighton.

Dorrington, R., Bradshaw, D., Bourne, D. and Karim, S.A. (2000) 'HIV Surveillance Results – Little Grounds for Optimism Yet', *South African Medical Journal*, 90(5): 452–3.

Dorrington, R., Bourne, D., Bradshaw, D., Laubscher, R. and Timaeus, I.M. (2001) *The Impact of HIV/AIDS on Adult Mortality in South Africa*. Johannesburg Medical Research Council Technical Report.

Dorrington, R. and Johnson, L. (2001) *The Ingredients and Impact of the HIV/AIDS Epidemic in South Africa and its Provinces* (Pretoria: UNICEF).

Doyle, P. (1996) Personal communication.

Drèze, J. and Sen, A. (1989) *Hunger and Public Action* (Oxford: Clarendon Press).

Duffield, M. (1996) 'The Symphony of the Damned: Racial Discourse, Complex Political Emergencies and Humanitarian Aid' (2 March). Occasional Paper, School of Public Policy, University of Birmingham.

Economist Intelligence Unit (1997) <http://database.townhall.com/heritage/index/country.cfm>

Edet, T. (1997) 'Cultural Politics, 1997, HIV/AIDS and Higher Education in Nigeria: Research and Policy Implications'. MA thesis, School of Development Studies, University of East Anglia, Norwich.

Egolf, B., Lasker, J., Wolf, S. and Potvin, L. (1992) 'The Roseto Effect: A 50-year Comparison of Mortality Rates', *American Journal of Public Health*, 82: 1,089–92.

Eliot, E. (1998) 'Changes in Mortality in Mumbai: Monitoring Mortality to Analyse the Spread of HIV', in P. Godwin (ed.), *The Looming Epidemic: The Impact of HIV and AIDS in India* (New Delhi: Mosaic Books), pp. 62–93.

Ellis, F. (2000) *Rural Livelihood Diversity in Developing Countries: Analysis, Policy, Methods* (Oxford: Oxford University Press).

Employment Bureau of Africa Limited (various years) *Report and Financial Statements for Year Ended 31 December*: 1984, 1989, 1994, 1998.

Epstein, H. (2001) 'Time of Indifference', *New York Review of Books* (12 April): 33–8.

FAOSTAT is an online statistical database on the FAO website. One can access and then interrogate it to compile sets of information. The website address for FAO is <http://www.fao.org>

Farmer, P. (1992) *AIDS and Accusation: Haiti and the Geography of Blame* (Berkeley, CA: University of California Press).

Farmer, P. (1996) 'Social Inequalities and Emerging Infectious Diseases', *Emerging Infectious Diseases*, 2(4) (October–December): 259–69.

Farmer, P. (1999) *Infections and Inequalities: The Modern Plagues* (Berkeley, CA, Los Angeles and London: University of California Press).

Feachem, R. and Jamison, D. (eds) (1991) *Disease and Mortality in Sub-Saharan Africa* (Washington, DC: World Bank).

Feldman, T.R. and Assaf, S. (1999) 'Social Capital: Conceptual Frameworks and Empirical Evidence: An Annotated Bibliography'. Social Capital Initiative Working Paper No. 5 (January) (Washington, DC: World Bank, Social Development, Family, Environmentally and Socially Sustainable Development Network).

Filmer, D. (1996) 'Socioeconomic Correlates of Risky Behavior: Results from the Demographic and Health Surveys' (publication forthcoming).

Fine, B. (1999) 'The Development State is Dead – Long Live Social Capital?', *Development and Change*, 30: 1–19.

Fiscella, K. and Franks, P. (1997) 'Poverty or Income Inequality as Predictor of Mortality: Longitudinal Cohort Study', *British Medical Journal*, 314: 1,724–32.

Fleming, A., Carballo, M., FitzSimons, D., Bailey, M., Mann, J. (eds), (1988*) The Global Impact of AIDS* (New York: Alan R. Liss Inc).

Food and Agriculture Organisation (FAO) (2000) 'The State of Food Insecurity in the World' <http://www.fao.org/docrep/x8200e/x8200e03.htm#P2_33>

Food and Agriculture Organisation, Geographical Information Early Warning System (FAO/GIEWS) <http://www.fao.org/WAICENT/faoinfo/economic/giews/english/fs/fs0011/FS0011.htm>

Food and Agriculture Organisation/UNAIDS (2001) *Sustainable Agricultural/Rural Development and Vulnerability to the AIDS Epidemic* <http://www.fao.org/WAICENT/OIS/PRESS_NE?PRESSENG/2000/pren0037.htm>

Foner, N. (1984) *Ages in Conflict: A Cross-cultural Perspective on Inequality Between Old and Young* (New York: Columbia University Press).

Foster, S.D. (1996) 'Socio-economic Impact of HIV/AIDS in Monze District Zambia'. PhD thesis, LSHTM.

Fox, A.J. (ed.) (1989) *Health Inequalities in European Countries* (Aldershot: Gower).

Frank, T. (2001) *One Market Under God: Extreme Capitalism, Market Populism and the End of Economic Democracy* (London: Secker and Warburg).

Fransen, L. and Whiteside, A. (1995) 'HIV and Rural Development: An Action Plan', *Considering HIV/AIDS in Development Assistance: A Toolkit* (Brussels: EC).

French, N., Mujugira, A., Nakiyingi, D., Mulder, E.N. and Gilks, J.C.F. (1999) 'Immunologic and Clinical Stages in HIV-1 Infected Ugandan Adults are Comparable and Provide no Evidence of Rapid Progression but Poor Survival with Advanced Disease', *Journal of Acquired Immune Deficiency Syndromes*, 22(5).

Furnivall, J. (1948) *Colonial Policy and Practice* (London: Routledge).

Garnett, G.P. and Anderson, R.M. (1992) 'No Reason for Complacency about the Potential Demographic Impact of AIDS' (26 May) (London: Imperial College, Parasite Epidemiology Research Group).

Garrett, L. (1995) *The Coming Plague: Newly Emerging Diseases in a World out of Balance* (New York and London: Penguin).

Garrett, L. (2000) *Betrayal of Trust: The Collapse of Global Public Health* (New York: Hyperion).

Gellman, B. (2000) 'The Turning Point that Left Millions Behind', *Washington Post*, 27 December.

General Assembly on HIV/AIDS (2001) (Special Session) Fifty-fifth Session Agenda Item 179, 'Review of the Problem of Human Immunodeficiency Virus/Acquired Immunodeficiency Syndrome in All its Aspects', Report of the Secretary-General (report dated 16 February 2001 downloaded).

Gilgen, D., Campbell, C., Williams, B., Taljaard, D. and MacPhail, C. (2000) *The Natural History of HIV/AIDS in South Africa: A Biomedical and Social Survey in Carletonville* (Johannesburg: Council for Scientific and Industrial Research).

Gilks, C.F., Haran, D. and Wilkinson, D. (1996) 'Coping with the Impact of the HIV Epidemic – The Hlabisa–Liverpool HIV Link', *South African Medical Journal*, 86(9) (September): 1,077–8.

Gillespie, S. (1989) 'Potential Impact of AIDS on Farming Systems: A Case Study from Rwanda', *Land Use Policy*, 6: 301–12.

Gist, Y. and Kinsella, K. (1998) *Gender and Aging: Mortality and Health* (October) (US Bureau of the Census, International Programs Center).

Gluckman, M. (1955*) Custom and Conflict in Africa* (Oxford: Blackwell).

Gould, D. (1980) *Bureaucratic Corruption and Underdevelopment in the Third World: The Case of Zaire* (New York and Oxford: Pergamon).

Government of Botswana (1995) *AIDS/STD Unit, 1995 HIV Sero-Prevalence Survey* (Gaborone: Ministry of Health).

Government of Botswana (1997) *National Development Plan 8, 1997/98–2002/3* (Gaborone: Ministry of Finance and Development Planning).

Government of Botswana (2000) 'The Impact of HIV/AIDS on Primary and Secondary Education in Botswana: Developing a Comprehensive Strategic Response'. Report of the 'HIV/AIDS and Education' Study Group (December), Ministry of Education, Government of Botswana and the Department for International Development, UK.

Government of Botswana/UNDP (1998) *Botswana Human Development Report 1997* (Gaborone).

Government of Malawi/World Bank (1998) *Malawi AIDS Assessment Study.* Report No. 17740 MAI (place/publisher not cited).

Government of Swaziland/Ministry of Education (1999). *Assessment of the Impact of HIV/AIDS on the Education Sector* (November). (Mbabane: Government of Swaziland).

Government of the United Republic of Tanzania, Ministry of Health (1992) *Annual Report of the National AIDS Control Programme and HIV/AIDS/STD Surveillance Report*, No. 7.

Gow, G. and Desmond, C. (forthcoming) *The Cost-effectiveness of Six Models of Care for Orphan and Vulnerable Children in South Africa.*

Gravelle, H. (1998) 'How Much of the Relation Between Population Mortality and Unequal Distribution of Income is a Statistical Artifact?', *British Medical Journal*, 316: 382–5.

Gray, G. (1998) 'Anti-retrovirals and their Role in Preventing Mother to Child Transmission of HIV-1', in *The Implications of Anti-retroviral Treatments* (Geneva: WHO/UNAIDS).

Gray, R.H., Serwadda, D., Wawer, M.J. et al. (1997) 'Reduced Fertility in Women with HIV Infection: A Population-Based Study in Uganda'. The Socio-Demographic Impact of AIDS in Africa Conference, International Union for the Scientific Study of Population and the University of Natal, Durban, February.

Gray, R., Wawer, M. J., Sewankambo, N. K., Serwadda, D., Kiwanuka, N., Wabwire Mangen, F., Li, C., Lutalo, T. and Quinn, T.C. (2000) Paper presented at the XIII International AIDS Conference, Durban South Africa, 9–14 July. (MoOrC193)

Greenhalgh, S. (1996) 'The Social Construction of Population Science: An Intellectual, Institutional, and Political History of Twentieth-Century Demography', *Comparative Studies in Society and History*, 38: 26–66.

Gregorio, D.I., Walsh, S.J. and Parturzo, D. (1997) 'The Effects of Occupation-based Social Position on Mortality in a Large American Cohort', *American Journal of Public Health*, 87(9): 1,472–5.

Grosskurth, H., Gray, R., Hayes, R., Mabey, D. and Wawer, M. (2000) 'Control of Sexually Transmitted Diseases for HIV-1 Prevention: Understanding the Implications of the Mwanza and Rakai Trials', *Lancet*, 355: 1,981–7.

Guardian (2001) 'New Crisis as AIDS Sweeps into Asia', 5 October.

Gubrium, J. (1973) *The Myth of the Golden Years* (Springfield: Thomas).

Gui, B. (2000) 'Beyond Transactions: On the Interpersonal Dimension of Economic Reality', *Annals of Public and Cooperative Economics*, 71: 139–69.

Haddad, L. and Gillespie, S. (2001) 'Effective Food and Nutrition Policy Responses to HIV/AIDS: What we know and what we need to know' *J. of International Development*, 13(4): 487–511.

Hall, R. (1996) *Empires of the Monsoon: A History of the Indian Ocean and its Invaders* (London: HarperCollins).

Hamers, F.M. (1997) Monograph of 'HIV Infection in Ukraine'. Mimeograph Draft Paper, European Centre for Epidemiological Monitoring of AIDS (27 March), Saint Maurice, France.

Harries, A.D., Maher, D. and Nunn, P. (1997) 'Practical and Affordable Measures for Protection of Health Care Workers from TB in Low Income Countries', *WHO Bulletin*, 75: 477–89.

Harriss, J. and De Renzio, P. (1997) '"Missing Link" or Analytically Missing?: The Concept of Social Capital', *Journal of International Development*, 9(7): 919–37.

Hartwig, G. and Patterson, D. (1978) *Disease in African History* (Durham, NC: Duke University Press).

Haslwimmer, M. (1994) *The Social and Economic Impact of HIV/AIDS on Nakambala Sugar Estate* (FAO, AGSP, January). Report included in T. Barnett (1994) *The Effects of HIV/AIDS on Farming Systems and Rural Livelihoods in Uganda, Tanzania and Zambia, a Summary Analysis of Case Studies from Research Carried Out in the Period July–September 1993*, FAO Project TSS/1 RAF/92/TO/A, Overseas Development Group, University of East Anglia for the FAO, Rome, Food and Agriculture Organisation of the United Nations.

Hayami, Y. and Ruttan, V. (1971) *Agricultural Development: An International Perspective* (Baltimore, MD: Johns Hopkins University Press).

Health Action Information Network (HAIN) 'Asian Women Facing Greater Risks' <www.hain.org/aidsaction5/women.html>

Health Action Information Network/National Economic and Development Authority/United Nations Development Programme (2000) *A Matter of Time: HIV/AIDS and Development in the Philippines* (July) (Pasig City, Philippines: DEV AIDS Project Secretariat, National Economic and Development Authority).

Health Systems Trust (1999) *South African Health Review* (Durban: Health Systems Trust).

Hethcote, H.W. and Yorke, J.A. (1984) 'Gonorrhoea: Transmission Dynamics and Control; Lecture Notes', *Biomath*, 56: 1–105.

HIV Vaccine Development Report (2000) (May) <http://www.niad.nih.gov/aids/vaccine/whsummarystatus.htm>

HM Government (2000) *Eliminating World Poverty: Making Globalisation Work for the Poor*. White Paper on International Development, presented to Parliament by the Secretary of State for International Development, Cm. 5006 (London: HMSO) <www.globalisation.gov.uk>

Hochschild, A. (1999) *King Leopold's Ghost* (London: Macmillan).

Hoogvelt, A. (2001) *Globalization and the Postcolonial World: The New Political Economy of Development* (2nd edn) (Basingstoke: Palgrave Macmillan).

Hooper, E. (1990) *Slim* (London: Bodley Head).

Hooper, E. (1999) *The River: A Journey Back to the Source of HIV and AIDS* (London: Allen Lane/Penguin Press).

Hoover, D.A. and MacPherson, M.F. (2000) 'Capacity Building Programmes – Facing the Reality of HIV/AIDS: Training, Managing and Motivating in the Circumstance of High HIV/AIDS Prevalence', in *HIV/AIDS in the Commonwealth 2000/01* (London: Kensington Publications Ltd).

Horton, R. (2000) 'How Sick is Modern Medicine?', *New York Review of Books*, XLVII(17) (2 November): 46–50.

Hunter, S. (2000) *Reshaping Societies: HIV/AIDS and Social Change: A Resource Book for Planning, Programs and Policy Making* (Glen Falls, NY: Hudson Run Press).

Hunter, S. and Fall, D. (1998) 'Community Based Orphan Assistance in Malawi: Demographic Crisis as Development Opportunity' (Unpublished draft, 13 March). (New York: UNICEF).

Hunter, S. and Williamson, J. (2000) *Children on the Brink 2000*, 'Executive Summary: Updated Estimates and Recommendations for Intervention' (Washington: USAID).

Hutton, W. and Giddens, A. (2000) *On the Edge: Living with Global Capitalism* (London: Jonathan Cape).

Hyden, G. (1983) *No Shortcuts to Progress: African Development Management in Perspective* (London: Heinemann).

Im-em, W. (1999) *Mortality Trends and Levels to Verify the AIDS Eepidemic in Thailand: Analysis from Death Registration Statistics, 1984–1997* (Nakom Pathom, Thailand: Institute for Population and Social Research, Mahidol University).

Institute of Security Studies (1999) 'Violence Against Women in Metropolitan South Africa', Monograph Series No. 41 (September).

Isaacman, A. and Roberts, R. (1995) *Cotton, Colonialism and Social History in Sub-Saharan Africa* (Portsmouth, NH, and London: Heinemann and James Curry).

Jacques, G. (1998) 'Back to the Future: AIDS, Orphans, and Alternative Care in Botswana', quoted in D. Rajaraman (2001) 'The Future of the Nation? HIV/AIDS and Orphans in Botswana'. Unpublished paper, Oxford, Queen Elizabeth House.

Janjaroen Wattana, S. (1998) 'The Impact of AIDS on Household Composition and Consumption in Thailand', in M. Ainsworth, L. Fransen and M. Over (eds) *Confronting AIDS: Evidence from the Developing World, Selected Background Papers for the World Bank Policy Research Report, 'Confronting AIDS: Public Priorities in a Global Epidemic'* (Brussels: European Commission), pp. 349–54.

Janz, N. and Becker, M. (1984) 'The Health Belief Model: A Decade Later', *Health Education Quarterly*, 11(1): 1–47.

Jeater, D. (1993) *Marriage, Perversion and Power: The Construction of Moral Discourse in Southern Rhodesia, 1894–1930* (Oxford: Clarendon Press).

Jones, C. (1996) 'The Microeconomic Implications of HIV/AIDS'. MA thesis (September), School of Development Studies, University of East Anglia.

JTK Associates (1999) 'Impact Assessment of HIV/AIDS on the Education Sector' (Mbabane, Swaziland: Ministry of Education).

Kaburu Bauni, E. (1990) 'The Changing Sexual Patterns of the Chogoria Peoples, Kenya'. Paper presented at the IUSSP/DANIDA Seminar on Anthropological Studies Relevant to the Sexual Transmission of HIV, Esbjerg.

Kaldor, M. (ed.) (2001) *Global Civil Society 2001* (Oxford: Oxford University Press).

Kaleeba, N., Kadowe, J.N, Lalinaki, D. and Williams, G. (2000) *Open Secret: People Facing up to HIV and AIDS in Uganda*. Strategies for Hope Series No. 15 (July) (London: ACTIONAID).

Kallings, L.O. and Vella, S. (2001) 'Access to HIV/AIDS Care and Treatment in the South of the World', *AIDS 2001*, 15: 1–3.

Kambou, G., Devarajan, S. and Over, M. (1992) 'The Economic Impact of AIDS in an African Country: Simulations with a Computable General Equilibrium Model of Cameroon', *Journal of African Economies*, 1(1): 109–30.

Kaplan, G.A., Pamuk, E.R., Lynch, J.W., Cohen, R.D. and Balfour, J.L. (1996) 'Income Inequality and Mortality in the United States: Analysis of Mortality and Potential Pathways', *British Medical Journal*, 312: 999–1,003.

Katzenellenbogen, J., Joubert, G. and Karim, S. (1997) *Epidemiology: A Manual for South Africa* (Cape Town: Oxford University Press).

Kawachi, I. and Kennedy, B.P. (1997a) 'Socioeconomic Determinants of Health: Health and Social Cohesion: Why Care about Income Inequality?', *British Medical Journal*, 314: 1,037–40.

Kawachi, I. and Kennedy, B.P. (1997b) 'The Relationship of Income Inequality to Mortality: Does the Choice of Indicator Matter?', *Social Science and Medicine*, 45: 1,121–7.

Kawachi, I., Kennedy, B.P., Lochner, K. and Prothrow-Smith, D. (1997) 'Social Capital, Income Inequality and Mortality', *American Journal of Public Health*, 87(9): 1,491–8.

Keim, C. (1995) 'Africa and Europe before 1900', in P.M. Martin and P. O'Meara (eds) *Africa* (Bloomington, IN: Indiana University Press; London: James Curry), pp. 115–34.

Kelly, M. (1998) *The Inclusion of an HIV/AIDS Component in BESSIP* (Lusaka, Zambia).

Kelly, M. (2000) 'The Encounter Between HIV/AIDS and Education'. Unpublished manuscript, Lusaka, Zambia.

Kimani, D. (2000) 'AIDS Drugs Still Too Expensive in Africa', *The East African* (Nairobi), 10 December.

Kilian, A.H.D., Gregson, S., Ndyanabangi, B., Walusaga, K., Kipp, W., Sahlmuller, G. et al. (1999) 'Reductions in Risk Behaviour Provide the Most Consistent Explanation for Declining HIV-1 Prevalence in Uganda', *AIDS 1999*, 13: 391–8.

Kinghorn, A. (1998) *Projections of the Cost of Antiretroviral Interventions to Reduce Mother to Child Transmission of HIV in the South African Public Sector* (Johannesburg: HIV Management Services).

Kinsella, K. and Ferreira, M. (1997) 'Aging Trends: South Africa'. International Brief, US Department of Commerce, Economics and Statistics Administration, US Bureau of the Census (October 1998): 1–6.

Kinsella, K. and Tauber, C. (1992–93) *An Ageing World II* (Washington, DC: US Department of Commerce, International Population Report).

Kippax, S. and Crawford, J. (1993) 'Flaws in the Theory of Reasoned Action', in D. Terry, C. Gallois and M. McAmish (eds) *The Theory of Reasoned Action: Its Application to AIDS-preventive Behaviour* (Oxford: Pergamon).

Kjekshus, H. (1996) *Ecology Control and Economic Development in East African History* (London: James Curry).

Kjekshus, H. (1977) *Ecology Control And Economic Development In East African History* (London: Heinemann Educational Books).

Klein, N. (1999) *No Logo: Money, Marketing and the Growing Anti-corporate Movement* (New York: Picador).

Konde-Lule, J.K. (1994) 'The Effects of Urbanization on the Spread of AIDS in Africa', *African Urban Quarterly*, 6(1–2).

Kongsin, S. (2001) 'The Economic Impact of HIV/AIDS Morbidity on Households in Upper-North Thailand: Phayao Case Study'. PhD thesis, London School of Hygiene and Tropical Medicine.

Kongsin, S. and Watts, C. (2000) 'Household Impact of AIDS in Thailand'. Lecture delivered to the Annual Policy Research Workshop on the Social and Economic Impact of HIV/AIDS, Overseas Development Group, University of East Anglia, Norwich, 7 June.

Kramer, S. (2001) 'HIV and AIDS: Getting Down to Business' (personal communication).

Kuper, L. and Smith, M.G. (eds) (1969) *Pluralism in Africa* (Berkeley and Los Angeles, CA: University of California Press).

Kuzio, T., Kravchuk, R. and D'Anieri, P. (2000) *State and Institution Building in Ukraine* (New York: St Martin's Press).

Kwaramba, P. (1998) 'The Socio-economic Impact of HIV/AIDS on Communal Agricultural Production Systems in Zimbabwe'. Working Paper No. 19, Economic Advisory Project (Harare: Friedrich Ebert Stiftung).

Kyewalyanga, F-X. S. (1976) *Traditional Religion, Custom and Christianity in Uganda* (Freiburg im Breisgau: Offsetdrückerei Johannes Krause).

Laslett, P. (1965) *The World We Have Lost* (London: Methuen).

Le Blanc, N., Meintel, D. and Piché, P. (1991) 'The African Sexual System: Comment on Caldwell et al.', *Population and Development Review*, 17(3) (September): 497–505.

Leclerc-Madlala, S. (1997) 'Infect One, Infect All: Zulu Youth Response to the AIDS Epidemic in South Africa', *Medical Anthropology*, 17(4): 363–80.

Leith, J. (2001) 'Representation, Resources and Resettlement as Development in Eastern Indonesia'. PhD thesis, School of Development Studies, University of East Anglia, Norwich.

Loewenson, R. and Whiteside, A. (1997) 'Social and Economic Issues of HIV/AIDS in Southern Africa. A Consultancy Report Prepared for SAfAIDS, Harare'. SAfAIDS Occasional Paper Series No. 2. (March) <http://www.iaen.org/impact/sfaids1.pdf>

Low-Beer, D., Stoneburner, R.L. and Mukulu, A. (1997) 'Empirical Evidence for the Severe but Localised Impact of AIDS on Population Structure', *Nature Medicine*, 3(5).

Low-Beer, D., Stoneburner, R., Whiteside, A. and Barnett, A. (2000) 'Knowledge Diffusion and Personalizing Risk: Key Indicators of Behavior Change in Uganda Compared to Southern Africa' (Abstract ThPeD5787). XIII International AIDS Conference, Durban, South Africa, 7–14 July.

Lundberg, M. and Over, M. (2000) 'Transfers and Household Welfare in Kagera'. Unpublished paper, School of Development Studies, University of East Anglia, Norwich.

McCubbin, H.I. (1979) 'Integrating Coping Behavior in Family Stress Theory', *Journal of Marriage and the Family*, 41(4): 237–44.

McCubbin, H.I. et al. (1980) 'Family Stress and Coping: A Decade of Review', *Journal of Marriage and the Family*, 42(4): 855–71.

MacGaffey, J. (ed.) (1991) *The Real Economy of Zaire: The Contribution of Smuggling and Other Unofficial Activities to National Wealth* (London and Philadelphia, PA: James Curry).

McGrew, R.E. (1985) *Encyclopedia of Medical History* (New York: McGraw-Hill).

McNeil, W.H. (1976) *Plagues and People* (Garden City, NY: Doubleday).

MacPherson, M.F., Hoover, D.A. and Snodgrass, D.R. (2000) *The Impact on Economic Growth in Africa of Rising Costs and Labor Productivity Losses Associated with HIV/AIDS*. CAER II Discussion Paper No. 79 (August) (Boston, MA: Harvard Institute of International Development).

Malindi, G. and Rosebery, W., (1998) Unpublished presentation on application of Ministry of Agriculture and Industry in Malawi (Durban).

Mamdani, M. (1975) 'Class Struggles in Uganda', *Review of African Political Economy*, 4 (November): 26–61.

Manderson, L. and Jolly, M. (eds) (1997) *Sites of Desire, Economies of Pleasure: Sexualities in Asia and the Pacific* (Chicago, Il: University of Chicago Press).

Mann J., Francis, H. et al. (1986) 'HIV Seroprevalence among Hospital Workers in Kinshasa, Zaire: Lack of Association with Occupational Exposure', *JAMA*, 256: 3,099–102.

Mann, J. and Tarantola, D. (eds) (1996) *AIDS in the World II* (Oxford and New York: Oxford University Press).

Mann, J., Tarantola, D. and Netter, T. (eds) (1992) *AIDS in the World* (Cambridge, MA: Harvard University Press).

Mann, J., Tarantola, D. and Netter, T. (eds) (1993) *A AIDS No Mundo* (Portuguese abridged and adapted version of *AIDS in the World*) (Rio de Janeiro: Abia, Relume Dumara), pp. 176–7.

Marseille, E., Kahn, J., Mmiro, F., Guay, L., Musoke, P., Flower, M. and Jackson, J. (1999) 'Cost Effectiveness of Single-dose Neviropine Regimen for Mothers and Babies to Decrease Vertical HIV-1 Transmission in sub-Saharan Africa', *Lancet*, 354: 803–8.

Mauss, M. (1925) 'Essai sur le don', *Année sociologique*, 1 (n.s.): 30–186.

Mbeki, T. (1998) Address, Pretoria, 9 October.

Mehrotra, S. and Jolly, R. (eds) (1997) *Development with a Human Face* (Oxford: Clarendon Press).

Menon, R., Wawer, M.J., Konde-Lule, J.K., Sewankambo, N.K. and Li, C. (1998) 'The Economic Impact of Adult Mortality on Households in Rakai District, Uganda', in M. Ainsworth, L. Fransen and M. Over (eds) *Confronting AIDS: Evidence from the Developing world, Selected Background Papers for World Bank Policy Research Report, 'Confronting AIDS: Public Priorities in a Global Epidemic'* (Brussels: European Commission).

Mercury (KwaZulu-Natal) (2001) 13 July.

Michael, K. (2000) 'HIV/AIDS and the Retail Sector', *AIDS Analysis Africa*, 9(6): 1999.

Mills, G. (2000) 'AIDS and the South African Military: Timeworn Cliché or Timebomb?', Konrad Adenauer Stiftung Occasional Papers, *HIV/AIDS: A Threat to the African Renaissance?* (Johannesburg) (June).

Mocroft, A., Miller, F.V., Chiesi, A., Blaxhult, A., Katlama, C., Clotet, B., Barton, S. and Lundgren, J.D. (2000) 'Virological Failure Among Patients on HAART from Across Europe: Results from the EuroSIDA Study', *Antiviral Therapy*, 5(2): 107–12.

Monitoring the AIDS Pandemic (2000) 'The Status and Trends of the HIV/AIDS Epidemic in the World'. Report from the MAP meeting, 5–7 July, Durban.

Monk, N. (2000) 'A Study of Orphaned Children and their Households in Luweero District, Uganda'. Research carried out for Association François-Xavier Bagnoud (AFXB) (February).

Monk, N. (2001) *Orphans and Vulnerable Children in India: An Assessment of the Vulnerability of India's Children, in Relation to the Social Impact of HIV/AIDS, from Research Carried Out in Rajasthan, Goa and Mumbai, September–December 2000* (Boston, MA: François-Xavier Bagnoud Foundation).

Montano, D. (1986) 'Predicting and Understanding Influenza Vaccination Behaviour: Alternatives to the Health Belief Model', *Medical Care*, 5: 438–53.

Morgan, S. (2000) 'Response for all AIDS Affected Children, not AIDS Orphans Alone', *AIDS Analysis*, 10(6) (March/April).

Morris, C., Burdge, D. and Cheevers, E. (2000) 'Economic Impact of HIV Infection in a Cohort of Male Sugar Mill Workers in South Africa', *Journal of South African Economics*, 68(5): 933–46.

Morris, G.J. and Potter, M. (1997) 'The Emergence of New Pathogens as a Function of Changes in Host Susceptibility', *Emerging Infectious Diseases*, 3(4) <http://www.cdc.gov.ncidod/eid/vol3no4/morris.htm>

Mulder, D. (1996) 'Disease Progression and Mortality Following HIV-1 Infection', in J. Mann and D. Tarantola (eds) *AIDS in the World II* (Oxford and New York: Oxford University Press).

Musagara, M., Okware, S. et al. (1989) Seroprevalence of HIV-1 in Rakai District, Uganda, Fourth International Conference on AIDS and Associated Cancers in Africa, Marseilles, poster 010, p. 117 of abstracts.

Mutangadura, G.B. (2000) 'Household Welfare Impacts of Adult Females in Zimbabwe: Implications for Policy and Program Development'. Paper presented at the AIDS and Economics Symposium, IAEN, Durban, 7–8 July.

Nahaylo, B. (1999) *The Ukrainian Resurgence* (Toronto: University of Toronto Press).

Nahaylo, B. (2000) *The Ukrainian Resurgence* (Toronto: University of Toronto Press).

Nampanya-Serpell, N. (2000) 'Social and Economic Risk Factors for HIV/AIDS-Affected Families in Zambia'. Paper presented at the AIDS and Economics Symposium, IAEN, Durban, 7–8 July, p. 1.

National AIDS Commission (2001) *National Strategic Framework for HIV/AIDS Activities in Uganda 2000/1 to 2006/6* (Kampala) <http://www.aidsuganda.org>

National AIDS Control Organisation (NACO) (1998) <http://www.naco.nic.in/1998>

National AIDS Control Organisation (2001) <http://www.naco.nic.in/> (March).

National AIDS Coordinating Agency (NACA), Botswana (2000) 'HIV Seroprevalence Sentinel Survey Amongst Pregnant Women and Men with Sexually Transmitted Disease. A Technical Report'. (AIDS/STD Unit) (December).

National Economic and Development Authority (NEDA) (2000) 'Living with HIV/AIDS: Case Study on Filipinos living with HIV/AIDS'. Produced by the Health Action Information Network for NEDA with the support of the UNDP.

National Institute of Allergy and Infectious Diseases <www.niaid.hih.gov>

National Intelligence Council (2000) 'The Global Infectious Disease Threat and its Implications for the United States, *National Intelligence Estimate, NIE 99-17D* (Washington, DC: NIC).

Navarro, V. (1998) 'Comment: Whose Globalization?', *American Journal of Public Health*, 88(5) (May): 742–3. <http://news.bbc.co.uk/hi/english/events/newnight/newsid_1274000/1274831.stm>

Nicholls, S., McLean, R., Theodore, K., Henry, R. and Camara, B. (2000a) 'Modelling the Macroeconomic Impact of HIV/AIDS on the English Speaking Caribbean: The Case of Trindad and Tobago and Jamaica'. Paper presented at the AIDS and Economics Symposium, IAEN, Durban, 7–8 July.

Nicholls., S., McLean, R.M., Theodore, K., Henry, R. and Camara, B. (2000b) 'Modelling the Macroeconomic Impact of HIV/AIDS in the English Speaking Caribbean', *Journal of South African Economics*, 68(5): 916–32.

Ntozi, J.P.M. (1997) 'Widowhood, Remarriage and Migration during the HIV/AIDS Epidemic in Uganda'. Paper presented at the Socio-Demographic Impact of AIDS in Africa Conference, International Union for the Scientific Study of Population and University of Natal, Durban, February.

Observer (2001) 22 April.

Ohmae, K. (1985) *Triad Power: The Coming Shape of Global Competition* (New York: The Free Press and Collier Macmillan).

Okiror, G., Opio, A., Musinguzi, J., Madraa, E., Tembo, G. and Carael, M. (1997) 'Change in Sexual Behaviour and Decline in HIV Infection Among Young Pregnant Women in Urban Uganda', *AIDS*, 11: 1,757–3.

Oldstone, M.B.A. (1998) *Viruses, Plagues and History* (Oxford: Oxford University Press), p. 109.

Oliver, R. (1991) *The African Experience* (London: Weidenfeld and Nicolson), pp. 122, 125.

Organisation for Economic Co-operation and Development (OECD) (1997) 'New Strategies for the Challenges Ahead: A Changing Development Co-operation' <http://www.oecd.org/dac/htm/stc/intro.htm>

Orroth, K.K., Gavyole, A., Todd, J., Mosha, F., Ross, D., Mwijarubi, E., Grosskurth, H. and Hayes, R.J. (2000) 'Syndromic Treatment of Sexually Transmitted Diseases Reduces the Proportion of Incident HIV Infections Attributable to These Diseases in Rural Tanzania', *AIDS 2000*, 14: 1,429–37.

Over, M. (1992) 'Macroeconomic Impact of AIDS in Sub-Saharan Africa'. Africa Technical Department, Population, Health and Nutrition Division, Technical Working Paper No. 3 (Washington, DC) (June).

Peters, K. and Richards, P. (1998) 'Why We Fight: Voices of Youth Combatants in Sierra Leone', *Africa*, 68(2): 56–78.

Petersen, W. and Petersen, R. (1985) *Dictionary of Demography: Multilingual Glossary* (Westport, CT, and London: Greenwood Press).

Philippines National AIDS Council (2000) *HIV/AIDS Country Profile, Philippines* (January) (Manila: Philippines National AIDS Council).

Public Health Laboratory Service (PHLS) (2000) <http://www.phls.co.uk> (February).

Polanyi, K. (1945) The Origins of Our Times: The Great Transformation (London: Victor Gollancz). <www.policyproject.com>

Portes, A. and Landolt, P. (1996) 'The Downside of Social Capital', *American Prospect*, 26 (May–June): 18–21, 94.

Portes, A. and Sensenbrenner, J. (1993) 'Embeddedness and Immigration: Notes on the Social Determinants of Economic Action', *American Journal of Sociology*, 98(6): 1,320–50.

Preston-Whyte, E. (1999) 'Reproductive Health and the Condom Dilemma in South Africa', in J.C. Caldwell et al. (eds) *Resistances to Behavioural Change to Reduce HIV/AIDS Infection* (Canberra: Health Transition Centre, Australian National University), pp. 139–55.

Presidential AIDS Advisory Panel (2001) <www.polity.org.za/govdocs/reports/aids/aidspanel.htm>

Putnam, R.D. (2000) *Bowling Alone: The Collapse and Revival of Amercian Community* (New York: Simon and Schuster).

Putnam, R.D. with Leonardi, R. and Nanetti, R.Y. (1993) *Making Democracy Work. Civic Traditions in Modern Italy* (Princeton, NJ: Princeton University Press).

Putzel, J. (1997) 'Accounting for the "Dark Side" of Social Capital: Reading Robert Putnam on Democracy', *Journal of International Development*, 9(7): 939–49.

Quattek, K. (2000) 'The Economic Impact of AIDS in South Africa: A Dark Cloud on the Horizon', Konrad Adenauer Stiftung Occasional Papers, *HIV/AIDS: A Threat to the African Renaissance?* (Johannesburg) (June). (First produced as an ING Barings Research Report and reprinted with their permission.)

Rajaraman, D. (2001) 'The Future of the Nation? HIV/AIDS and Orphans in Botswana'. Unpublished paper, Oxford, Queen Elizabeth House. <www.reliefweb.int/IRIN>

Republic of Botswana (1997), *National Development Plan 8, 1997/98 – 2002/2003* (Gaborone: Ministry of Finance and Development Planning).

Republic of South Africa, Department of Justice (1927) *Immorality Act Five* (Pretoria: Government Printer).

Richards, P. (1985) *Indigenous Agricultural Revolution: Ecology and Food Production in West Africa* (London: Hutchinson).

Richards, P. (1993) 'Cultivation: Knowledge or Performance?', in M. Hobart (ed.) *An Anthropological Critique of Development: The Growth of Ignorance* (London: Routledge).

Ridley, M. (2000) *Genome: The Autobiography of a Species in 23 Chapters* (New York: HarperCollins).

Roberts, B. (1999) 'Apartheid Forces Spread AIDS', *Mail and Guardian* Online, 12 November <http://www.mg.co.za/mg/za/archive/99nov/12novam-news.html#aids>

Roberts, M., Rau, B. and Emery, A. (1996) 'Private Sector AIDS Policy: Businesses Managing AIDS, A Guide for Managers' (Arlington, VA: Family Health International AIDSCAP) <www.fhi.org/en/aids/aidscap/aidspub/policy/psapp>

Robinson, J. (1964) *Economic Philosophy* (Garden City, NY: Doubleday).

Rogaly, B., Biswas, J., Coppard, D., Rafique, A., Rana, K. and Sengupta, A. (2001) 'Seasonal Migration and Welfare/Illfare in Eastern India: A Social Analysis'. Unpublished paper, School of Development Studies, University of East Anglia, Norwich.

Rogaly, B. and Coppard, D. (2001) '"They Went to Eat, Now They Go to Earn": The Changing Meanings of Seasonal Migration from Purulia District in West Bengal, India'. Paper for the Workshop on Social Relations and

Well-Being in South Asia, School of Development Studies, University of East Anglia, 23–24 March.

Rogers, E.M. (1995) *Diffusion of Innovations* (4th edn) (New York: The Free Press).

Ross, L., Johnson, M., DeMasi, R., Liao, Q., Graham, N., Shaefer, M. and St Clair, M. (2000) 'Viral Genetic Heterogeneity in HIV-1 Infected Individuals is Associated with Increasing Use of HAART and Higher Viraemia', *AIDS*, 14(7): 813–19.

Rossi, M.M. and Reijer, P. (1995) 'Prevalence of Orphans and their Geographical Status'. Research Report for the AIDS Department, Catholic Diocese of Ndola.

Rothschild, D. and Harbeson, J.W. (1981) 'Rehabilitation in Uganda', *Current History*, 80(463) (March).

Rowley, J.T., Anderson, R.M. and Ng, T.W. (1990) 'Reducing the Spread of HIV Infection in Sub-Saharan Africa: Some Demographic and Economic Consequences', *AIDS*, 4: 47–56.

Rugalema, G.H.R. (1999) 'Adult Mortality as Entitlement Failure: AIDS and the Crisis of Rural Livelihoods in a Tanzanian Village'. PhD thesis, Institute of Social Studies, The Hague (September).

Rugalema, G.H.R. (2000) 'Coping Strategies: A Global Concept for a Global Epidemic'. Unpublished paper, first presented as a lecture in the series 'HIV/AIDS: The First Epidemic of Globalisation', School of Development Studies, University of East Anglia, Norwich (June).

Salt, H., Boyle, M. and Ives, J. (1990) 'HIV Prevention: Current Health Promoting Behaviour Models for Understanding Psychosocial Determinants of Condom Use', *AIDS Care*, 1(2): 69–75.

Schoepf, B.G., (1988), 'Women, AIDS and Economic Crisis in Central Africa', *Canadian Journal of African Studies*, 22(3): 625–44.

Schoepf, B.G. (1991) 'Political Economy, Sex and Cultural Logics: A View from Zaire', *African Urban Quarterly*, 6(1–2): 27–38.

Schoepf, B.G. (1992) 'Women at Risk: Case Studies from Zaire', in G. Herdt and S. Lindenbaum (eds) *In the Time of AIDS: Social Analysis, Theory and Method* (Newbury Park, CA: Sage).

Schoepf, B.G. (1993) 'Faire face au Sida: une situation nouvelle pour la jeunesse africaine', in V. d'Almeida-Topor and C. Coquery-Vidrovitch et al. (eds) *Les jeunes en Afrique, Vol. 2, La Politique et la Ville* (Paris and Montreal: L'Harmattan).

Schoepf, B. and Engundu, W. (1991) 'Women's Trade and Contributions to Household Budgets in Kinshasa', in J. MacGaffey (ed.) *The Real Economy of Zaire: The Contribution of Smuggling and Other Unofficial Activities to National Wealth* (London and Philadelphia, PA: James Curry), pp. 124–51.

Schönteich, M. (1999) 'AIDS and Age: SA's Crime Time Bomb', *AIDS Analysis Africa*, 10(2) (August/September).

Schoub, B.D. (1999) *AIDS and HIV in Perspective: A Guide to Understanding the Virus and its Consequences* (2nd edn) (Cambridge: Cambridge University Press).

Scrimshaw, N. and SanGiovanni, J. (1997) 'Synergism of Nutrition, Infection and Immunity: An Overview', *Amercian Journal of Clinical Nutrition*, 66 (Supplement): S464–7.

Sen, A.K. (1985) *Commodities and Capabilites* (Amsterdam: North Holland).

Sen, A. (1987) *Gender and Cooperative Conflicts* (Helsinki, Finland: World Institute for Development Economics Research).

Sen, A. (1997) *On Economic Inequalities* (expanded edition with a substantial annexe by J. Foster and A. Sen) (Oxford: Clarendon Press).

Sen, A. and Sengupta, S. (1983) 'Malnutrition of Rural Children and Sex Bias', *Economic and Political Weekly*, 19.

Sennett, R. and Cobb, J. (1973) *The Hidden Injuries of Class* (New York: Alfred Knopf).

Serwadda, D., Gray, R., Wawer, M.J., Sewankambo, N.K., Kiwanuka, N. and Kelly, R. (2000a) 'Potential Efficacy of Male Circumcision for HIV Prevention in Rakai, Uganda'. XIII International AIDS Conference, Durban, South Africa, 7–14 July.

Serwadda, D., Gray, R., Wawer, M.J., Sewankambo, N.K., Kiwanuka, N., Wabwire-Mangen, F., Li, C., Lutalo, T. and Quinn, T.C. (2000b) 'Rakai, Uganda: HIV Incidence Associated with Male Circumcision in a Population-based Cohort, and HIV Acquisition/Transmission Associated with Circumcision and Viral Load in Discordant Couples'. XIII International AIDS Conference, Durban, South Africa, 7–14 July.

Serwadda, D., Sewankambo, N., Lwegaba, A., Carswell, J. et al. (1985) 'Slim Disease: A New Disease in Uganda and its Association with HTLV-III Infection', *Lancet*, 2(2): 849–52.

Setel, P. (1996) 'AIDS as a Paradox of Manhood and Development in Kilimanjaro, Tanzania', *Social Science and Medicine*, 43(8): 1,169–78.

Setel, P. (1999a) *A Plague of Paradoxes: AIDS, Culture and Demography in Northern Tanzania* (Chicago, IL: University of Chicago Press).

Setel, P. (1999b) 'Local Histories of Sexually Transmitted Diseases and AIDS in Western and Northern Tanzania', in P. Setel, M. Lewis and M. Lyons (eds) *Histories of Sexually Transmitted Diseases and HIV/AIDS in Sub-Saharan Africa, Contributions in Medical Studies, No. 44* (Westport, CT, and London: Greenwood Press), pp. 119–42.

Setel, P., Lewis, M. and Lyons, M. (eds) (1999) *Histories of Sexually Transmitted Diseases and HIV/AIDS in Sub-Saharan Africa, Contributions in Medical Studies, No. 44* (Westport, CT, and London: Greenwood Press).

Sewankambo, N.K., Gray, R.H., Ahmad, S. et al. (2000) 'Mortality Associated with HIV Infection in Rural Rakai District, Uganda', *AIDS 2000*, 14: 2,391–400.

Shell, R. (2000) 'Halfway to the Holocaust: The Economic, Demographic and Social Implications of the AIDS Pandemic to the Year 2010 in the Southern African Region', Konrad Adenauer Stiftung Occasional Papers, *HIV/AIDS: A Threat to the African Renaissance?* (Johannesburg) (June), pp. 7–27.

Shell, R.C. and Zeitlin, R. (2000) 'POSITIVE OUTCOMES: The chances of acquiring HIV/AIDS during the school-going years in the Eastern Cape, 1990-2000', *Population Research Unit 26* (Grahamstown, South Africa: Rhodes University).

Shilts, R. (1987) *And the Band Played On: Politics, People and the AIDS Epidemic* (New York: St Martin's Press).

Simon, J., Rosen, S., Whiteside, A., Vincent, J. and Thea, D. (2000) *The Response of African Businesses to AIDS, in the Commonwealth Secretariat, HIV/AIDS in the Commonwealth 2000/01* (London: Kensington Publications) pp. 72–7. <www.sirius.com>

Smith, J. (1995) 'The Socioeconomic Impact of HIV/AIDS on Zambian Business'. Unpublished paper prepared for and with the support of the Commonwealth Development Corporation, London.

Soonthorndhada, A. (2000) 'Context and Patterns of Sexuality and Sexual Risk-taking among Young People: Implication for Aids Prevention in Thailand'.

PhD thesis, School of Development Studies, University of East Anglia, Norwich.

South African Government (1967) General Circular No. 25.

South African Medical Council (2000) 'HIV Surveillance – What Grounds for Optimism?', *South African Medical Journal*, 90(11) (November): 1,062–4.

Southall, A. (1980) 'Social Disorganisation in Uganda: Before, During and After Amin', *Journal of Modern African Studies*, 18: 627–56.

Stanecki, K.A. (2000) 'AIDS in the 21st Century', *World Population Profile 2000* (US Census Bureau).

Steinberg, M., Kinghorn, A., Soderlund, N., Schierhout, G. and Conway, S. (2000) 'HIV/AIDS – Facts, Figures and the Future', *South African Health Review*.

Stillwaggon, E. (2000) 'HIV Transmission in Latin America: Comparison with Africa and Policy Implications', *South African Journal of Economics*, 68(5): 985–1,011.

Stine, G.J. (2001) *AIDS Update 2001: An Annual Overview of Acquired Immune Deficiency Syndrome* (New Jersey: Prentice Hall).

Stoneburner, R.L. and Low-Beer, D. (2000) 'Analyses of HIV Trend and Behavioral Data in Uganda, Kenya, and Zambia: Prevalence Declines in Uganda Relate More to Reduction in Sex Partners than Condom Use' (Abstract ThOrC734). XIII International AIDS Conference, Durban, South Africa, 7–14 July.

Stover, J. and Way, P. (1998a) 'Projecting the Impact of AIDS on Mortality', *AIDS*, 12 (Supplement 1): S29–39.

Stover, J and Way, P.O. (1998b) 'Impact of Interventions on Reducing the Spread of HIV in Africa: Computer Simulation Applications', *African Journal of Medical Practice*, 2: 110–20.

Sugden, R. (2000) 'Team Preferences', *Economics and Philosophy*, 16: 175–204.

Sunter, C. (1987) *The World and South Africa in the 1990s* (Cape Town: Human and Rousseau Tafelberg).

Swarms, R.L. (2001) 'AIDS Drug Battle Deepens in Africa' <www.globaltreatment-access.org/content/press_releases/a01/030801_NYT_ GENERICS.html>

Swaziland Ministry of Health and Social Welfare (2000) *Seventh HIV Sentinel Serosurveillance Report Year 2000* (Mbabane, Swaziland: Ministry of Health and Social Welfare, Swaziland National AIDS/STDs Programme) (October).

Swaziland National AIDS/STDs Programme (1998) *Sixth HIV Sentinel Surveillance Report 1998* (Mbabane, Swaziland: Ministry of Health and Social Welfare) (September).

Swazi Observer (2001) 22 April.

Swazi Times (1994–99) Bereavement Notices, 1 July 1994 to 30 June 1999. <www.tfgi.com>

Thangpet, S. (2001) 'The Impact of HIV/AIDS on Community-based Resource Management: A Case Study of an Indigenous Irrigation System in Northern Thailand'. Unpublished paper (July), Overseas Development Group, University of East Anglia, Norwich.

Thea, D., Rosen, S., Vincent, J.R., Singh, G. and Simon, J. (2000) 'Economic Impact of HIV/AIDS in Company A's Workforce', Session D14 (11 July), XIII International AIDS Conference, Durban, 7–14 July.

Thomas, P. (2001) *Big Shot: Passion, Politics and the Struggle for an AIDS Vaccine* (New York: Perseus).

Timaeus, I.M. (1998) 'Impact of the HIV Epidemic on Mortality in Sub-Saharan Africa: Evidence from National Surveys and Censuses', *AIDS*, 12 (Supplement 1): S15–27.

Tomlinson, R. (2000) 'Time to Rethink Housing Policy', *Mail and Guardian*, 18 October.

Topouzis, D. (2000) 'Review and Analysis of Approaches to Measuring the Impact of HIV/AIDS on the Agricultural Sector in Africa'. Draft paper prepared for the African Development Forum, Addis Ababa, December.

Uganda AIDS Commission <http://www.aidsuganda.org/>

Uganda AIDS Commission (1993) *Annual Report* (Kampala: Government of Uganda).

Ukraine Government, Ministry of Health, The Project (2000) 'Strategic Planning Process in the Ukraine for a National Response to HIV/AIDS in 2000–2003', *HIV/AIDS in the Ukraine: Situation Analysis* (March–May) (Kyiv: Ukraine Government).

Ukraine Statistical Annual (1995) (Kyiv: Technika).

UNAIDS <http://www.unaids.org>

UNAIDS country epidemiological fact sheets <http://www.unaids.org/hivaidsinfo/statistics/june00/fact_sheets>

UNAIDS (1999a) *Level and Flow of National and International Resources for the Response to HIV/AIDS* (Geneva: UNAIDS).

UNAIDS (1999b) *Acting Early to Prevent AIDS: The Case of Senegal*. UNAIDS Best Practice Collection (June) (Geneva: UNAIDS).

UNAIDS (2000a) *Democratic Republic of the Congo Epidemiological Fact Sheet on HIV/AIDS* (Geneva: UNAIDS) <http://www.unaids.org/hivaidsinfo/statistics/june00/fact_sheets/pdfs/demrepcongo.pdf>

UNAIDS (2000b) *India Epidemiological Fact Sheet* (Geneva: UNAIDS).

UNAIDS (2000c) *Epidemiological Facts Sheets*: Laos, Vietnam and Thailand (Geneva: UNAIDS).

UNAIDS (2000d) *Nigeria Epidemiological Fact Sheet on HIV/AIDS* (Geneva: UNAIDS) <http://www.unaids.org/hivaidsinfo/statistics/fact_sheets/pdfs/Nigeria_en.pdf>

UNAIDS (2000e) *Philippines Epidemiological Fact Sheet on HIV/AIDS*, Update (Geneva: UNAIDS).

UNAIDS (2000f) *Report on the Global HIV/AIDS Epidemic* (June) (Geneva: UNAIDS) <http://www.unaids.org/hivaidsinfo/statistics/june00/fact_sheets/>

UNAIDS (2000g) *AIDS Epidemic Update* (December) (Geneva: UNAIDS).

UNAIDS (2000h) *The Business Response to HIV/AIDS: Impact and Lessons Learned* (Geneva: UNAIDS).

UNAIDS/Pan American Health Organisation/WHO (1998) *Cuba: Epidemiological Fact Sheet on HIV/AIDS and Sexually Transmitted Diseases* (UNAIDS) <www.unaids.org>

UNICEF (2000) *The Progress of Nations* (New York: UNICEF).

UNICEF/UNAIDS/WHO/HTP/MSF Project (2001) *Sources and Prices of Selected Drugs and Diagnostics for People Living with AIDS* (May).

United Nations (UN) (1996) *Demographic Indicators, 1950–2050 (1996 Revision)* (New York: UN, Population Division) <http://www.wri.org/wr-98-99/001-ptn2.htm>

United Nations Development Programme (UNDP) Aids facts <www.undp.org.ws/HIV/aidsfacts.htm>

United Nations Development Programme (UNDP) (various years) *Human Development Report*: 1996, 1997, 1998, 1999, 2000 (New York: Oxford University Press).

United States Bureau of the Census (forthcoming) *World Population Profile 2000* (Washington DC).

United States Bureau of the Census, International Programs Center, Health Studies Branch, HIV/AIDS Surveillance Data Base CD #623510.

United States Center for Disease Control (1981) *Morbidity and Mortality Weekly Report* (5 June) (Atlanta, GA: US Center for Disease Control).

Van der Vliet, V. (2000) 'New Light on the Origin of AIDS' (published in the electronic newsletter *PulseTrack*).

Van Doorslaer, E., Wagstaff, A., Bleichrodt, H., Calonge, S., Gerdtham, U-G., Gerfin, M. et al. (1997) 'Income-related Inequalities in Health: Some International Comparisons', *Journal of Health Economics*, 16(1): 93–112.

Van Griensven, G.J.P., Surasiengsunk, S. and Panza, A. (1998) *The Use of Mortality Statistics as a Proxy Indicator for the Impact of the AIDS Epidemic on the Thai Population* (Bangkok: Institute of Population Studies, Chulalongkorn University) Institute of Population Studies Publication no 267/98.

Van Rensburg, E.J. (2000) 'The Origin of HIV', *South African Journal of Science*, 96(6) (June): 267–69.

Velkoff, V.A. and Lawson, V.A. (1998) 'Gender and Aging: Caregiving'. International brief, US Department of Commerce, Economics and Statistics Administration, Bureau of Census (December).

Voelker, R. (2000) 'Setting Priorities and Budgets to Fight Against Global AIDS', *JAMA*, 284(21) (6 December).

Wallace, R. (1991a) 'Travelling Waves of HIV Infection on a Low Dimensional "Socio-geographic" Network', *Social Science and Medicine*, 32: 122–33.

Wallace, R. (1991b) 'Social Disintegration and the Spread of AIDS: Thresholds for Propogation Along Sociogeographic Networks', *Social Science and Medicine*, 33: 122–37.

Wallace, R. (1993) 'Social Disintegration and the Spread of AIDS – II: Meltdown of Sociogeographic Structure in Urban Minority Neighbourhoods', *Social Science and Medicine*, 37(7): 887–96.

Wallace, R. and Fullilove, M. (1991) 'AIDS Deaths in the Bronx 1983–1988: spatiotemporal analysis from a sociogeographic perspective', *Environmental Planning*, A 23, 1,701.

Wallace, R., Fullilove, M. and Flisher, A. (1996) 'AIDS, Violence and Behavioral Coding: Information Theory, Risk Behaviour and Dynamic Process on Core-Group Sociogeographic Networks', *Social Science and Medicine*, 43(3): 339–52.

Wallace, R., Fullilove, M., Fullilove, R., Gould, P. and Wallace. D. (1994) 'Will AIDS be Contained Within US Minority Urban Populations?', *Social Science and Medicine*, 39(8) (October): 1,051–62.

Wallace, R. and Wallace, D. (1990) 'Origins of Public Health Collapse in New York City: The Dynamics of Planned Shrinkage, Contagious Urban Decay and Social Disintegration', *Bulletin of the New York Academy of Medicine*, 66: 57–75.

Wallace, R. and Wallace, D. (1995) 'US Apartheid and the Spread of AIDS to the Suburbs: A Multi-city Analysis of the Political Economy of Spatial Epidemic Threshold', *Social Science and Medicine*, 41(3): 333–45.

Walton, D.J. (1987) Letter to S. Cross, 2 September.

Watts, M. (1983) *Silent Violence: Food, Famine and Peasantry in Northern Nigeria* (Berkeley, CA: University of California Press).

Watts, S. (1997) *Epidemics and History: Disease, Power and Imperialism* (New York and New Haven, CT: Yale University Press).

Wawer, M.J., Sewankambo, N.K., Serwadda, D., Quinn, T.C., Paxton, L.A., Kiwanuka, N., Wabwire-Mangen, F., Li, C., Lutalo, T., Nalugoda, F., Gaydos, C.A., Moulton, L.H., Meehan, M.O., Ahmed, S. and Gray, R.H. (1999) 'Control of sexually transmitted disease for AIDS prevention in Uganda: a randomised community trial' (Rakai Project Study Group), *Lancet*, 353(9,152): 525–35.

Weekly Mail and Guardian (2000) <www.mg.co.za> 15 October.

Welsh, F. (2000) *A History of South Africa* (London: HarperCollins).

Went, R. (2000) *Globalization: Neoliberal Challenge, Radical Response* (London: Pluto Press).

White, K.L. (1991) *Healing the Schism: Epidemiology, Medicine and the Public's Health* (Berlin: Springer-Verlag).

Whiteside, A.W. (1986) 'Some Aspects of Labour Relationships Between the Republic of South Africa and Neighbouring States. Part I: Legislation and Agreements, and Part II: Economic Implications', HSRC Investigation into Manpower Issues: Manpower Studies No. 5, Pretoria.

Whiteside, A. (1998) 'Far-reaching Legislation in the Philippines', *AIDS Analysis Asia*, 4(3) (May).

Whiteside, A., Desmond, C., King, J. and Tomlinson, J. (2000) 'Evidence of AIDS Mortality from an Alternative Source. Swaziland Case Study', *AIDS Analysis Africa*, 1(5).

Whiteside, A. and FitzSimons, D. (1992) 'The AIDS Epidemic, Economic, Political and Security Implications', *Conflict Studies 251*, Research Institute for the Study of Conflict and Terrorism.

Whiteside, A. and Sunter, C. (2000) *AIDS: The Challenge for South Africa* (Cape Town: Human and Rousseau Tafelberg).

Whiteside, A. and Wood, G. (1994) *Socio-Economic Impact of HIV/AIDS in Swaziland* (Mbabane: Ministry of Economic Planning and Development).

Wilkinson, R.G. (ed.) (1986) *Class and Health: Research and Longitudinal Data* (London: Tavistock).

Wilkinson, R.G. (1996) *Unhealthy Societies: The Afflictions of Inequality* (London: Routledge).

Wilkinson, R.G. (1997) 'Health Inequalities: Relative or Absolute Material Standards?', *British Medical Journal*, 314: 591–5.

Wilkinson, R.G. (1999a) 'Income Inequality, Social Cohesion and Health: Clarifying the Theory. A Reply to Muntaner and Lynch', *International Journal of Health Services*, 29(3): 525–43.

Wilkinson, R.G. (1999b) 'Health, Hierarchy and Social Anxiety', in N.E. Adler, M. Marmot, B.S. McEwen and J. Stewart (eds) *Socioeconomic Status and Health in Industrial Nations: Social, Psychological and Biological Pathways*. Annals of the New York Academy of Sciences, Vol. 896, pp. 48–63.

Wilkinson, R.G., Kawachi, I. and Kennedy, B. (1998) 'Mortality, the Social Environment, Crime and Violence', *Sociology of Health and Illness*, 20(5): 578–97.

Williams, A. (1998) '"Abantu Abaafa!" [People are Dying!]: Old Age in Contemporary Uganda'. PhD thesis, University of Queensland, Australia.

Williams, J-C. (1972) *Patrimonialism and Political Change in the Congo* (Stanford, CA: Stanford University Press).

Wills, S. (1996) *Plagues: Their Origins, History and Future* (London: Flamingo).

Winnicott, D.W. (1965) *The Maturational Process and the Facilitative Environment* (New York: International Universities Press).

Woolcock, M. (1999) 'Managing Risk, Shock, and Opportunity in Developing Economies: The Role of Social Capital' (Development Research Group, 2 August) (Washington, DC: World Bank).

World Bank, website on climate change <http://worldbank.org/html/extdr/climchng/afrclim.htm>

World Bank, website on confronting aids <http://www.worldbank.org/aids-econ/confront/present/lima/sld009.htm>

World Bank (various years*) World Development Report*: 1993, 1998, 1999, 2000, 2001 (New York: Oxford University Press).

World Bank (1981) *Accelerated Development in Sub-Saharan Africa* (The Berg Report) (New York: Oxford University Press).

World Bank (1996) *Poverty in the Ukraine*, Report No.15602-UA, Country Operations Division II, Country Department IV, European and Central Asia Region (27 June) (Washington, DC: World Bank).

World Bank (1997a) *Confronting AIDS: Public Priorities in a Global Epidemic*. A World Bank Policy Research Report (New York and Oxford: Oxford University Press for the World Bank, European Commission and UNAIDS).

World Bank (1997b) *Global Development Finance 1997* (Washington, DC: World Bank).

World Bank (1998) *World Development Report 1998* (Washington, DC: World Bank; Oxford: Oxford University Press).

World Bank (2000a) *Can Africa Claim the 21st Century?* (Washington, DC: World Bank).

World Bank (2000b) *World Development Indicators, 2000* (New York: Oxford University Press).

World Bank (2000/01) *World Development Report: Attacking World Poverty* (New York: Oxford University Press).

World Bank, Social Monitor Thailand (2000) *Thailand's Response to AIDS 'Building on Success, Confronting the Future'* (Bangkok: World Bank, November).

World Health Assembly, Fortieth (1987) *Global Strategy for the Prevention and Control of AIDS, Resolution*, WHA40.26, Document E/1987/109, Twentieth Plenary Meeting, 15 May.

World Health Organisation (WHO) (2000) *The World Health Report 2000: Health Systems – Improving Performance* (Geneva: WHO).

World Health Organisation (2001) 'Initiative on HIV/AIDS and Sexually Transmitted Infections', *Safe and Effective Use of Antiretroviral Treatments in Adults with a Particular Reference to Resource-Limited Settings* (January) (Geneva: WHO).

Yach, D. and Bettcher, D. (1998) 'The Globalization of Public Health, I: Threats and Opportunities'; 'The Globalization of Public Health, II: The Convergence of Self-Interest and Altruism', *American Journal of Public Health*, 88(5): 735–41.

Zack-Williams, A.B. (1999) 'Child Soldiers in the Civil War in Sierra Leone'. Paper presented at the United Kingdom Development Studies Association Conference, 12–14 September, University of Bath.

Index

The Association
François-Xavier Bagnoud

The Association François-Xavier Bagnoud was founded in 1989 to promote the concept of health and human rights, especially of children and the most disadvantaged peoples in innovative and non-traditional ways. A Swiss-based international NGO, FXB, as it is called, looked for the most creative partners to join with it in a new mission to help AIDS orphans and vulnerable children, oppressed sex workers and their families, children with HIV/AIDS, street children, and all destitute children fallen through society's safety net.

Purposely, avoiding traditional models of intervention, FXB received its direction from its founder, Albina du Boisrouvray, who herself fashioned its projects and chose its implementors. She supported the work of the late Dr Jonathan Mann who pioneered the concept that where people are poor and oppressed and deprived of human rights, pandemics such as AIDS thrive and poverty abounds, demonstrating the inextricable link between health and human rights.

FXB develops and promotes the concept of health and human rights in a number of ways. Early on, it created the FXB Center for Health and Human Rights at Harvard University as the first major educational institution to focus its efforts on developing this paradigm with Dr Mann as its first director. At the same time, FXB has been supporting for over a decade the FXB Center at the University of Medicine and Dentistry of New Jersey to operate an innovative prevention and care programme for inner-city children infected by AIDS; to develop and implement an international training programme which has already benefited over 100 health care workers dealing with HIV/AIDS prevention all around the world; and to support research for a vaccine to treat individuals living with AIDS.

FXB equally develops and supports innovative programmes focusing particularly on HIV/AIDS prevention and treatment throughout the world. For example, in India, it catalysed the development of an Indian NGO, FXB India, with its own national board. The same model was followed in Colombia, Thailand, Uruguay and Uganda. In other countries such as Bolivia, Brazil, Myanmar, Rwanda and South Africa, FXB partnered with local actors to develop its own community-based projects with minimal overhead to care for these children. In Europe, FXB has pioneered the concept of comprehensive palliative care at home for individuals at the end of life in Switzerland and in France, and is looking to expand this innovative concept in developing countries, particularly where AIDS is ravaging populations.

FXB is difficult to characterise since it is an evolving non-traditional movement with a purpose that allocates all resources to the work and to local capacity-building. Since FXB is comprised of a foundation, a Swiss-based international NGO and community-based organisations in a number of developing countries, it is able to work on many levels to achieve its objectives. In this sense, it is a social entrepreneur that hopes to move traditional aid to more effective models through example and advocacy. Nevertheless, FXB works within existing structures and is an NGO recognised by the UN ECOSOC. Supported by the FXB Foundation, it also raises funds to extend its work.

NEWMARKET PUBLIC LIBRARY

NEWMARKET PUBLIC LIBRARY